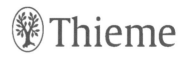

Pediatric Audiology Casebook

Second Edition

Jane R. Madell, PhD, FAAA, CCC-A/SLP, LSLS Cert AVT
Director
Pediatric Audiology Consulting
New York, New York

Carol Flexer, PhD, FAAA, CCC-A, LSLS Cert AVT
Consultant in Pediatric Audiology
Distinguished Professor Emeritus, Audiology
School of Speech-Language Pathology and Audiology
The University of Akron
Akron, Ohio

Jace Wolfe, PhD, CCC-A
Director of Audiology
Hearts for Hearing Foundation
Adjunct Assistant Professor
Department of Audiology
University of Oklahoma Health Sciences Center
Oklahoma City, Oklahoma

Erin C. Shafer, PhD, FAAA, CCC-A
Professor
Department of Audiology and Speech-Language Pathology
College of Health and Public Service
University of North Texas
Denton, Texas

Thieme
New York • Stuttgart • Delhi • Rio de Janeiro

Library of Congress Cataloging-in-Publication Data

Names: Madell, Jane Reger, editor. | Flexer, Carol Ann, editor. | Wolfe, Jace, editor. | Schafer, Erin C., editor.

Title: Pediatric audiology casebook / [edited by] Jane R. Madell, Carol Flexer, Jace Wolfe, Erin C. Schafer.

Description: Second edition. | New York : Thieme, [2019] | Includes bibliographical references.

Identifiers: LCCN 2018038410 (print) | LCCN 2018038971 (ebook) | ISBN 9781626234048 (ebook) | ISBN 9781626234031 (pbk.) | ISBN 9781626234048 (eBook)

Subjects: MESH: Hearing Disorders diagnosis | Child | Infant | Hearing Disorders therapy | Case Reports

Classification: LCC RF291.5.C45 (ebook) | LCC RF291.5.C45 (print) | NLM WV 271 | DDC 618.92/09789dc23

LC record available at https://lccn.loc.gov/2018038410

© 2020 Thieme Medical Publishers, Inc.
Thieme Publishers New York
333 Seventh Avenue, New York, NY 10001 USA
+1 800 782 3488, customerservice@thieme.com

Thieme Publishers Stuttgart
Rüdigerstrasse 14, 70469 Stuttgart, Germany
+49 [0]711 8931 421, customerservice@thieme.de

Thieme Publishers Delhi
A-12, Second Floor, Sector-2, Noida-201301
Uttar Pradesh, India
+91 120 45 566 00, customerservice@thieme.in

Thieme Publishers Rio de Janeiro, Thieme Publicações Ltda.
Edifício Rodolpho de Paoli, 25º andar
Av. Nilo Peçanha, 50 – Sala 2508,
Rio de Janeiro 20020-906 Brasil
+55 21 3172-2297 / +55 21 3172-1896
www.thiemerevinter.com.br

Cover design: Thieme Publishing Group
Typesetting by DiTech Process Solutions

Printed in Germany by CPI books, Leck   5 4 3 2 1

ISBN 978-1-62623-403-1

Also available as an e-book:
eISBN 978-1-62623-404-8

Important note: Medicine is an ever-changing science undergoing continual development. Research and clinical experience are continually expanding our knowledge, in particular our knowledge of proper treatment and drug therapy. Insofar as this book mentions any dosage or application, readers may rest assured that the authors, editors, and publishers have made every effort to ensure that such references are in accordance with **the state of knowledge at the time of production of the book.**

Nevertheless, this does not involve, imply, or express any guarantee or responsibility on the part of the publishers in respect to any dosage instructions and forms of applications stated in the book. **Every user is requested to examine carefully** the manufacturers' leaflets accompanying each drug and to check, if necessary in consultation with a physician or specialist, whether the dosage schedules mentioned therein or the contraindications stated by the manufacturers differ from the statements made in the present book. Such examination is particularly important with drugs that are either rarely used or have been newly released on the market. Every dosage schedule or every form of application used is entirely at the user's own risk and responsibility. The authors and publishers request every user to report to the publishers any discrepancies or inaccuracies noticed. If errors in this work are found after publication, errata will be posted at www.thieme.com on the product description page.

Some of the product names, patents, and registered designs referred to in this book are in fact registered trademarks or proprietary names even though specific reference to this fact is not always made in the text. Therefore, the appearance of a name without designation as proprietary is not to be construed as a representation by the publisher that it is in the public domain.

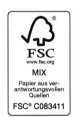

Contents

Foreword

The complete audiologist generates valid quantitative data, makes accurate diagnoses, uses hearing instruments to bring auditory capacity to its highest possible level and maintain it there over the widest possible range of listening conditions, instructs so as to ensure optimal use of equipment and effective control of communication environments and situations, and provides counseling to help the one with hearing loss adjust to the residual deficits of hearing function. The professional expertise of the complete audiologist lies not so much in dealing with hearing loss in people, as it does in helping people who have hearing loss. Reaching this state requires integration of knowledge from many disciplines and application of this knowledge to the development of clinical skills. Relevant disciplines include such things as acoustics, hearing science, speech science, psychoacoustics, psychology, human development, geriatrics, hearing impairment, hearing instrument technology, and counseling. Many years of study and experience are required; indeed, the process should never end. Of course, the aspiring audiologist can learn a lot from lectures, standard text books, practicum experiences, journal articles, short courses, and conference presentations. But the information gained has limited value without the essential ingredient of mentoring—learning at the feet (or elbow) of a master. How refreshing it is to see a text that dispenses with exposition and makes the experiences of master clinicians available to the reader—student and seasoned practitioner alike. This collection of new case studies in the second edition of the Pediatric Audiology Casebook, compiled by Jane R. Madell, Carol Flexer, Jace Wolfe, and Erin C. Schafer, makes the learning experiences of numerous accomplished clinicians available. I see this second edition as a giant leap in the provision of access to mentorship.

Arthur Boothroyd, PhD
Emeritus Professor of Speech and Hearing Sciences
City University of New York
Scholar in Residence
School of Speech, Language, and Hearing Sciences
San Diego State University
Distinguished Visiting Scientist
The House Ear Institute

Preface

Many experienced clinicians and students found the first edition of the Pediatric Audiology Casebook extremely helpful for understanding a wide variety pediatric cases. Indeed, problem-based learning (PBL) is a most effective pedagogical paradigm. Therefore, this 2nd edition was written to further facilitate independent analysis and problem-solving, using 64 new cases, including

- Basic and complex diagnostic cases.
- Management of technologies (hearing aids, cochlear implants, Baha, and RM systems).
- Vestibular issues.
- Management of auditory development.

Clinicians and students alike will benefit from reading each new case in this second edition, even if they are not directly involved with the particular issue. By reading cases in an area in which we do not practice, we may recognize issues in our patients that might require referral. For example, even if vestibular issues are not a primary area of practice, if we see a "clumsy" child, or a child with a wide gait, we should consider making a referral for a vestibular evaluation. In fact, the cases in this book demonstrate that many children with hearing loss, more than we would ever imagine, also have vestibular issues.

Perusal of technology cases and cases describing misdiagnosis leads one to quickly recognize that if the child is not progressing as expected, always suspect technology problems first.

By reading the auditory management cases, among others, the audiologist may recognize other issues in children they are seeing, including sensory processing issues, sensory integration issues, autism, etc. By recognizing concomitant concerns in our children, audiologists can offer them the best holistic management.

The goal for managing pediatric cases is to have very high expectations for what a child with a hearing loss is capable of achieving in life. To reach these high expectations, the first step is to make sure that the hearing loss is properly diagnosed, including obtaining accurate information about the degree, type, and progression of hearing loss. Next, we must be absolutely certain that the child has the best auditory brain access through their technologies, to maximize development of their auditory neural centers. We can never assume that the child has good acoustic access unless we document carefully the detection of every single speech sound and evaluate speech perception at soft speech levels, at distances (across the room using a normal voice level), and in noise. Therefore, functional evidence must be obtained to verify the child's auditory brain access of information, and to document their auditory development.

Audiologists have a pivotal and a collaborative role in managing today's infants and children who experience auditory issues. Families and other professionals cannot succeed in their job of developing the child's listening, spoken language, literacy, and learning until we have completed our ongoing task of maximizing auditory functioning. This book is designed to assist in that regard.

We cannot thank enough the wonderful authors who contributed their experience, wisdom, and insights to this second edition. They are amazing professionals who generously give of their time and energy on a daily basis, to children with hearing and vestibular issues and their families.

Jane R. Madell, PhD, FAAA, CCC-A/SLP, ABA, LSLS Cert. AVT
Carol Flexer, PhD, FAAA, CCC-A, LSLS Cert. AVT
Jace Wolfe, PhD, FAAA, CCC-A
Erin C. Schafer, PhD, FAAA, CCC-A

Acknowledgments

The first edition of the Pediatric Audiology Casebook was developed to complement the 2nd edition of the Pediatric Audiology textbook. That dynamic duo was so well-received that we were excited to develop a second edition of the Pediatric Audiology Casebook, with all new cases, to complement the 3rd edition of the Pediatric Audiology textbook.

Another sixty-one authors gave of their time, effort, and wisdom, grown from experience, to write new and expanded cases for this book. We are grateful for their contributions of time, knowledge, and expertise. It has been a privilege to work with them.

We would like to thank our families who have for many years put up with us spending heaps of time doing audiology things and not always being home. We thank our amazingly supportive spouses, Rob Madell, Pete Flexer, Lynnette Wolfe, Michael Schafer; our equally amazing children, Jody, Josh, Heather, Hillari, David, Hayden, Harper, Henley, Avery, and Keira; our children in-laws, James, Dawn, Joe, Josh, and Hilary; and the most special group of grandchildren, Eva, Rose, Trixie, Yehuda, Rachel, Yishai, Libby, Tikva, Rebekah, Binyamin, Jak, Yonah, Aitza and Miriam and those still to come (from whom we continue to learn every day.)

Everyone who contributed to this book has been able to do so because of what they have learned from wonderful audiologists, auditory-verbal therapists, listening and spoken language specialists, educators, and physicians who came before us and helped set the stage for work with infants and children—women and men who believed that anything was possible for children with hearing loss.

We would all know much less than we do were it not for the wonderful families who gave us the honor of allowing us to work with them, and we cannot thank them enough.

And finally, we would like to thank our publisher, Thieme, for having faith in us, and our editors, Kenny Chumbley, Elizabeth Palumbo, and Keith Palumbo who have helped us find our way through these new editions. We dedicate this book to all of them.

Jane R. Madell, PhD, FAAA, CCC-A/SLP, LSLS Cert. AVT
Carol Flexer, PhD, FAAA, CCC-A, LSLS Cert. AVT
Jace Wolfe, PhD, FAAA, CCC-A
Erin C. Schafer, PhD, FAAA, CCC-A

Contributors

Joni Alberg, PhD
Consultant
Yale Alberg & Associates
Raleigh, North Carolina

Tracey Ambrose, AuD, CCC-A
Audiologist
Hearing and Speech
Children's National Health system
Washington, DC

Katherine Maloney (Anderson), MA, CCC-SLP
Speech-Language Pathologist
Speech-Language Pathology: Health and Human Services
University of Toledo
Toledo, Ohio

Kimberly Auerbach, AuD, CCC-A
Senior Audiologist
Audiology Department
Hackensack University Medical Center
Hackensack Meridian Health Network
Hackensack, New Jersey

Marlene Bagatto, AuD, PhD
Assistant Professor
School of Communication Sciences & Disorders
National Centre for Audiology
Western University
London, Ontario, Canada

Christi M. Barbee, AuD, CCC-A, F-AAA
Assistant Professor
University of Oklahoma Health Sciences Center
Oklahoma City, Oklahoma

Marc Bennett MD, MMHC
Associate Professor
Department of Otolaryngology
Vanderbilt Medical Center
Nashville, Tennessee

Lindi Berry, AuD, CCC-A
Audiologist
Clinical Manager of Audiology
Texas Health Care
Fort Worth, Texas

Lori A. Beutler-Pakulski, PhD, CCC-A
Professor
School of Intervention and Wellness
The University of Toledo
Toledo, Ohio

Amy Lynn Birath, AuD, CCC-A/SLP, FAAA, LSLS Cert. AVEd
Pediatric Audiologist/Speech Language Pathologist
The Moog Center for Deaf Education
St. Louis, Missouri

Kenneth A. Bodkin, AuD, PASC
Manager
Hackensack-Meridian Health
Hackensack University Medical Center
Joseph M. Sanzar Children's Hospital
Hackensack, New Jersey

Jane A. Burton, AuD, CCC-A
Auditory neuroscience researcher
Neuroscience
Vanderbilt University
Nashville, Tennessee

Catherine Cronin Carotta, EdD, SLP-CCC
Associate Director Center for Childhood Deafness,
    Language, and Learning
Boys Town National Research Hospital
Omaha, Nevada

Aubrey Chesner, AuD., CCC-A
Audiologist
Fort Worth Independent School District
Fort Worth, Texas

Lisa Vaughan Christensen, AuD
Audiology Program Manager
Cook Children's Medical Center
Fort Worth, Texas
Keller, Texas

Jackie L. Clark, PhD
Clinical Professor
UT Dallas and U. Witwatersrand
UT Dallas/Callier Center
Dallas, Texas

Rollen M. Cooper, MS, LSLS Cert AVEd
Director of Early Intervention
Child's Voice
Wood Dale, Illinois

Lisa S. Davidson, PhD
Associate Professor
Department of Otolaryngology
Washington University School of Medicine
Director of Audiology Outcomes
CID – Central Institute for the Deaf
St. Louis, Missouri

Michele DiStefano, AuD, CCC-A
Clinical Audiologist
The Center for Hearing and Communication
New York, New York

William Michael Douglas
Assistant Director/Principal
Mama Lere Hearing School
Vanderbilt University Medical Center
Nashville, Tennessee

Elizabeth M. Fitzpatrick, PhD AUD (C), LSLS, Cert AVT
Associate Professor
University of Ottawa
Ottawa, Ontario, Canada

Carol Flexer, PhD, FAAA, CCC-A, LSLS Cert AVT
Consultant in Pediatric Audiology
Distinguished Professor Emeritus, Audiology
School of Speech-Language Pathology and Audiology
The University of Akron
Akron, Ohio

David R. Friedmann, MD
Assistant Professor of Otolaryngology
Division of Otology, Neurotology, and
   Skull Base Surgery
Department of Otolaryngology – Head and
   Neck Surgery
NYU Cochlear Implant Center
New York University School of Medicine
New York, New York

Hilary Gazeley, AuD
Audiologist
Koss Cochlear Implant Program
Department of Otolaryngology and Communication
   Sciences
Medical College of Wisconsin
Milwaukee, Wisconsin

Danielle Glista, PhD
Research Professor
The University of Western Ontario
The National Centre for Audiology
London, Ontario, Canada

Janet E. Green, AuD
Audiologist
Department of Otolaryngology
NYU Langone Health
New York, New York

Lindsay M. Hanna, M.S., CCC-SLP, LSLS Cert. AVT
Speech Language Pathologist
Hearts for Hearing
Oklahoma City, Oklahoma

Kelsey Hatton, AuD, CCC-A
Audiologist
Vanderbilt University Medical Center
Vanderbilt Bill Wilkerson Center
Medical Center East, South Tower
Nashville, Tennessee

Marianne Hawkins, MClSc
Research Associate
National Centre for Audiology
Western University
London, Ontario, Canada

Joan G. Hewitt, AuD
Pediatric Audiologist
Project TALK, Inc.
Encinitas, California

Tessa Hixon, MS
Speech-Language Pathologist
Hearts for Hearing
Oklahoma City, Oklahoma

Meredith A. Holcomb, AuD, CCC-A
Clinical Assistant Professor
Clinical Director, Cochlear Implant Program
Department of Otolaryngology – Head and
   Neck Surgery
Division of Audiology
Medical University of South Carolina
Charleston, South Carolina

Shawna Jackson, AuD
Callier Center for Communication Disorders
University of Texas at Dallas
Dallas, Texas

Kristen Janky, Aud, PhD
Director
Vestibular & Balance Laboratory
Coordinator
Vestibular Clinical Services
Clinical Vestibular Laboratory
Boys Town National Research Hospital
Omaha, Nevada

Andrew B. John, PhD
Associate Professor
Department of Communication Sciences and Disorders
College of Allied Health
University of Oklahoma Health Sciences Center
Oklahoma City, Oklahoma

Margaret A. Kenna, MD, MPH
Professor of Otolaryngology
Harvard Medical School
Department of Otolaryngology and Communication
  Enhancement
Boston Children's Hospital
Boston, Massachusetts

Darius Kohan, MD, PC
Division Chief Otology/Neurotology
Lenox Hill Hospital
Manhattan Eye Ear Nose Throat Hospital
Northwell Health System
Associate Professor of Otolaryngology
NYU School of Medicine
New York, New York

Michelle L. Kraskin, Aud, CCC-A
Assistant Director
Hearing and Speech Department
Weill Cornell Medicine
New York, New York

Meghan Kuhlmey, AuD, CCC-A
Assistant Professor of Audiology at CUMC
Department of Otolaryngology – Head & Neck Surgery
Columbia University Irving Medical Center
New York, New York

Cathryn A. Luckoski, MS, MBA, CCC-A
Center Coordinator for Clinical Education
Clinical Audiologist
Rehabilitation Services
St. Vincent Hospital and Healthcare Services
Indianapolis, Indiana

Stacey R. Lim, AuD, PhD
Assistant Professor of Audiology
Central Michigan University
Department of Communication Disorders
Health Professions Building
Mt. Pleasant, Michigan

Jane R. Madell, PhD, FAAA, CCC-A/SLP, LSLS Cert AVT
Director
Pediatric Audiology Consulting
New York, New York
Brooklyn, New York

Laurel A. Mahoney, AuD, CCC-A
Senior Audiologist
Department of Otolaryngology
NYU School of Medicine
New York, New York

**Josephine Marriage, BSc speech science,
  MSc Audiology, PhD**
Clinical Scientist
Audiology and Hearing Aid Dispenser
Chear Ltd
Research Associate
Department of Psychology
University of Cambridge
Shepreth, Royston Herts, United Kingdom

Devin L. McCaslin, PhD
Director
Vestibular and Balance Program
Mayo Clinic
Rochester, Minnesota

Shelley R. Moats, AuD, PASC
Executive Director
Little Ear Hearing Center
Louisville, Kentucky

Cynthia C. Morton, PhD
William Lambert Richardson Professor of Obstetrics,
  Gynecology, and Reproductive Biology
Department of Obstetrics and Gynecology
Brigham and Women's Hospital
Professor of Pathology
Harvard Medical School
Chair in Auditory Genetics
Manchester Center for Audiology and Deafness
University of Manchester
Manchester, United Kingdom
Boston, Massachusetts

Karen Muñoz, EdD
Communicative Disorders and Deaf Education
Utah State University
Logan, Utah

Elizabeth Musgrave, AuD, CCC-A
Audiologist
Hearts for Hearing
Oklahoma City, Oklahoma

Homira Osman, PhD, AuD
Post-Doctoral Clinical/Research Fellow
The Hospital for Sick Children
Collaborative Program in Neuroscience
University of Toronto
Toronto, Canada

Catherine V. Palmer, PhD
Associate Professor
Department of Communication Science and Disorders
Department of Otolaryngology
University of Pittsburgh
Pittsburgh, Pennsylvania

Bari Pham, AuD
Audiologist
Cook Children's Northeast Center Rehab
Hurst, Texas

Cache Pitt, AuD, CCC-A
Clinical Associate Professor
Clinical Education Coodinator
Utah State University
Logan, Utah

Diego Preciado, MD, PhD
Professor with tenure
Vice Chair of Pediatric Otolaryngology
Division of Pediatric Otolaryngology
Children's National Medical Center
Washington, DC

Elizabeth Preston, AuD, CCC-A
Pediatric Cochlear Implant Audiologist
Audiology Clinic Manager
Clinical Instructor
The Children's Cochlear Implant Center at UNC
UNC School of Medicine
Durham, North Carolina

Kristi Reed, AuD
Audiologist
Cook Children's Medical Center
Fort Worth, Texas

Amy McConkey Robbins, MS, CCC-SLP, LSLS Cert. AVT
Speech-Language Pathologist
Communication Consulting Services
Indianapolis, Indiana

Tommie L. Robinson, Jr. PhD, CCC-SLP
Board Certified Specialist-Fluency Disorders
Chief
Division of Hearing and Speech
Director
Scottish Rite Center for Childhood Language Disorders
Children's Hearing and Speech Center
Children's National Health System
Associate Professor of Pediatrics
The George Washington University School of Medicine and
    Health Sciences
Washington, DC

J. Thomas Roland, Jr., MD
Mendik Foundation Chairman
Department of Otolaryngology – Head and Neck Surgery
NYU School of Medicine
Professor of Otolaryngology and Neurosurgery
Co-Director
NYU Cochlear Implant Program
Co-director NYU NF2 Center
NYU Langone Health
New York, New York

Patricia Roush, AuD
Professor
Department of Otolaryngology
University of North Carolina at Chapel Hill
Chapel Hill, North Carolina

Katherine Marie Schaars, AuD
Doctor of Audiology
Cook Children's Health Care System
Fort Worth, Texas

Erin C. Schafer, PhD, FAAA, CCC-A
Professor
Department of Audiology and Speech-Language Pathology
College of Health and Public Service
University of North Texas
Denton, Texas

Susan Scollie
Associate Professor
Western University
National Centre for Audiology
Faculty of Health Sciences
London, Ontario, Canada

Andi Seibold, AuD
Owner and Pediatric Audiologist
Little Ears Audiology, PLLC
Keller, Texas

Brett Shonebarger, AuD
Pediatric Audiologist
McLane Children's Specialty Clinic
Baylor Scott & White Health
Temple, Texas

William Shapiro, AuD
Executive Secretary to L. Dade Lunsford, MD
Lars Leksell Professor of Neurological Surgery
Distinguished Professor
University of Pittsburgh
Director, Center for Image Guided Neurosurgery
Director, Neurosurgery Residency Program
UPMC Presbyterian
Pittsburgh, Pennsylvania

Jun Shen, PhD, FACMG
Clinical Molecular Geneticist
Department of Pathology
Brigham and Women's Hospital
Harvard Medical School
Boston, Massachusetts

Jeffrey L. Simmons, AuD
Cochlear Implant Clinic Coordinator
Center for Childhood Deafness, Language, and Learning
Boys town National Research Hospital
Omaha, Nevada

Cui Song, MD
Associate Professor
Department of Endocrinology and Genetic Metabolic
    Diseases
Children's Hospital of Chongqing Medical University
Chongqing Key Laboratory of Pediatrics
Chongqing, China

Neil Sperling, MD
Affiliate Assistant Professor
Department of Otolaryngology
Weill Cornell Medical College
New York, New York

Meredith Spratford, AuD, CCC-A
Staff Research Audiologist
Boys Town National Research Hospital
Audibility, Perception and Cognition Laboratory
Omaha, Nevada

Casey J. Stach, AuD
Audiologist
University of Michigan
Cochlear Implant Program
Ann Arbor, Michigan

Shelby L. Stephenson, AuD
Audiologist
Hearts for Hearing
Oklahoma City, Oklahoma

Darcy L. Stowe, MS ccc-SLP, LSLS Cert AUT
Director of Listening and Spoken Language
Hearts for Hearing
Oklahoma City, Oklahoma

Jessica Renee Sullivan, PhD
Assistant Professor
University of West Georgia
Carrolton, Georgia

Marie T. Tan
Research Assistant
Wellesley College
Department of Pathology
Brigham and Women's Hospital
Harvard Medical School
Wellesley, Massachusetts

Linda M. Thibodeau, PhD
Professor
Doctorate of Audiology Program
University of Texas at Dallas
Dallas, Texas

Jennifer Tunnell, AuD, PASC
Audiology Manager
Mayo Clinic Health System
Mankato, Minnesota

Dawn Violetto, AuD, FAAA, CCC/A
Director of Audiology
Child's Voice
Wood Dale, Illinois

Andrea D. Warner-Czyz, PhD, CCC-A
Associate Professor
Department of Behavioral and Brain Sciences
The University of Texas at Dallas
Richardson, Texas

Jennifer Lynn Naylor Wilk, AuD, CCC-A
Audiologist
Callier Center for Communication Disorders
The University of Texas at Dallas
Dallas, Texas

Jace Wolfe, PhD, CCC-A
Director of Audiology
Hearts for Hearing Foundation
Adjunct Assistant Professor, Audiology
University of Oklahoma Health Sciences Center and
   Salus University
Oklahoma City, Oklahoma

Rose Wright, AuD, CCC-A
Audiologist
Dun Laoghaire
Dublin, Ireland

Lori Zitelli, AuD
Audiology Department
UPMC
University of Pittsburgh
Pittsburgh, Pennsylvania

Teresa A. Zwolan, PhD
Clinical Professor
Director Cochlear Implant Program
University of Michigan
Department of Otolaryngology
Ann Arbor, Michigan

1 Managing Mild Hearing Loss

Jane R. Madell

1.1 Clinical History and Description

Jamie is entering second grade. Jamie's mother brings him for an audiological evaluation and reports the history. Pregnancy and birth histories are normal. Early development was within normal limits. There is no significant medical history and no history of middle ear disease. In kindergarten and first grade, Jamie seemed to be struggling with some aspects of academic learning, and his teachers are concerned. Hearing testing was recommended as a way to begin identifying the problem(s). His mother's observation at home is that hearing is not a concern.

1.2 Audiologic Testing

Jamie was cooperative, and testing was accomplished with good reliability. Results indicated a mild sensorineural hearing loss, bilaterally. See ▶ Fig. 1.1 and ▶ Table 1.1.

Tympanograms were within normal limits, bilaterally. The audiologist reported to Jamie's mother that hearing sensitivity was at very mild hearing loss levels, and therefore, no additional services were needed at this time. It was recommended that Jamie return for reevaluation in 1 year.

1.3 Questions for the Reader

1. Do you agree with the audiologist's diagnosis and recommendation? Why?
2. Is additional testing needed? If yes, what testing is needed?

1.4 Discussion of Questions

1. **Do you agree with the audiologist's diagnosis and recommendation? Why?**
   No, we disagree with the audiologist. Jamie does not have normal hearing. Normal hearing sensitivity for children is 15 dB HL or better at all frequencies in both ears. Jamie is, in fact, demonstrating a mild hearing loss. Research over the years has indicated that a "mild" hearing loss can have substantial negative effects on language development, academic learning, and the advancement of social skills.[1,2,3,4]

2. **Is additional testing needed? If yes, what testing is needed?**
   Testing is not complete. Because speech reception thresholds were obtained at higher than normal levels, speech perception testing was conducted at loud levels. Testing speech perception at loud levels is not predictive of how Jamie's brain will be receiving auditory information at normal and soft conversational levels typical of hearing in everyday situations. With his current thresholds at around 30 dB HL, it is likely that Jamie will have a difficult time hearing soft speech, which will have a negative effect on hearing at a distance, overhearing conversations (thereby reducing incidental learning), and hearing comments of peers during classroom discussions.

Table 1.1 Speech perception testing under earphones

	Right ear	Left ear
Speech reception threshold	30 dB HL	30 dB HL
Speech perception: 40 dB SL (70 dB HL)	84%	88%

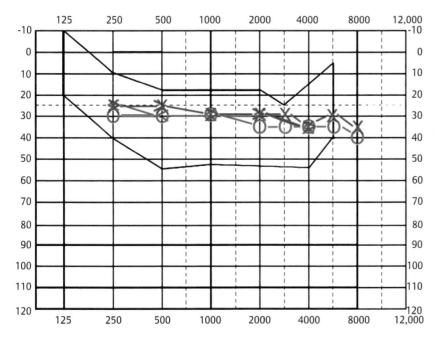

Fig. 1.1 Initial audiologic evaluation. O, right ear air conduction; X, left ear air conduction; <, right ear bone conduction; >, left ear bone conduction.

Additional audiologic testing should include speech perception testing in sound field, at normal and at soft conversational levels, and in quiet and in competing noise. Once Jamie's hearing loss is confirmed, and especially since there are academic concerns, a complete speech and

language evaluation should be considered, as well as a psychoeducational evaluation to identify any areas of academic weakness that could benefit from therapy/intervention.

1.5 Additional Testing

Jamie returned for additional speech perception testing. See ▶ Table 1.2.

1.6 Additional Questions for the Reader

1. What does sound-field speech perception testing indicate about Jamie's hearing?

1.7 Discussion of Additional Questions

1. What does sound-field speech perception testing indicate about Jamie's hearing?
   Speech perception testing suggests that Jamie is going to be struggling to hear in the classroom. While his brain is receiving auditory information at a normal conversational level in quiet, his speech perception is poor for soft speech and for speech in noise. We would expect that language learning will be affected and that this hearing loss will have a significant negative effect on classroom learning.

1.8 Recommended Treatment

Jamie has a mild, bilateral sensorineural hearing loss. Because a mild hearing loss can negatively affect all aspects of learning, a hearing aid evaluation should be recommended.

Table 1.2 Sound-field speech perception testing

	Sound field (%)
50 dB HL (average conversational-level speech)	76
35 dB HL (soft conversational-level speech)	46
50 dB HL + 5 SNR (four-talker speech babble)	54

SNR, signal to noise ratio

With appropriately fit hearing aids, Jamie's brain should have more access to conversational language (especially from peers) and to academic learning.[5] In addition:
- Jamie would benefit from a remote microphone system for use in school. A personal, wearable, remote microphone system should be recommended.
- As with any child who is identified with hearing loss, Jamie should have a speech-language-listening evaluation by a practitioner who is knowledgeable about language and auditory development for children with hearing loss.
- As with any child identified with a hearing loss, Jamie should be referred for a psychoeducational evaluation to determine if there are any academic delays that need to be addressed.
- The family would benefit from contact with other families with similar hearing loss to provide support.

References

[1] Bess FH, Dodd-Murphy J, Parker RA. Children with minimal sensorineural hearing loss: prevalence, educational performance, and functional status. Ear Hear. 1998; 19(5):339–354
[2] Bess FH, Hornsby BWY. Commentary: listening can be exhausting—fatigue in children and adults with hearing loss. Ear Hear. 2014; 35(6):592–599
[3] Fitzpatrick EM, Whittingham J, Durieux-Smith A. Mild bilateral and unilateral hearing loss in childhood: a 20-year view of hearing characteristics, and audiologic practices before and after newborn hearing screening. Ear Hear. 2014; 35(1):10–18
[4] Tharpe AM. Unilateral and mild bilateral hearing loss in children: past and current perspectives. Trends Amplif. 2008; 12(1):7–15
[5] McCreery RW, Bentler RA, Roush PA. Characteristics of hearing aid fittings in infants and young children. Ear Hear. 2013; 34(6):701–710

2 Newborn Follow-up

Christi Barbee and Andrew B. John

2.1 Clinical History and Description

Marissa, a 3-month-old female infant, was born full-term with no complications. She was referred to us because she did not pass her newborn hearing screening in either ear. Per parental report, Marissa's mother and maternal grandmother both have hearing loss which began in childhood. Marissa's mother and father accompanied her to the appointment and expressed concerns that Marissa was not responding to sounds. Specifically, she did not seem to startle or wake up in response to loud sounds.

2.2 Audiologic Testing

Otoscopy indicated clear canals for both ears. Tympanometry, using a 1,000-Hz probe tone, indicated normal middle ear pressure and compliance for both ears. Auditory brainstem response (ABR) testing was conducted (► Table 2.1).

2.3 Questions for the Reader

1. What other testing do you think should have been included in this appointment?
2. What recommendations would you make for Marissa's family?
3. When should Marissa's next hearing evaluation be scheduled?
4. How would you counsel Marissa's parents regarding their concerns about her hearing?

2.4 Discussion of Questions

1. **What other testing do you think should have been included in this appointment?**
   To help rule out the possibility of a cookie-bite hearing loss configuration, it would have been helpful to have otoacoustic emissions testing, or to have included both 1,000 and 2,000 Hz frequency-specific ABR measurements. In addition, acoustic reflex thresholds would be a useful and objective cross-check measure.

2. **What recommendations would you make for Marissa's family?**
   Due to Marissa's family history of hearing loss, we recommended a genetic evaluation. We also counseled Marissa's parents to verbalize often with her, including reading aloud to her daily.

Table 2.1 Auditory brainstem response thresholds obtained at initial appointment (3 months of age)

	Auditory brainstem response		
	Click (db nHL)	500 Hz (db nHL)	4,000 Hz (db nHL)
Right ear	20	20	20
Left ear	20	20	20

3. **When should Marissa's next hearing evaluation be scheduled?**
   We recommended reevaluating Marissa's hearing at 6 months of age or sooner if changes in her hearing were noted. We expected that VRA would be possible around 6 months of age, but not much earlier.

4. **How would you counsel Marissa's parents regarding their concerns about her hearing?**
   In addition to encouraging Marissa's parents to verbalize with her and read aloud to her often, we provided the parents with information on age-appropriate speech, language, and hearing milestones.

2.5 Additional Testing

At 6 months of age, Marissa returned for audiometric and otoacoustic emissions testing. During this appointment, her parents reported that Marissa was now responding consistently to sounds. Visual reinforcement audiometry (VRA) in soundfield suggested hearing within normal limits for at least the better-hearing ear. Marissa responded consistently to both speech and warbled tones. She fatigued to the task before ear-specific audiometric thresholds could be obtained using insert earphones. Tympanometry showed normal middle ear pressure and compliance in both ears. Distortion product otoacoustic emissions (DPOAEs) revealed present responses with normal absolute amplitudes from 1,000 to 8,000 Hz for both ears. Marissa's parents reported that, after her initial hearing test at 3 months of age, Marissa began responding to sounds (► Fig. 2.1; ► Table 2.2).

2.6 Additional Questions for the Reader

1. Are the behavioral results obtained at the 6-month follow-up appointment consistent with the objective results obtained during this and the initial appointment?
2. Were ear-specific measures obtained at this appointment?
3. Is there still any reason to be concerned that Marissa may have a disorder of hearing?

2.7 Discussion of Additional Questions

1. **Are the behavioral results obtained at the 6-month follow-up appointment consistent with the objective results obtained during this and the initial appointment?**
   Behavioral results matched well with ABR and OAEs test results, at least in the better-hearing ear. Marissa's responses to tones and speech were very consistent in the soundfield.

2. **Were ear-specific measures obtained at the six-month follow-up appointment?**
   Yes, OAEs were measured in each ear separately at this appointment. This is important as a child with a unilateral hearing loss might respond at low presentation levels in soundfield because signals were heard only in the better ear.

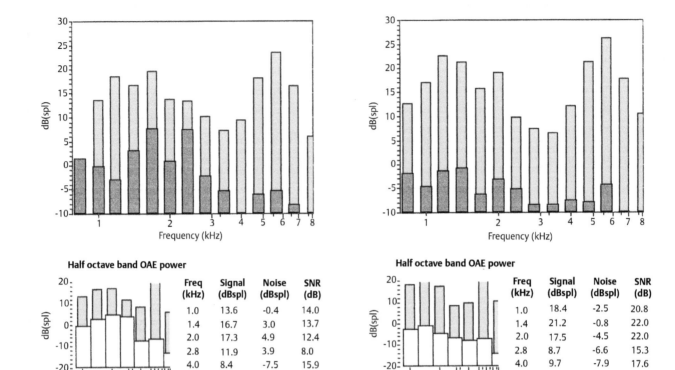

Fig. 2.1 Results of distortion product otoacoustic emission (DPOAE) testing at follow-up appointment.

Table 2.2 Soundfield speech detection and warble-tone thresholds obtained at follow-up appointment (6 months of age)

	SDT	500 Hz	1,000 Hz	2,000 Hz	4,000 Hz
Soundfield	20	20	20	20	20

Note: Testing was not attempted at presentation levels below 20 dB HL. SDT, speech detection threshold.

However, ear-specific behavioral testing, using ear-insert earphones, should be performed at the next test session.

3. **Is there still any reason to be concerned that Marissa may have a disorder of hearing?**

Our test results suggest that Marissa has hearing sensitivity within normal limits at 6 months of age. The reason for her referral from the newborn hearing screening program is not indicated, but it may have reflected a transient conductive hearing loss due to vernix in the ear canals or other environmental obstacle to obtaining a successful hearing screening result. However, coupled with the family history of childhood hearing loss, there is reason for Marissa's parents, doctor, and audiologist to remain vigilant about changes in her hearing and development of speech and language. The results reported here do not rule out progressive postnatally

developing sensorineural hearing loss, auditory processing disorder, or other subtle pathology.

2.8 Recommended Treatment

Hearing evaluations every 6 months until 3 years of age were recommended, or sooner if parents noted a decrease in response to sounds. Genetic evaluation was recommended due to the positive family history of hearing loss.

2.9 Outcome

Marissa's parents were relieved to know that, at this time, Marissa seems to be responding well to sound. Her parents received information on speech-language and hearing milestones, and plan to follow up with hearing evaluations.

Suggested Reading

[1] American Speech-Language-Hearing Association. Newborn Hearing Screening (Practice Portal). Available at: www.asha.org/Practice-Portal/Professional-Issues/Newborn-Hearing-Screening. Accessed 2016

[2] American Academy of Pediatrics, Joint Committee on Infant Hearing. Year 2007 position statement: principles and guidelines for early hearing detection and intervention programs. Pediatrics. 2007; 120(4):898–921

3 Probable Enlarged Vestibular Aqueduct and Hearing Loss in a 6-Year-Old Child

Jessica Sullivan and Homira Osman

3.1 Clinical History and Description

Luis was diagnosed with profound sensorineural hearing loss in his right ear at birth via brainstem auditory evoked response testing. Distortion product otoacoustic emissions were absent from 750 to 4,000 Hz for the right ear. The left ear demonstrated normal hearing at birth. His parents reported that his hearing was evaluated approximately every 6 months consistently from the time of diagnosis at an outside facility (▶ Fig. 3.1). Luis was not fitted with any type of amplification given the severity of hearing loss in the right ear. Luis's parents did not enroll him in any early intervention services as they felt he was demonstrating consistent responses to their voice and to sounds in the environment. At the age of 4 years, Luis's parents began to suspect a change in his hearing. On the date of this exam, case history revealed normal birth history and developmental milestones, including speech and language. His parents reported no permanent childhood hearing loss in their family. An audiologic evaluation revealed that the hearing in the left ear had dropped to a moderate to moderately severe sensorineural hearing loss (▶ Fig. 3.2). The hearing in the right ear was stable as a profound sensorineural hearing loss. His pure-tone average (PTA) of 60 dB HL (hearing level) in the left ear was within 5 dB of his speech reception threshold (SRT). An SRT was unable to be obtained at the equipment limits for the right ear. Tympanograms were type A$_S$ bilaterally, showing reduced compliance of the eardrum mobility bilaterally.

Luis was referred for close monitoring of his hearing. Audiologic thresholds at the 1- and 3-month follow-up appointments were consistent with the thresholds on audiogram 2. His parents reported no fluctuations in hearing or dizziness. Luis was fitted with a digital behind-the-ear hearing aid for the left ear. Initially, he did not wear his hearing aid consistently, but eventually he was wearing his hearing aid for close to 9 hours per day. According to his audiologist, the hearing aid was fitted to prescribed targets using real ear measures. An aided word recognition score of 68% using the NU-CHIPS (Northwestern University-Children's Perception of Speech) recorded test materials was obtained, but no aided thresholds were measured. Additionally, Luis began to use a remote microphone (RM) system at school, and his mother reported benefit from the RM system when it was used. Luis has been using successfully a digital behind-the-ear hearing aid since that time.

At the age of 5 years, Luis described spinning vertigo, usually in the morning before he got out of bed. He reported the spinning vertigo to occur as frequently as twice a month. His parents reported that Luis easily became sick in the car. Luis was referred to a multidisciplinary clinic to explore the etiology of his hearing loss. As part of this clinic, a computed tomography (CT) scan of the temporal bone was ordered.

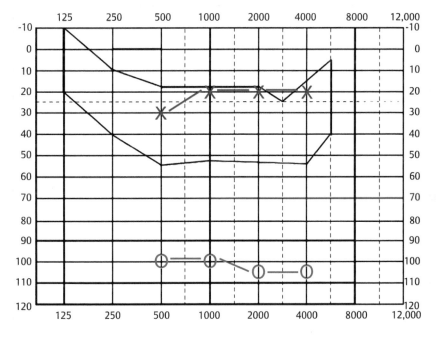

Fig. 3.1 Results at the diagnostic brainstem auditory evoked response test (age 5 weeks). O, right ear air conduction; X, left ear air conduction.

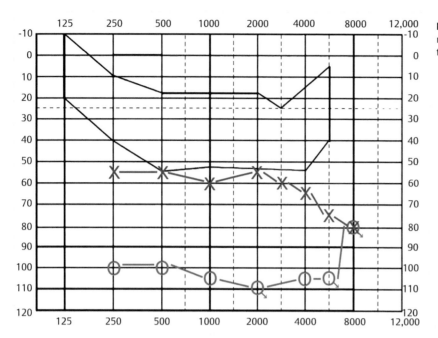

Fig. 3.2 Pure-tone test results (age 4.2 years). O, right ear air conduction; X, left ear air conduction; Arrows, no response.

3.1.1 Question: What is the probable diagnosis? What findings led you to this conclusion?

A CT scan of his temporal bones indicated enlarged vestibular aqueducts for both ears, with the right (4.0 mm) being larger than the left (1.6 mm). Following a discussion with the physician and audiologist, Luis's family was given information about cochlear implants.

3.2 Cochlear Implant Candidacy Evaluations

At this initial appointment through the cochlear implant program, Luis received a complete hearing evaluation. Otoscopy revealed clear ear canals bilaterally. No vestibular episodes were reported. Tympanograms were type A bilaterally, showing no evidence of middle ear pathology. Pure-tone thresholds had worsened since his previous testing approximately 6 months before. Previous testing yielded moderate to moderately severe sensorineural hearing loss, and current testing was consistent with a severe to profound sensorineural hearing loss (▶ Fig. 3.3). Programming changes were made to Luis's hearing aid. The hearing aid was fitted to prescribed targets using real ear measures, but the output was slightly lower than the targets for the mid- to high-frequency range. It was recommended that Luis return for an aided audiologic evaluation.

Aided warble thresholds were obtained (▶ Fig. 3.4). Aided word recognition (NU-CHIPS, recorded) performance was 16% correct in the left ear with a 45 dB HL presentation level. This is a significant decrease from the last evaluation (▶ Fig. 3.2). A few weeks following this appointment, Luis's family met with an otologist and aural habilitation specialist.

3.3 Outcome

At present, Luis, age 6 years, continues to use the hearing aid in his left ear and an RM system at school. Luis's parents are very interested in cochlear implants and are awaiting a decision from the cochlear implant program team. His parents would like for him to be implanted in both ears prior to the new school year. They have started services with an aural habilitation specialist at the hospital.

3.4 Questions for the Reader

1. How prevalent is enlarged vestibular aqueduct (EVA) disease in children?
2. Is Luis a good candidate for a cochlear implant?
3. Would you recommend one or two cochlear implants in this case?
4. What would an aural habilitation plan consist of postimplant?
5. What other recommendations would you suggest for this family?

3.5 Discussion of Questions

1. **How prevalent is EVA disease in children?**
   It is estimated that 5 to 15% of children with a sensorineural hearing loss have EVA. Most children with EVA will have some degree of hearing loss and a small portion of them will also have vestibular function issues. Alemi and Chan[1] conducted a systematic review of 23 studies and found that progressive sensorineural hearing loss was found in 39.6% of ears (1,115 with enlarged vestibular aqueduct) and only 12% were associated with head trauma. In addition, EVA has been associated with a genetic disorder (Pendred's syndrome) that causes early onset of hearing loss in children. Children with

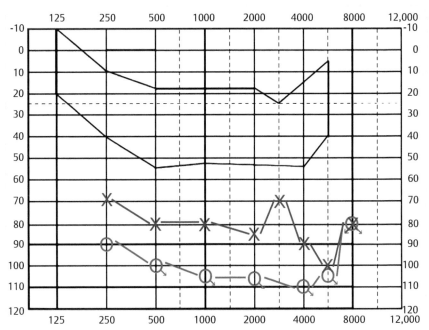

Fig. 3.3 Unaided pure-tone test results for cochlear implant candidacy (age 5 years). O, right ear air conduction; X, left ear air conduction; Arrows, no response.

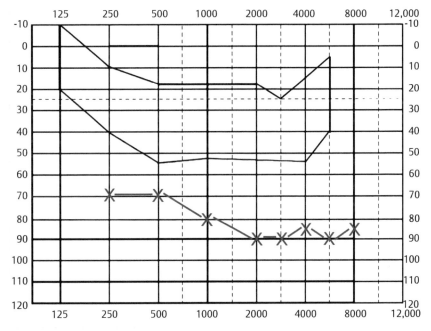

Fig. 3.4 Aided pure-tone test results for cochlear implant candidacy (age 5.1 years). X, left ear air conduction.

Pendred's syndrome have progressive hearing loss, and that usually occurs bilaterally.

2. **Is Luis a good candidate for a cochlear implant?**
   Luis is a good candidate for a cochlear implant, and it is reasonable to consider bilateral implantation. He has already had a hearing aid trial and is familiar with the benefits of using amplification in the left ear. He has a supportive family unit that would support him through the process of getting the implant. Bichey et al[2] found an improvement in quality of life associated with cochlear implantation in postlingually deafened patients with EVA. Additionally, Miyamoto et al[3]

found that pediatric and adult cochlear implant users had improved speech and auditory outcomes.

3. **Would you recommend one or two cochlear implants in this case?**
   Even though there he has only worn amplification on the left ear, we would recommend implanting both ears. The left ear is predicted to provide the best outcome. Luis had a period of normal hearing in the left ear, and has worn a hearing aid, resulting in less auditory deprivation than the right. There could be an increase in localization abilities.

4. **What would an aural habilitation plan consist of postimplant?**

Postimplantation, it is important begin to develop self-advocacy skills so Luis can explain to his peers how the implant works. To begin, it is imperative to teach Luis how to handle communication breakdowns and to use appropriate repair strategies.

In addition, it is important that he participates in auditory training to help use his implant effectively. Furthermore, it is important to have time where he has auditory training for each ear alone during each session. Because of his age, we would suggest a combination of analytical and synthetic exercises to facilitate language development. Analytic exercises use training stimuli, such as phonemes and syllables, while synthetic exercises may involve training with sentences and stories. For example, an analytic activity might be to discriminate between /k/ and /g/ or one versus two syllables. A synthetic activity might involve the child listening to a short passage and then recalling specific details from the story.

In terms of his academic progress, we would request a language evaluation (e.g., Oral Written Language Scales [OWLS]) to determine his language needs and to help develop appropriate goals based on the results. If he demonstrates a need, then his individualized education program (IEP) and/or 504 plan would be revised as needed.

5. **What other recommendations would you suggest for this family?**

If Luis returned to our center, we would want to work with his school audiologist to make sure all of his needs are being met in terms of additional hearing assistance technologies (e.g., RM system) for school and extracurricular activities. Also, we would discuss any additional accommodations that would facilitate his learning in the classroom, such as preferential seating, frequent checks for understanding by his teacher, and repeated instructions based on his IEP and/or 504 services. It is important to monitor Luis as he progresses through school because children with hearing loss have difficulties with speech recognition in noise, especially as academic demands increase.

References

[1] Alemi AS, Chan DK. Progressive hearing loss and head trauma in enlarged vestibular aqueduct: a systematic review and meta-analysis. Otolaryngol Head Neck Surg. 2015; 153(4):512–517

[2] Bichey BG, Hoversland JM, Wynne MK, Miyamoto RT. Changes in quality of life and the cost-utility associated with cochlear implantation in patients with large vestibular aqueduct syndrome. Otol Neurotol. 2002; 23(3):323–327

[3] Miyamoto RT, Bichey BG, Wynne MK, Kirk KI. Cochlear implantation with large vestibular aqueduct syndrome. Laryngoscope. 2002; 112(7, Pt 1):1178–1182

4 Being Mindful of "Mild"

Meredith Spratford

4.1 Clinical History and Description

Sam is a 5-year-old who was enrolled in a longitudinal study of outcomes of children with hearing loss (Outcomes of Children with Hearing Loss, OCHL).[1] Records indicate that Sam referred on the newborn hearing screen in both ears, and the family was given a written recommendation for a follow-up rescreen by 4 weeks of age. Medical records from his pediatrician do not mention a referral on the newborn hearing screen or any hearing-related follow-up until age 14 months when Sam presented with otitis media. He received bilateral tympanostomy tubes at 18 months after experiencing chronic middle ear effusion. Sam's mother reported that he was fitted with hearing aids (HAs) at age 3 years and was not enrolled in early intervention services due to his late confirmation of hearing loss.

4.2 Audiologic Testing

At Sam's 5-year-old research visit, pure-tone thresholds were obtained using ER-3A insert earphones with good reliability using conventional audiometry and video reinforcement (i.e., Sam saw a picture appear on a computer monitor each time he responded to the stimuli). As seen in ▶ Fig. 4.1, hearing thresholds corresponded to normal hearing at 250 Hz, gently sloping to a moderately severe hearing loss at 8,000 Hz in both ears. When aided, he obtained 72% correct on the Phonetically-Balanced Kindergarten (PBK) speech recognition test in quiet. Sam wore behind-the-ear HAs that were verified with simulated real-ear speech mapping and measured

real-ear-to-coupler differences, as part of the OCHL protocol.[1] His HAs were well-fitted to DSL v.5 targets and provided appropriate aided audibility (see ▶ Table 4.1 for measures of unaided and aided speech intelligibility index [SII]) for his degree of hearing loss.[2]

As part of the OCHL test battery, Sam's mother was interviewed about the amount of hours and consistency of Sam's daily HA use across varying situations using the Hearing Aid Checklist (found online at www.ochlstudy.org).[3] She reported that he wore HAs 7 hours each day at school, but never in outside-of-school settings, including at home and over summer vacation. Furthermore, she reported that Sam had been without his HAs for 2 to 3 months in the past year because they were lost and needed to be replaced.

4.3 Speech and Language Testing

A battery of standardized measures[1] was performed to assess aspects of Sam's speech and language development (▶ Fig. 4.2). Findings showed that Sam performed below average compared to normative standards on tests of articulation, receptive vocabulary, expressive grammar, and global language. Common articulation errors included substituting /dz/

Table 4.1 Unaided and aided speech intelligibility measures at input levels of 50 and 65 dB SPL

	Unaided SII	Aided SII-50	Aided SII-65
Right	64	87	92
Left	76	93	93

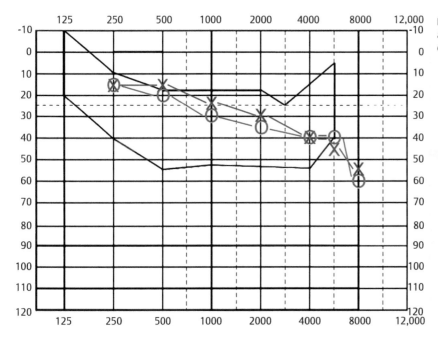

Fig. 4.1 Air conduction thresholds for the right and left ears. O, right ear air conduction; X, left ear air conduction.

Speech and Language Measures	Below Average 55 70 85	Average 100 115	Above Average 130 145
Articulation	X		
Receptive vocabulary	X		
Expressive grammar	X		
Global language	X		
Phonological processing & memory	X		

Fig. 4.2 Standard scores on speech and language measures. Standard scores between 85 and 115 indicate the average range of performance for the normative samples.

for fricatives ("jipper" for "zipper"). He demonstrated difficulty using morphological markers involving /s/, as well as irregular plurals and irregular past tense. On the measure of global language, he had difficulty on items that required him to understand complex language concepts (e.g., point to all of the items you do *not* need to dress this doll). He also had below average scores on phonological processing and memory tasks, which are considered important preliteracy skills.

4.4 Questions for the Reader

1. Does Sam's aided speech recognition score of 72% on the PBK test seem appropriate based on his degree of hearing loss and aided speech mapping results?
2. What factors potentially contributed to Sam's lack of HA use at home?
3. What strategies could you use to encourage Sam's family to increase HA use at home?
4. Do you think Sam's limited HA use contributed to his language skills being below average? If so, how will you use this information to encourage consistent HA use?

4.5 Discussion of Questions

1. **Does Sam's aided speech recognition score of 72% on the PBK test seem appropriate based on his degree of hearing loss and aided speech mapping results?**
   Based on speech mapping findings, the majority of the long-term average speech spectrum was audible to Sam through his HAs. Sam's score on the PBK test (72%) fell below the 25th percentile of performance compared to other peers with HAs in the OCHL study.[4] The mismatch between aided SII measures and his actual performance leads us to believe factors other than audibility contributed to his lower-than-expected speech recognition ability. Sam's language and/or memory abilities may be affecting his speech recognition performance.
2. **What factors potentially contributed to Sam's lack of HA use at home?**
   In a recent report,[3] families who have younger children, children with milder losses, and mothers with lower levels of maternal education reported lower amounts of daily HA use for their children. Furthermore, parents of children with mild hearing loss were less likely to report consistent use of amplification in the home and across other situational contexts. After a late confirmation of hearing loss and fitting of HAs, Sam's

mother may have seen him developing language and responding to sound without HAs. Among other possible reasons for nonuse at home, Sam's mother could feel that his mild hearing loss is inconsequential and does not warrant the use of HAs at home. Or, she could see that Sam benefits from the HAs, but is worried about losing them again and the financial burden of replacement, thus restricting HA use to supervised situations at school. Exploring Sam's mother's perception of his hearing loss and the benefit from HAs might reveal underlying reasons for not using the HAs at home.

3. **What strategies could you use to encourage Sam's family to increase HA use at home?**
   Understanding family-related factors that contribute to Sam's lack of HA use at home will help address family concerns and provide guidance with appropriate informational and support counseling. Because Sam was unable to participate in early intervention due to a late confirmation of hearing loss, consider that Sam's mother may be missing some of the information and skills, as well as emotional support, which promote HA use. An often overlooked component of device use is self-efficacy for managing the HAs, which families typically learn about and become comfortable with during early intervention. For families who did not experience early intervention, additional mentored, hands-on practice with the HAs may support self-confidence in managing the technology for both the parent and child and increase device use. Without an understanding of the implications of hearing loss for the child's language and learning, parents may not see a need for wearing HAs. Experiential learning opportunities, such as hearing loss simulations that include distant speech or speech in noise and/or reverberation, may help parents internalize the critical contributions of HAs to their child's speech perception and language learning.[5] Providing an opportunity to obtain advice from other parents who have children who wear HAs may also help Sam's mother with the emotional and practical support needed to navigate a path to full-time HA use.

   Another strategy is to complete situational consistency ratings with Sam's mother at regular audiology visits. The audiologist can address any discrepancies between data logging and parent-reported use or consistency ratings in an open dialogue about recent challenges or progress with HA use. From these discussions, manageable, situation-specific goals can be created. A quality-over-quantity goal (wearing HAs in supervised situations that are language-rich, such as during meals or when reading books together) would be an appropriate first step when encouraging Sam's family to initiate HA use at home.

4. **Do you think Sam's limited HA use contributed to his language skills being below average? If so, how will you use this information to encourage consistent HA use?**
Sam's limited amount of daily HA use could have contributed to his language delay. According to a recent study,[6] children with mild hearing loss who wear their amplification for greater amounts of time on a daily basis have better receptive vocabulary and expressive grammar skills compared to children with lower amounts of device use. Among others, these were two skill areas in which Sam showed delays that potentially could have been lessened with consistent access to auditory-linguistic information.

It is important to communicate to Sam's mother that his HAs are providing optimal audibility and benefit for understanding speech and developing literacy and academic skills—when they are worn. Connecting inconsistent HA use to Sam's lower-than-expected language abilities may further help Sam's mother understand the importance of providing optimal auditory access at home. Without consistent use of HAs, Sam may continue to struggle in elementary school with reading, comprehension, and complex social language, which could have implications for his long-term academic success and relationships with friends.

4.6 Final Diagnosis and Recommended Treatment

Sam's inconsistent auditory experience—having a late age at HA fit and not wearing HAs full-time—likely contributed to his delayed language skills.[7] In order to educate the family on the importance of treating mild hearing loss,[6] we need to first openly explore the family's perception of hearing loss and benefits of HAs. Afterward, we may provide appropriate informational and support counseling, which may include emphasizing the positive effects of full-time HA use on language development, sharing simulations of hearing loss, and creating collaborative goals for improving device use outside of school based on consistency ratings and data logging over time.

4.7 Outcome

At Sam's 6-year-old research visit, his mother again reported HA use at school only. His global language score was still

depressed, and he struggled most with grammar and social aspects of language. Auditory access via well-fitted amplification that is worn consistently helps many children who are hard of hearing develop age-appropriate language skills over time.[7] Compared to children whose language improved with full-time HA use and optimal aided audibility, Sam's language remained delayed compared to his peers.

Children with mild hearing loss are at risk for low HA use and potentially persistent delays in language. It is critical that audiologists and other communication/educational interventionists provide supports that relate the importance of treating mild hearing loss during times of language growth and development, especially when early intervention is missed. Reinforcing full-time HA use from many perspectives (pediatrician, speech language pathologist, teacher, audiologist, parent–parent support group) may help encourage the family to achieve full-time device use and help Sam optimize his potential for improving his future language and academic outcomes.

References

[1] Tomblin JB, Walker EA, McCreery RW, Arenas RM, Harrison M, Moeller MP. Outcomes of children with hearing loss: Data collection and methods. Ear Hear. 2015; 36 Suppl 1:14S–23S

[2] Bagatto MP, Moodie ST, Malandrino AC, Richert FM, Clench DA, Scollie SD. The University of Western Ontario pediatric audiological monitoring protocol (UWO PedAMP). Trends Amplif. 2011; 15(1):57–76

[3] Walker EA, Spratford M, Moeller MP, et al. Predictors of hearing aid use time in children with mild-to-severe hearing loss. Lang Speech Hear Serv Sch. 2013; 44(1):73–88

[4] McCreery RW, Walker EA, Spratford M, et al. Speech recognition and parent ratings from auditory development questionnaires in children who are hard of hearing. Ear Hear. 2015; 36 Suppl 1:60S–75S

[5] Haggard RS, Primus MA. Parental perceptions of hearing loss classification in children. Am J Audiol. 1999; 8(2):83–92

[6] Walker EA, Holte L, McCreery RW, Spratford M, Page T, Moeller MP. The influence of hearing aid use on outcomes of children with mild hearing loss. J Speech Lang Hear Res. 2015; 58(5):1611–1625

[7] Tomblin JB, Harrison M, Ambrose SE, Walker EA, Oleson JJ, Moeller MP. Language outcomes in young children with mild to severe hearing loss. Ear Hear. 2015; 36 Suppl 1:76S–91S

Suggested Reading

[1] Fitzpatrick EM, Durieux-Smith A, Gaboury I, Coyle D, Whittingham J. Communication development in early-identified children with mild bilateral and unilateral hearing loss. Am J Audiol. 2015; 24(3):349–353

[2] Lewis DE, Valente DL, Spalding JL. Effect of minimal/mild hearing loss on children's speech understanding in a simulated classroom. Ear Hear. 2015; 36(1):136–144

5 Minimal/Mild Bilateral Hearing Loss

Marlene Bagatto

5.1 Clinical History and Description

Following a bilateral refer result on her newborn hearing screening, Abby was routed to an audiologist for an assessment. There is no report of a family history of permanent childhood hearing loss, and Abby does not have any associated risk indicators for late-onset or progressive hearing loss.

5.2 Audiologic Testing

Frequency-specific auditory brainstem responses (ABRs) were obtained from each ear using air- and bone-conducted stimuli when she was 8 weeks old. Abby's ear canals were clear, middle ears were functioning normally, and otoacoustic emissions were essentially absent in both ears. The audiologist confirmed a mild bilateral sensorineural hearing loss (▸ Fig. 5.1). Following the completion of the audiological assessment, the results and potential impact on Abby's development were explained to her parents.

The Early Hearing Detection and Intervention (EHDI) program in which Abby is involved includes mild hearing loss levels within its target population. Therefore, Abby has the opportunity for intervention and monitoring of her mild bilateral hearing loss (MBHL). Hearing aids were discussed with the family as part of the intervention program, in addition to communication development and family support. Abby's parents declined to pursue hearing aids at the time of hearing loss confirmation, but accessed communication development and family support.

5.3 Additional Audiologic Testing and Monitoring

Regular monitoring of Abby's hearing thresholds and auditory development was conducted. Visual reinforcement audiometry (VRA) was performed at a variety of frequencies using insert earphones at 5 and 10 months of age. Results were similar to the ABR assessment. In addition, the LittlEARS Auditory Questionnaire[1] was completed by Abby's parents to monitor her auditory development. As illustrated in ▸ Fig. 5.2, Abby was demonstrating age-appropriate auditory development milestones. She was also developing normally in all other aspects, as reported by her parents and other team members.

During the early months of life when Abby was not yet walking, she was home with a caregiver and no siblings. Hearing aids remained an intervention option for Abby, but her parents chose not to pursue them initially. With the arrival of a baby sister and Abby's attendance at daycare in the coming months, Abby's parents were motivated to proceed with hearing aids. She received her first pair of hearing aids at 18 months of age. With some perseverance by her parents to ensure consistent use, Abby is now a full-time hearing aid wearer and continues to meet speech, language, and auditory development milestones.

5.4 Questions for the Reader

1. What challenges might audiologists experience when recommending hearing aids for an 2-month-old infant who has been identified with an MBHL?

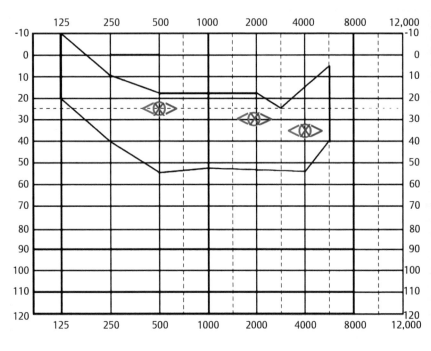

Fig. 5.1 Hearing levels obtained from frequency-specific ABR that have been corrected using nHL to estimated hearing level (eHL) corrections. O, right ear air conduction; X, left ear air conduction; <, right ear bone conduction; >, left ear bone conduction.

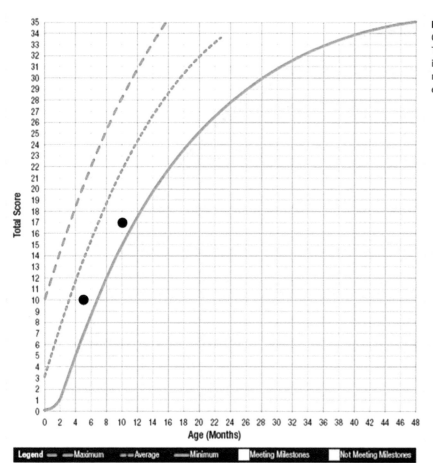

Fig. 5.2 Abby's scores on the LittlEARS Auditory Questionnaire at 5 months and 10 months of age. The filled circles are in the nonshaded region indicating she is meeting auditory development milestones for her age. (Score sheet from Bagatto et al[10]; www.dslio.com.)

2. What additional measures could the audiologist obtain to further understand Abby's hearing levels and the appropriateness of hearing aids?
3. What characteristics about Abby and her family are important to consider when discussing hearing aid intervention?
4. Why might Abby's parents have been reluctant to proceed with hearing aids in the initial stages?

5.5 Discussion of Questions

1. **What challenges might audiologists experience when recommending hearing aids for a 2-month-old infant who has been identified with an MBHL?**
Available consensus-based and evidence-based protocols and guidelines have consistently recommended the selection of amplification for children with MBHL on a case-by-case basis[2] with consideration for whether the degree of hearing loss could interfere with normal development.[3] This is because there is a lack of clear evidence that hearing aid use benefits *all* infants with MBHL.[4,5] Without the obvious benefits of hearing aid use consistently noted in children with more significant degrees of hearing loss, it is challenging for audiologists working with families to state clear hearing aid recommendations for every child with MBHL. Additionally, the impact of MBHL in infants in real-world situations is often undetectable, and families decide that the resources necessary for pursuing hearing aids (e.g., financial, time) are not beneficial in the early months of life. If they pursue hearing aids, even on a trial basis, their usefulness is often not noticeable and usage declines.

From a technical standpoint, for many infants initially assessed using frequency-specific ABR, the minimum test levels are limited to about 25 or 30 dB nHL for a variety of reasons. This limits the ability to assess the true threshold from ABR for some frequencies, and VRA is often pursued when the child is developmentally capable (e.g., 5–6 months of age). For an appropriate hearing aid fitting, ear- and frequency-specific thresholds are required and may not be confirmed until the child is a few months older, given the limitations of ABR threshold estimation at low levels. The motivation of the family and need for accurate hearing aid intervention make recommending a hearing aid to a 2-month-old infant with MBHL challenging.

2. **What additional measures could the audiologist obtain to further understand Abby's hearing levels and the appropriateness of hearing aids?**
The external ear canals of infants and young children are significantly smaller than those of adults,[2,6] and the size changes as the child grows. This growth has substantial implications when defining accurate hearing levels as well as when measuring hearing aid output in devices that are calibrated with reference to an average adult ear canal. It is therefore essential to measure the real-ear-to-coupler difference (RECD) in infants with MBHL and use this measurement

13

to convert the audiogram (referenced in dB HL) to sound pressure level.[7] This will provide a more accurate description of the infant's hearing levels that can be directly compared to hearing aid output on an SPL scale (▸ Fig. 5.3).

Small infant ears can also impact the desired earmold acoustics of a potential hearing aid fitting for an infant with MBHL. In cases like Abby's, her ear canals were too small to accommodate vents in the earmolds, which may interfere with the hearing aid benefit necessary in the high-frequency region due to upward spread of masking, as well as decrease localization abilities. In addition to RECD measures, simulated or coupler-based real-ear verification should be conducted with various speech inputs to assess the output of the hearing aids to be provided. This may demonstrate that minimal hearing aid gain is required and it could interact with the low-level hearing aid noise floor. Therefore, the infant's hearing levels should be defined in SPL by measuring the RECD and the hearing aid prescription characteristics and appropriateness of the fitting should be considered.

3. **What characteristics about Abby and her family are important to consider when discussing hearing aid intervention?**

Learning about Abby beyond her hearing levels is necessary when discussing hearing aid intervention with her family. The presence of additional conditions may be a factor in her parents' decision to pursue hearing aids. Although Abby is healthy, if she had a medical condition requiring frequent visits to a variety of health professionals, her parents may feel that they are not able to also manage hearing aids. On the other hand, depending on the other condition (e.g., low vision), hearing aids may be vital for development.

Mobility and the environment are other significant considerations for hearing aid use in infants with MBHL. An infant in a quiet home with a caregiver will likely have speech available to her if presented in close range and at a reasonable level. Infants in daycare, where it may be difficult for caregivers to offer optimal communication strategies, may require some support from an assistive listening device. Another important consideration is the family context and their readiness to apply

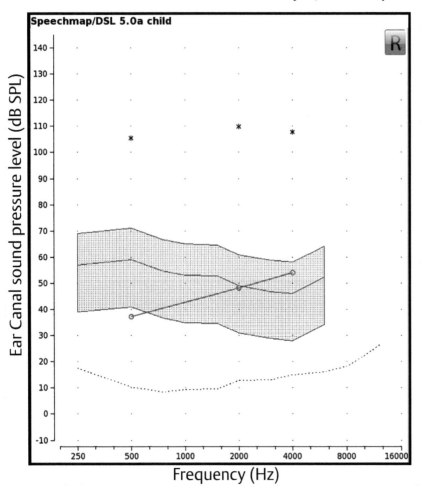

February 23, 2016 02:31pm

Fig. 5.3 Audiogram (dB HL) converted to dB SPL (open circles) for Abby's right ear. Her left ear thresholds are similar. The dashed line represents normal hearing in dB SPL. The shaded region is the unaided long-term average speech spectrum for conversational speech which is mostly audible to Abby without hearing aids.

the hearing aids for Abby. Factors within and surrounding the family may make it difficult for them to follow through with the intervention, despite the best intentions. Therefore, a family-centered approach to hearing aid intervention is vital when working with infants with MBHL.[8]

4. **Why might Abby's parents have been reluctant to proceed with hearing aids in the initial stages?**

The impact of an MBHL in an infant is not obvious in the real world. Therefore, the need to pursue expensive hearing aids, which require time and perseverance, may not be considered worthwhile for parents at this young age. Although the potential impact of Abby's MBHL would have been explained to her parents, a "wait and see" approach is a common decision for parents, especially in the absence of a clear recommendation offered from current protocols and guidelines. The quiet family home and interaction with an in-home caregiver likely contributed to the decision to support Abby's language development using good communication strategies in lieu of technology at the early stage. Although the family was motivated to monitor Abby's hearing and development closely, their incentive to pursue hearing aids at the early stages was likely impacted by these factors.

5.6 Diagnosis and Recommended Treatment

Frequency-specific ABR assessment at 2 months of age confirmed an MBHL. Subsequent VRA assessments using insert earphones revealed stable hearing levels. Developmental monitoring (including speech, language, auditory milestones) described typical development. When the family was ready to proceed, binaural behind-the-ear hearing aids with standard earmolds were provided to Abby when she was 18 months of age. The devices were fitted using measured RECD values to DSL v5.0 Child Targets following recommended protocols.[9,10] Speech and language development as well as hearing levels, aided function, and ear canal acoustics are monitored regularly.

5.7 Outcomes

The LittlEARS and PEACH were administered as part of an EHDI outcome measurement protocol.[8,9] Hearing aid fitting details, such as the speech intelligibility index and RECD, are gathered to inform the interpretation of the outcome measures. Abby is demonstrating typical auditory performance while wearing the hearing aids and is developing speech and language skills appropriate for her age. Recently, her parents noted that she may be bothered by noise in the daycare setting. They were not interested in pursuing a remote microphone system at this time, so noise management was activated within Abby's hearing aids following recommended protocols.[11]

Suggested Readings

[1] Bagatto MP, Tharpe AMT. Decision support guide for hearing aid use in infants and children with minimal/mild bilateral hearing loss. In: Northern J, ed. A Sound Foundation through Early Amplification: 6th International Conference Proceedings. Stafa: Phonak AG; 2014:145–151

References

[1] Tsiakpini L, Weichbold V, Kuehn-Inacker H, Coninx F, D'Haese P, Almadin S. LittlEARS Auditory Questionnaire. Innsbruck, Austria: MED-EL; 2004

[2] Bagatto MP, Scollie SD, Seewald RC, Moodie KS, Hoover BM. Real-ear-to-coupler difference predictions as a function of age for two coupling procedures. J Am Acad Audiol. 2002; 13(8):407–415

[3] American Academy of Audiology. American Academy of Audiology Pediatric Amplification Guidelines. 2013. Available at: http://audiology-web.s3.amazo-naws.com/migrated/PediatricAmplificationGuidelines.pdf_539975b3e7e9f1.74471798.pdf

[4] Lewis DE, Valente DL, Spalding JL. Effect of minimal/mild hearing loss on children's speech understanding in a simulated classroom. Ear Hear. 2015; 36(1):136–144

[5] Walker EA, Holte L, McCreery RW, Spratford M, Page T, Moeller MP. The influence of hearing aid use on outcomes of children with hearing loss. J Speech Lang Hear Res. 2015; 58(5):1611–1625

[6] Feigin JA, Kopun JG, Stelmachowicz PG, Gorga MP. Probe-tube microphone measures of ear-canal sound pressure levels in infants and children. Ear Hear. 1989; 10(4):254–258

[7] Seewald RC, Scollie SD. Infants are not average adults: Implications for audiometric testing. Hear J. 1999; 52(10):64–, 66, 69, 70, 72

[8] Bagatto MP, Moodie ST. Relevance of the International Classification of Functioning, Health and Disability: Children & Youth Version in Early Hearing Detection and Intervention Programs. Semin Hear. 2016; 37(3):257–271

[9] Bagatto M, Moodie S, Brown C, et al. Prescribing and verifying hearing aids applying the AAA Pediatric Amplification Guideline: Protocols and outcomes from the Ontario Infant Hearing Program. J Am Acad Audiol. 2016; 27:188–203

[10] Bagatto MP, Moodie ST, Malandrino AC, Richert FM, Clench DA, Scollie SD. The University of Western Ontario Pediatric Audiological Monitoring Protocol (UWO PedAMP). Trends Amplif. 2011; 15(1):57–76

[11] Scollie S, Levy C, Pourmand N, et al. Fitting noise management signal processing applying the AAA Pediatric Amplification Guideline: Updates and protocols. J Am Acad Audiol. 2016; 27:237–251

6 Management of Mild/Moderate Mixed Hearing Loss in a 2-Year-Old

Josephine Marriage

6.1 Clinical History and Description

Adam is 2.1 years old. His parents requested a hearing assessment because his speech is difficult to understand. Adam did not have a newborn hearing screening, as his parents declined it at birth. Adam has around 100 words, mostly used as single words but with very poor speech clarity. His vowels are stable, but he has very few consonants.

He is prone to colds and congestion. His family history includes Adam's father having a mild to moderate hearing loss for which he has had no management.

6.2 Audiologic Testing

Tympanometry has flat traces in both ears. On otoscopy, the eardrums are red and vascular, giving an appearance of effusion behind both ear drums (▶ Table 6.1; ▶ Fig. 6.1).

Speech discrimination testing with live voice presentation and no lip-reading using the items of the McCormick toy test needed levels of 55 to 60 dBA in quiet for Adam to identify familiar objects. Of note, the McCormick toy test is a speech recognition test that consists of 14 objects (i.e., toys) that correspond to 14 different words with vowel pairs: cup/duck, shoe/spoon, horse/fork, man/lamb, tree/key, plate/plane, and house/cow. The child names each item, if able, as each is taken out of a box. The tester then says each of the 14 words and asks the child to point to the corresponding item with no lip-reading cues. Voice level is reduced and monitored using a sound level meter (and avoiding eye-pointing cues from looking at target item). The lowest level at which the child consistently identifies 80% of words correctly is recorded in dBA from the sound level meter reading.

6.3 Questions for the Reader

1. What type of hearing loss does Adam have?
2. What intervention would you suggest for him, if any?
3. How would you describe his cochlear hearing levels?
4. What is the potential likelihood that Adam's hearing loss will negatively influence his spoken language development?
5. Make a comment about his current language level and any indications of his cognitive level.

6.4 Discussion of Questions

1. **What type of hearing loss does Adam have?**
   Bilateral, moderate mixed (conductive and sensorineural) hearing loss.

Table 6.1 Conditioned play audiometry in sound field

500 Hz	1,000 Hz	2,000 Hz	4,000 Hz
40 db HL	40 db HL	50 db HL	60 db HL

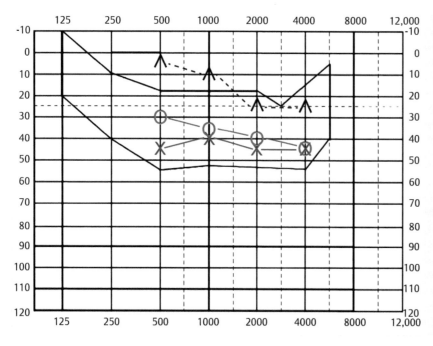

Fig. 6.1 Initial conditioned audiogram under insert earphones. O, right ear air conduction; X, left ear air conduction; Λ, unspecified bone conduction.

2. **What intervention would you suggest for him, if any?**
Possibilities include
- Air conduction hearing aid fitting.
- Bone conduction processor coupled to a soft headband.
- ORL intervention to remove conductive component.
- Watch and wait for a specified period.

3. **How would you describe his cochlear hearing levels?**
Mild sloping sensorineural hearing loss (SNHL). Recall that there tends to be an artefact of -10 to -15 dB on unmasked bone conduction at 4,000 Hz.

4. **What is the potential likelihood that Adam's hearing loss will negatively influence his spoken language development?**
The unaided speech intelligibility index (SII) score (measured for speech presented at 65 dB SPL) for this extent of hearing loss is less than 40%. That is, Adam is able to hear less than 40% of speech information spoken at an average conversational voice level. This reduction in hearing of conversational-level speech would negatively impact his opportunities for speech and language learning.

5. **Make a comment about his current language level and any indications of his cognitive level.**
He has 100 words (only understood in context), which is broadly age-appropriate at 2.1 years; however, he is not putting two or more words together, which should be beginning at this age. Adam is able to perform a conditioned play audiogram for separate ears using air conduction and bone

conduction at 2.1 years of age, which suggests good cognitive and interactive attention.

6.5 Additional Testing

Adam was fitted binaurally with behind-the-ear (BTE) hearing aids on soft-shell earmolds. He regularly asked for the hearing aids to be put in his ears.

Two months later, Adam was seen by an otolaryngology (ORL) surgeon for removal of his adenoids and insertion of pressure equalization (PE) tubes. His hearing responses were reported to have improved, but his speech clarity continued to be poor. He stopped using his BTE hearing aids once the conductive component was improved.

At 2.5 years of age, another audiogram was completed with results shown in ▶ Fig. 6.2.

Speech discrimination using the items of the McCormick toy test needed levels of 37 to 46 dBA without lip-reading.

6.6 Additional Questions for the Reader

1. Describe the hearing loss that Adam has now.
2. Does he require additional hearing management, and if so, why?
3. What are the possible reasons that parents might choose not to have a hearing screen at birth for their child?
4. How has Adam's speech discrimination score improved following PE tube insertion?

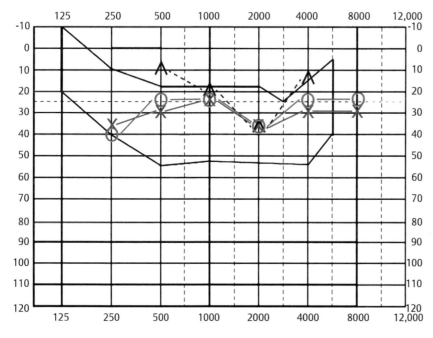

Fig. 6.2 Post PE-tube audiogram. O, right ear air conduction; X, left ear air conduction; Λ, unspecified bone conduction.

6.7 Discussion of Additional Questions

1. **Describe the hearing loss that Adam has now.**
   Mild bilateral SNHL.

2. **Does he require additional hearing management, and if so, why?**
   Adam has very poor speech clarity, though he has good inter-action and vocabulary. He has missed a good deal of experi-ence in hearing speech around him. He may benefit from enhanced speech clarity from well-fitted amplification at this important learning time. His unaided SII score is 63% on the right and 67% on the left. Speech perception would be even poorer for soft speech, which means that he would be at risk for receiving acoustic cues that support incidental learning, and as a result, he will miss a great deal.

3. **What are the possible reasons that parents might choose not to have a hearing screening at birth for their child?**
   There are many possible reasons including possible concern that there may be hearing loss, which they want more time to come to terms with. Adam's father has a mild to moderate hearing loss for which he receives no management.

4. **How has Adam's speech discrimination score improved following PE tube insertion?**
   He is able to recognize words at reduced (softer) presenta-tion levels through hearing alone. However, this speech test can be performed reasonably well by hearing the vowels of the words, rather than the consonants, as it has seven pairs of words, such as cup and duck or shoe and spoon. If the child hears "oo," he has a 50% chance of selecting the correct item from shoe or spoon, despite not hearing the consonants. The speech test needs to be sensitive to the speech features appropriate to the developmental level of the child.

6.8 Final Diagnosis and Recommended Treatment

Adam has a mild high-frequency SNHL with delayed speech clarity. A trial of hearing aids was recommended to improve consonant discrimination with speech testing to confirm bene-fit and satisfactory performance.

6.9 Outcome

Adam was fitted with bilateral BTE hearing aids. He would not wear full-shell earmolds, as these restricted his hearing of environmental sounds. He was therefore changed to size 0 open slim-tube fittings, which he has worn consistently from 2.7 years of age without any problems. His speech clarity is improving with speech therapy.

Suggested Readings

[1] Aided SII score: Available at: http://www.audiologyonline.com/articles/20q-baby-steps-following-verification-783

[2] Margolis RH, Eikelboom RH, Johnson C, Ginter SM, Swanepoel W, Moore BC. False air-bone gaps at 4 kHz in listeners with normal hearing and sensorineu-ral hearing loss. Int J Audiol. 2013; 52(8):526–532

[3] Use of open fittings in children. Available at: http://www.asha.org/SIG/06/

7 Behavioral Hearing Evaluation: 2-Year-Old Girl

Jennifer Wilk

7.1 Clinical History and Description

Caroline, age 2 years, 3 months, was seen for a hearing evaluation due to parental concerns of limited expressive vocabulary and multiple articulation errors. She was born at 39 weeks of gestation via repeat cesarean section following an uneventful pregnancy. Caroline passed her newborn hearing screen at birth, which was an automated auditory brainstem response (ABR) screener with a click presented at 35 dBnHL. There is a known family history of hearing loss that includes her two older sisters. The oldest sister was identified at 6 years old and the middle sister was identified at 2.5 years old, both with moderate, cookie-bite sensorineural hearing loss. Because of her family history of hearing loss in early childhood, a tone burst ABR evaluation was performed when Caroline was 7 months old, which indicated normal hearing sensitivity for 500 and 4,000 Hz in each ear. Periodic behavioral audiometric testing was recommended to monitor hearing sensitivity every 6 months until age 3, but the family was unable to keep her previously scheduled appointments. There is no significant history of middle ear fluid or ear infections. Per parental report, Caroline has spontaneous speech, but most utterances are unintelligible. Her family can distinguish less than 12 words without context cues.

7.2 Audiologic Testing

Otoscopic inspection revealed clear, dry external auditory canals bilaterally. Tympanometry indicated normal tympanic membrane compliance with normal middle ear pressure peak (type A tympanograms) bilaterally. Visual reinforcement audiometry (VRA) in sound field indicated a mild to moderate hearing loss for 500 to 4,000 Hz, with a "cookie-bite" configuration, in at least the better hearing ear (▶ Fig. 7.1).

A speech awareness threshold was obtained at 25 dB HL in at least the better hearing ear. Ear-specific testing was attempted but not completed due to patient's refusal to wear supra-aural headphones.

Distortion product otoacoustic emission (DPOAE) testing was completed, bilaterally, with robust responses present for the 3,000 to 8,000 Hz bilaterally, indicating normal outer hair cell function for the frequency range tested in each ear. DPOAEs were absent for 750 to 2,000 Hz in each ear, which is consistent with sound-field thresholds of the better hearing ear.

7.3 Questions for the Reader

1. When the child was seen for a tone burst ABR evaluation at 7 months old, what additional testing would you have obtained?

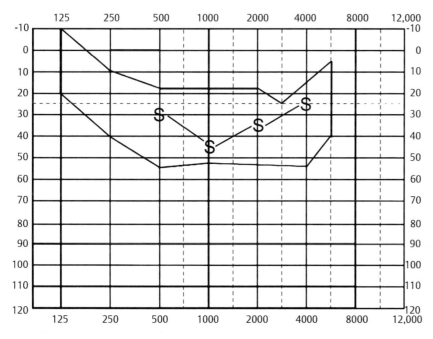

Fig. 7.1 A speech awareness threshold was obtained at 25 dB HL in at least the better hearing ear. Ear-specific testing was attempted but not completed due to patient's refusal to wear supra-aural headphones. S, soundfield air conduction.

2. When counseling Caroline's parents on today's results, what key points would you emphasize?
3. Would you recommend any additional audiometric testing for Caroline?
4. What other recommendations or referrals would you suggest?

7.4 Discussion of Questions

1. **When the child was seen for a tone burst ABR evaluation at 7 months old, what additional testing would you have obtained?**
Because of the family history of a cookie-bite sensorineural hearing loss, thresholds for 1,000 and 2,000 Hz tone bursts should have been obtained. DPOAEs testing should also have been performed. During behavioral evaluations every 6 months, the DPOAEs could have been an additional monitoring tool.

2. **When counseling Caroline's parents on today's results, what key points would you emphasize?**
When testing with loud speakers in the sound field, we are testing both ears together. The results indicate the best hearing. Today's evaluation indicates a significant hearing loss in at least the better hearing ear. Her hearing may be the same in each ear, or the other ear's hearing loss may be worse. The degree and configuration of her hearing loss is consistent with her older siblings' hearing loss. This type of hearing loss will have a significant negative impact on her receptive and expressive language development, as well as her reading development because the hearing loss is interfering with auditory information/knowledge reaching her brain.

3. **Would you recommend any additional audiometric testing for Caroline?**
Based on her age and temperament, a two-person VRA/conditioned play audiometry evaluation, or possibly play audiometry, should be scheduled as soon as possible to attempt ear-specific audiometric testing with insert earphones. A threshold ABR evaluation under sedation could also be recommended to obtain estimated ear-specific, air- and bone-conduction thresholds for 500 to 4,000 Hz in each ear. Even though the family has two older children with hearing loss, the parents may be in denial or shock that this child also has a hearing loss. She passed her newborn hearing screen at birth. A threshold ABR evaluation at 7 months old indicated normal hearing sensitivity in each ear. In stressing the importance of obtaining ear-specific thresholds to aid in the programming of amplification, the family doubted their child's ability to respond reliably during behavioral testing. This family agreed to return the next day for a sedated ABR evaluation.

4. **What other recommendations or referrals would you suggest?**
During the appointment, the need to return for ear-specific audiometric testing and immediate hearing aid fitting was stressed to the family. A consultation with an otologist (or otolaryngologist) was scheduled for the same day as the follow-up testing. Also, a referral for a speech-language evaluation through a private therapist or the state's program for infants and toddlers (Part C of IDEA) should be scheduled as soon as possible. In the formal report and during the subsequent visits, it was recommended that the child follow up with her pediatrician. Genetic testing and an ophthalmology referral are also warranted. Information on a parent-to-parent support group should be provided to lend support.

7.5 Key Points

- Children who have risk factors for hearing loss (such as a family history of hearing loss like the child in this case study) should undergo routine audiologic monitoring throughout childhood.
- Audiologic assessment should utilize the cross-check principle. When an audiogram cannot be reliably obtained via behavioral assessment, the audiologist should consider evaluating otoacoustic emissions across a broad frequency range (e.g., 750–8,000 Hz), the ABR to tone bursts for at least three tone burst frequencies (e.g., 500, 2,000, and 4,000 Hz), and acoustic admittance measures including tympanometry and acoustic reflex assessment.
- Test procedures should be modified as needed based on the patient's case history and unique needs. In the case of this child, tone burst ABR assessment should have been conducted at 1,000 and 2,000 Hz, because her siblings both had cookie-bite hearing loss.
- Audiologists should provide the family with a clear description of test results, the implications of test results, and the subsequent recommendations necessary to optimize the child's auditory brain development and outcomes.

8 "Well-Baby" Burt

Tracey Ambrose, Tommie L. Robinson Jr., and Diego Preciado

8.1 Clinical History and Description

Burt was born full term via vaginal delivery weighing 7.10 lb. Mother received prenatal care. There were no infections or complications during pregnancy. There was no exposure to cigarettes, drugs, alcohol, or medications. There were no postbirth complications.

Burt failed the initial newborn hearing screening (NHS) using automated auditory brainstem response (AABR) and hospital follow-up screen 2 weeks later, bilaterally. At that time, he was referred for follow-up testing at an audiology clinic where he passed a transient-evoked otoacoustic emission (TEOAE) hearing screen for each ear (▶ Fig. 8.1).

8.2 Results/Recommendations

No hearing loss risk factors were identified in birth/medical history. Burt was discharged from audiological follow-up with "Pass" results, bilaterally.

8.3 Pediatrician Referral for Hearing Loss Risk Factor: Parental Concerns, Speech/Language Developmental Delay (16 months)

Burt returned to audiology clinic at 16 months of age with concerns about speech/language delay. His parents expressed concerns about his hearing ability noting that he did not respond consistently to his name/simple commands.

No reliable behavioral results were obtained at the evaluation, as patient reliability was deemed fair-poor (▶ Fig. 8.2). It is not clear if response reliability was fair-poor due to inability to maintain a reliable conditioning bond for speech or tonal

stimuli, or due to underlying pathology. Immittance was consistent with normal tympanic membrane mobility and absent ipsilateral acoustic reflex screening in both ears. Distortion product otoacoustic emissions (DPOAEs) were present in both ears. There were concerns regarding his inability to condition to behavioral testing and the absence of acoustic reflexes in the presence of normal middle ear function. The results were reviewed with his parents and uncle. A recommendation was made to have Burt return for repeat behavioral testing in 6 to 8 weeks at an appointment time at which he may be more likely to be alert, attentive, and cooperative. The possibility of a sedated auditory brainstem response (ABR) evaluation was discussed to determine hearing status in both ears if limited results are obtained at the next audiological evaluation.

8.4 Early Intervention Assessment for Speech/ Language Developmental Delay Concerns Completed (16 Months)

The early learning accomplishment profile was completed (▶ Table 8.1).

Recommendations to the family included the following:
- Narrate all activities. Talk about everything he sees, touches, and hears.
- Sing songs and do actions with the songs, encourage him to clap, pat, stomp, etc.
- Consider follow-up with a developmental pediatrician.

8.5 Neurodevelopment Clinic for Autism Evaluation (17 Months)

Burt was seen for evaluation at the neurodevelopment clinic *new patient visit (NPV) evaluation.*

Screening Results:

Enter Manual Screening Results

	Screen Type	Facility	Screener	Ear	Result	Test Time	Test	In	Ov
view	Outpatient Screen	Children's National Medical Center		R	Pass	10/15/2015 12:00:00 PM	OAE	M	
view	Outpatient Screen	Children's National Medical Center		L	Pass	10/15/2015 12:00:00 PM	OAE	M	
view	Outpatient Screen	Prince George's Hospital Center		L	Refer	09/11/2015 12:00:00 PM	AABR	M	!
view	Outpatient Screen	Prince George's Hospital Center		R	Refer	09/11/2015 12:00:00 PM	AABR	M	!
view	Birth Screen	Prince George's Hospital Center		R	Refer	08/31/2015 12:00:00 AM	AABR	M	
view	Birth Screen	Prince George's Hospital Center		L	Refer	08/31/2015 12:00:00 AM	AABR	M	
view	Birth Screen	Prince George's Hospital Center		R	Refer	08/30/2015 12:00:00 AM	AABR	M	
view	Birth Screen	Prince George's Hospital Center		L	Refer	08/30/2015 12:00:00 AM	AABR	M	

Fig. 8.1 Rescreen follow-up for failed newborn hearing screening at hospital: (2 months old).

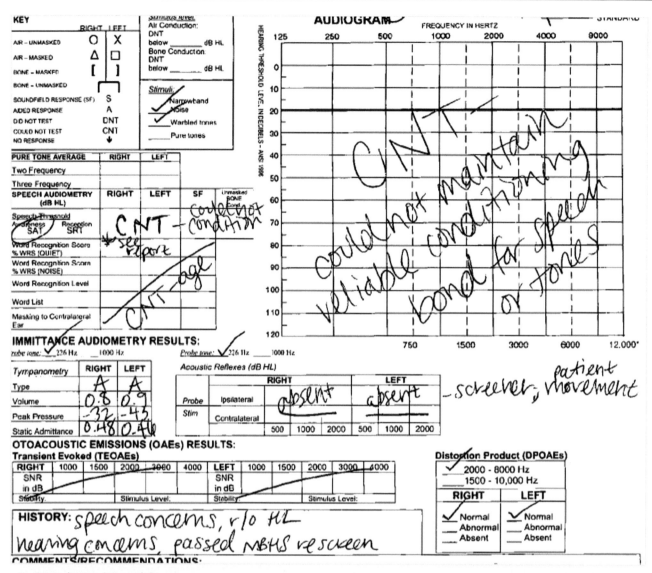

Fig. 8.2 Audiogram (16 months).

Table 8.1 The early learning accomplishment profile scores

Developmental domain	Age equivalent in months
Cognitive thinking	8
Communication	4
Social	7
Self-care	15
Fine motor	12
Gross motor	15

Mother reported concern that Burt is not speaking yet. His parents first became concerned when he was a year old. His parents were also concerned about Burt's hearing.

His parents reported that if Burt wants something, he will bring it to his parents. He started pointing at objects about 1 month ago. He also will grab their hands and show them to what he wants. He waves bye-bye. Mother is concerned that Burt does not hear her. He does not consistently respond to his name. If his parents tap his shoulder to get his attention, he will turn to them. If he can see his parents and they tell him to come to them, he will do so. Burt does not seem to notice loud noises such as the vacuum cleaner. His parents felt that he makes good eye contact with them, but at times can be shy. Burt loves to play with his older brother. His parents denied any repetitive movements or use of objects. Burt does not have any sensitivity to lights or textures. He loves to play with different types of toys, especially blocks, puzzles, and cars. At home, his parents speak English to him and his brother. They also speak their native language of Yoruba. Burt's parents have not had concerns for autism.

His developmental history included concerns about early speech development. There was no history of regression. In terms of early milestones, his parents felt that he developed a little slower than his older brother. Burt had torticollis around 7 to 8 months, and after it resolved, he was able to sit up on his own at 7 to 8 months and crawled at 10 months. He stood alone at 11 months and walked at 11 months. He ran at 14 months. Burt had not said any words by 17 months of age. He started following simple commands at about 16 months of age. For example, if his mother asked him to drop his diaper in the trash, he would do it. Burt is able to scribble. He is using an open cup and sippy cup. His parents read to Burt every day.

Burt lives at home with his mother, his father, and his 3-year-old brother. He had an early intervention evaluation and he started early intervention services shortly thereafter. An individual family service plan (IFSP) was established. He was found to be eligible for early intervention services due to 25% delay in development.

8.6 Audiologic Results/ Recommendation

Test results today were consistent with previous results obtained, indicating fair-poor behavioral test reliability with present DPOAEs, normal middle ear function, and absent acoustic reflexes, bilaterally (▶ Fig. 8.3). Due to inability to rule out hearing loss and/or retrocochlear pathology, Burt was referred for ABR testing. Due to his age/activity level, and inability to maintain natural sleep state for ABR testing, an anxiolytic agent was administered for testing. Burt's pediatrician medically cleared him for medication. Anxiolytic drugs work on the central nervous system to treat anxiety and insomnia. The main classes of drugs are benzodiazepines and barbiturates. ABR testing was completed at 18 months (▶ Fig. 8.4).

Electrodes were placed on the high forehead and on the left and right mastoid regions. An air-conducted click stimulus using rarefaction and condensation polarities were employed in a one-channel system. Reliability was good.

8.6.1 Click Stimulus Right Ear

Rarefaction and condensation polarities were employed at 80 and 90 dB normal hearing level (nHL). A reversal of the cochlear microphonic was noted with inversion of stimulus polarity. No measurable neural responses were present.

8.6.2 Click Stimulus Left Ear

Rarefaction and condensation polarities were employed at 90 dB nHL and waves III and V were measured. Response at 60 dB nHL is inconclusive, but may suggest response through the pathway up to the level of the cochlear nucleus.

8.7 Auditory Brainstem Response Test Results/Recommendations

ABR and DPOAE results indicate normal or near-normal cochlear function and absent or abnormal auditory pathway transduction. The results indicate hearing loss to be retrocochlear or involving dysfunction at the level of the inner hair cells, bilaterally. ABR is a test of the auditory system and cochlear (auditory) nerve function to produce a synchronous response to stimulus up to the level of the brainstem. Behavioral audiometric testing should be attempted to fully assess the entire auditory system, including cognition of sound and to support today's findings.

Burt was referred to an ear, nose, and throat (ENT) physician for medical evaluation. It was also recommended that Burt undergo behavioral audiology assessment after medical clearance is obtained and in no more than 1 month.

8.8 Ear, Nose, and Tongue Evaluation and Recommendations

Burt's physical examination was within normal limits. The ENT physician recommended MRI assessment of the auditory system and a hearing aid trial. The ENT physician also suggested consideration of cochlear implantation if no benefit was obtained from the hearing aids.

8.9 MRI Completed (19 Months)

Technique: 3-T MRI. Sagittal spoiled gradient recalled (SPGR) T1, axial and coronal fat-saturated T2, axial T2 fluid-attenuated inversion recovery (FLAIR), and postcontrast coronal T1 cube images of the brain. Axial fiesta, axial T2, axial T1, and postcontrast axial T1-weighted images through the internal auditory canals.

Contrast: 1.6-mL IV Gadavist.

8.9.1 Impression

- Abnormal hyperintense signal in the cochlea bilaterally on precontrast T1-weighted images and T2 FLAIR images, consistent with sequela of prior hemorrhage or infection, and likely related to the provided history hearing loss.
- Structurally normal cochlea. Normal course and caliber of the cochlear nerves.
- Malformation of cortical development involving the deep left lateral sulcus, likely polymicrogyria.
- Focal gliosis and volume loss involving the deep left posterior frontal white matter. Evidence of old hemorrhage and adhesions in the left lateral ventricular choroid plexus. Together, findings likely represent sequela of remote grade 4 germinal matrix hemorrhage.

8.10 Questions to the Reader

1. What is the audiological diagnosis for this patient?
2. What is the prognosis for this patient?
3. What concerns do we have for his speech/ language development and communication impact in the future?
4. What type of audiological intervention will likely yield his best outcome and why?

8.11 Discussion of Questions

1. **What is the audiological diagnosis for this patient?**
   Bilateral retrocochlear pathology.

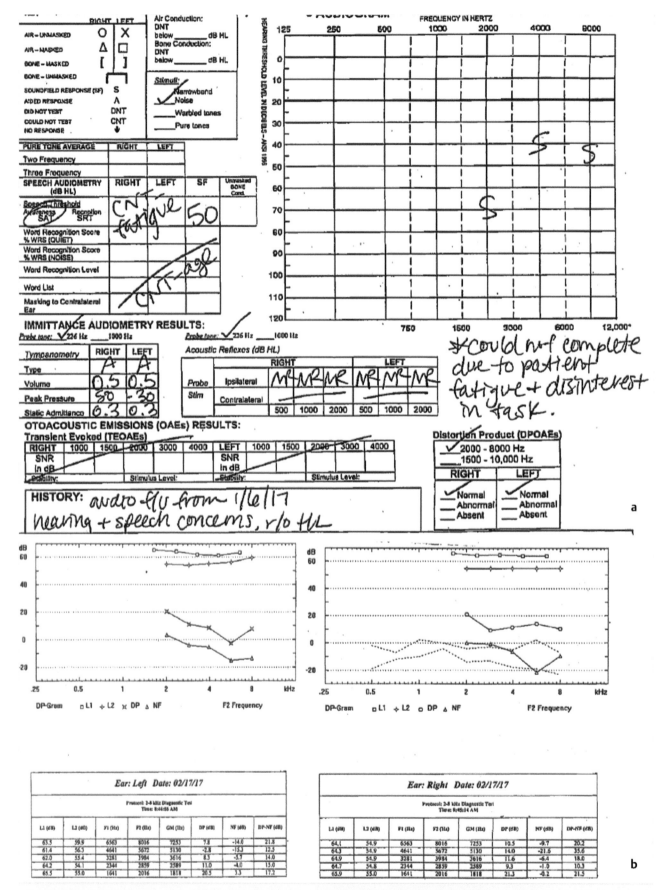

Fig. 8.3 **(a)** Repeat audiogram and distortion product otoacoustic emissions (DPOAEs; 17 months). **(b)** DPOAEs: 2 to 8 kHz.

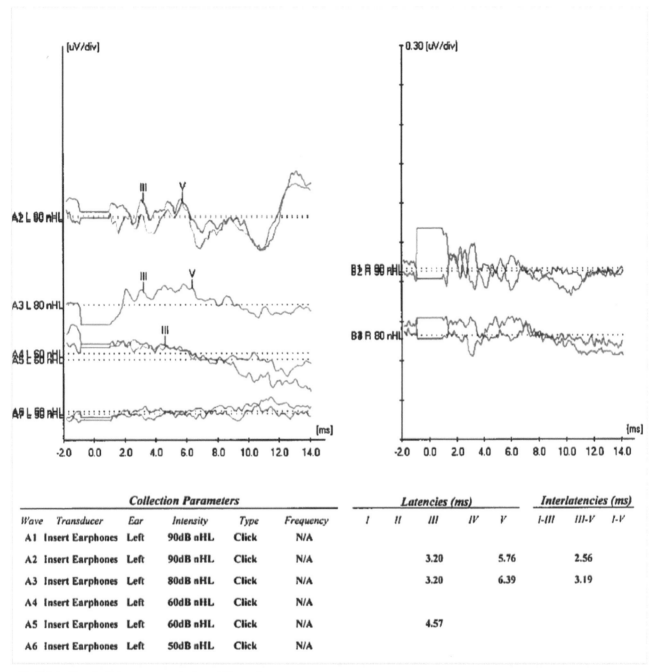

Fig. 8.4 Auditory brainstem response testing at 18 months.

2. **What is the prognosis for this patient?**

    With retrocochlear involvement, no guarantees can be made for auditory outcome. Hearing aid trial should be attempted; however, with normal structural cochlea and eighth nerve and abnormal sound reception/perception, prognosis for sufficient benefit is *not good*. As noted on MRI results: "findings likely represent sequela of remote grade 4 germinal matrix hemorrhage." The intraventricular hemorrhage (IVH) grading system created by Burstein et al in 1979 utilizes the measurement of subependymal germinal matrix and the ventricles. A grade 4 is consistent with an intraventricular rupture and hemorrhage into the surrounding white matter. IFSP assessment suggests that cognitive-thinking and communication are the most affected areas.

3. **What concerns do we have for his speech/ language development and communication impact in the future?**

    What we know from stroke victims with damage in a similar area of the brain as Burt's MRI findings is that if both Wernicke's and Broca's areas are affected it will likely result in global aphasia. That means Burt may never be able to communicate with full sentences—receptive or expressive language.

    Currently, Burt's speech and language skills are delayed in all domains, thus potentially impacting his future academic and social performance. It is imperative that Burt be enrolled in speech and language therapy addressing his vocabulary, auditory awareness, speech discrimination/association, and ability to process/comprehend information. Expressive language and articulation skills will be impacted also, so he will need therapy in these areas as well. It may be helpful to use a total communication approach since benefit from hearing technology is limited at this time. A team approach to managing his communication disorder is warranted.

4. **What type of audiological intervention will likely yield his best outcome and why?**

Cochlear implants. A cochlear implant is an electronic medical device that uses electrodes to directly stimulate the eighth (auditory) nerve in the inner ear and bypass damaged inner ear components. A hearing aid trial should be completed to determine if any benefit is obtained, but considering previous behavioral results, unlikely to achieve sufficient benefit with amplification for speech development. Traditional amplification cannot aid in obtaining synchronous firing of auditory nerve like a cochlear implant does. Start with unilateral implantation to determine benefit. Left ear is likely better candidate due to ABR results suggesting some level of synchronous response in the auditory system. Because multiple problems are occurring in the auditory pathway, it is unknown how the patient will respond to treatment of cochlear implantation. If benefit is obtained from initial cochlear implant, a sequential implant would be recommended. The left ear was chosen for implantation due to the ABR response suggesting some level of synchronous response.

8.12 Diagnosis and Recommended Treatment

The diagnosis made for Burt is a bilateral retrocochlear pathology with normal cochlea structure and eighth nerve but abnormal signal transduction and neurological involvement. The treatment plan for Burt included the following:

- Complete hearing aid trial for 3 months.
- Complete monthly assessment with Infant-Toddler Meaningful Auditory Integration Scale (IT-MAIS) measurement tool and behavioral testing once a month for the 3 months.
- Intensive speech-language-listening therapy.
- With no benefit from amplification, Burt is a candidate for cochlear implantation. Begin with unilateral implantation to ascertain benefit.
- Enroll in rigorous aural habilitation program and enforce importance of parent participation in speech/language development.

What we can learn from Burt's case is the importance of NHS technology and assessment. Even though Burt was a well baby and had no hearing loss risk factors, OAEs were not a sufficient measure of his auditory system, particularly after a refer result on AABR testing. Early diagnosis and intervention would have benefitted him immensely, as has been proven in countless research, emphasizing the importance of evaluating the entire auditory pathway in all our assessments.

9 Child with Late-Onset Mild to Moderate Hearing Loss

Elizabeth M. Fitzpatrick

9.1 Clinical History and Description

Dylan was a full-term baby who was first seen for a diagnostic audiologic assessment at age 10 months in the audiology clinic at the local pediatric hospital. He passed the newborn hearing screen, which was conducted in the birthing hospital using automated otoacoustic emission testing. However, based on the provincial newborn hearing screening protocol, he was placed on a surveillance list due to a family history of hearing loss. Dylan was referred to audiology at 10 months of age.

9.2 Audiologic Testing

Parents indicated that Dylan was babbling and understanding speech, and they expressed no concerns about his hearing at their initial visit to audiology. The first audiologic assessment was completed using sound-field audiometry as Dylan, at 10 months of age, would not tolerate earphones. Results suggested that hearing was within normal limits in the better ear with thresholds obtained at 15 to 20 dB HL at 500 to 4,000 Hz, using visual reinforcement audiometry (VRA). Distortion product otoacoustic emissions (DPOAEs) were present at normal levels in each ear, and tympanometry results showed normal middle ear function in each ear (type A tympanograms). Acoustic reflexes were not obtained at that time. Consistent with the newborn hearing screening protocol, given the risk indicator of family hearing loss, Dylan's parents were counselled to return for a reassessment in 1 year unless concerns developed prior to that time.

As recommended, Dylan's parents returned for a reassessment of his hearing when he was 23 months of age. They indicated that there were no concerns about his hearing or other areas of development. Again, the assessment involved sound-field testing, as Dylan would not accept earphones. However, this time, thresholds obtained using VRA techniques suggested a likely mild hearing loss in the better ear at 30 and 35 dB HL at 500 and 1,000 Hz. The full sound-field audiogram is displayed in ▶ Fig. 9.1. Bone conduction testing could not be completed. Tympanometry results showed normal middle ear function, and DPOAEs were present at normal levels in each ear. Given the borderline nature of the hearing loss, a 6-month follow-up assessment was recommended.

When Dylan returned to the clinic at age 2 years, 6 months, his parents indicated that he was producing several words and was starting to combine words. At this assessment, reliable individual ear information was obtained using a combination of VRA and play audiometry. The results revealed a mild to moderate sensorineural hearing loss in each ear, with a "cookie-bite" configuration, as shown in ▶ Fig. 9.2. Acoustic immittance results continued to indicate normal middle ear function, and the parents reported no history of otitis media. At the end of the session, parents were counselled regarding the potential negative impact of the hearing loss on auditory and language development, and binaural hearing aids were recommended. Parents appeared quite hesitant about using amplification, and indicated that they needed additional time to reflect and to observe Dylan's development because they felt he was hearing well in everyday situations.

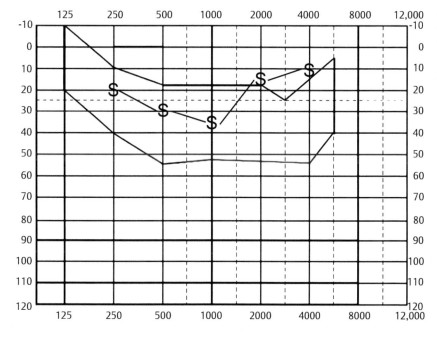

Fig. 9.1 First full sound-field audiogram obtained using VRA at 23 months of age. S, soundfield air conduction.

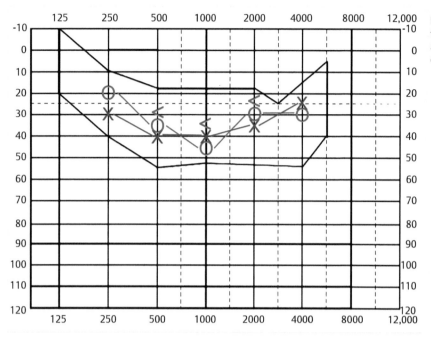

Fig. 9.2 First audiogram with individual ear information at age 2 years, 6 months. O, right ear air conduction; X, left ear air conduction; <, right ear bone conduction.

Parents also had an opportunity to briefly meet a listening and spoken language (LSL) specialist in the same audiology clinic to discuss speech and language development. The LSL and audiologist discussed with parents the potential negative effects of even a mild degree of hearing loss on listening and language development. Parents were encouraged to return to audiology within the next 3 months for further assessment and follow-up, or sooner if they wished to proceed with amplification.

Reassessment in audiology occurred approximately 6 months later, shortly after Dylan's third birthday. Audiometric thresholds obtained in each ear were essentially the same as those recorded at the previous appointment, consistent with a mild to moderate sensorineural hearing loss with a "cookie-bite" configuration. The benefits of amplification were again reviewed with parents, but they declined to proceed, indicating that they found Dylan's language development to be on track and that they had no concerns about his development. The family did agree to attend intervention sessions with an LSL specialist in the audiology clinic. These sessions occurred at approximately monthly intervals and focused on language stimulation and parent guidance. Language scores documented at age 3 years, 2 months on the Preschool Language Scale showed both auditory comprehension (standard score 108) and expressive communication (standard score 110) to be well aligned with the test norms of an average standard score of 100 for children with normal hearing. However, a speech assessment using the Goldman-Fristoe Test of Articulation 2 (GFTA-2) sounds-in-words subtest showed Dylan to be scoring at the 14th percentile (standard score of 74), considerably below the average score expected for his age group. An important component of the sessions with the LSL specialist involved parent guidance on all aspects of LSL development. Throughout the process, parents were counselled regarding the potential negative effects of the hearing loss on speech and language and on related areas such as social communication and reading skills.

Audiologic reassessment at age 3 years, 8 months indicted that the hearing loss was stable and, although parents were not willing to proceed with hearing aids, they did indicate they would consider the use of remote microphone technology in school when Dylan started kindergarten within a few months.

Approximately a year later, with parental consent, a classroom audio distribution system (CADS) was installed in Dylan's classroom. At about this time, by age 5, Dylan's mother expressed concern that he was experiencing difficulty in some listening situations, particularly in group activities in the presence of background noise (e.g., at parties and play groups). The benefits of hearing aids and a personal listening device for school were revisited as parents seemed more motivated to try amplification. By the end of kindergarten, parents agreed to a trial period with one hearing aid during the summer vacation. A loaner hearing aid was fitted to the left ear but seemed to be used inconsistently and was returned at the end of a 2-month trial period. However, by age 6, his mother indicated that she and the classroom teacher had observed some advantages of the CADS at school. Dylan's mother expressed feeling more concerned that Dylan was struggling to hear in group learning situations and that the hearing loss would affect his ability to learn to read. Loaner hearing aids were again available through the clinic for a binaural fitting, and were programmed through real-ear measurements applying the Desired Sensation Level prescription method based on the audiogram in ▶ Fig. 9.3. After a 2-month trial period, where Dylan reportedly used the hearing aids more consistently, parents reported that they observed differences in some listening situations. Dylan's family subsequently indicated that they would like to proceed with purchasing their own hearing aids.

9.3 Questions for the Reader

1. Why was this child's hearing loss identified late despite screening at birth?

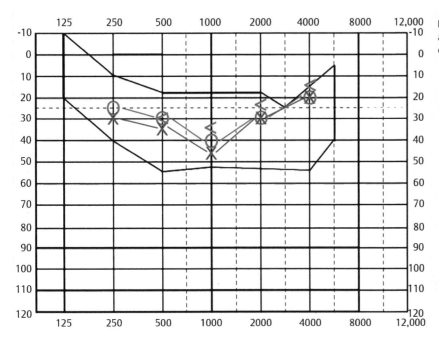

Fig. 9.3 Audiogram at time of hearing aid fitting at age 6 years. O, right ear air conduction; X, left ear air conduction; <, right ear bone conduction.

2. What might account for the parent's hesitation about proceeding with hearing aids when the child was age 2 years, 6 months, despite audiologic results, which showed a permanent bilateral, mild to moderate hearing loss?
3. What factors seem to have influenced the decision to consider amplification?
4. Although this child's language development remains on par with his peers, the audiology clinic recommended the services of an LSL specialist. Why?

9.4 Discussion of Questions

1. **Why was this child's hearing loss identified late despite screening at birth?**
   The child passed the initial screening at birth and presented with normal hearing in at least one ear based on sound-field audiologic test results at 10 months of age. Therefore, this child seems to present with late-onset hearing loss, which was identified at age 2 years, 3 months.

2. **What might account for the parent's hesitation about proceeding with hearing aids when the child was age 2 years, 6 months, despite audiologic results, which showed a permanent bilateral, mild to moderate hearing loss?**
   The impact of a hearing loss of primarily mild degree may not be obvious to parents. That is, with this hearing loss, the child's brain had access to speech sounds across the speech spectrum in quiet situations. He had developed some words and was responding to his name and other acoustic information in the environment, essentially appearing to "hear" normally. In particular, for these parents, it may be even more difficult, as the child appears to have started life with hearing within normal limits based on the screen and

first audiologic results. It is possible that this late-onset hearing loss was progressive, which can make it even more challenging for parents to notice the impact of the hearing loss. Furthermore, the presence of normal or near-normal hearing for the first 2.5 years of life, coupled with the mild-moderate degree of hearing loss, may account for the scores in language, which are comparable to those of his age-mates.

Research has shown that there is frequently a delay between diagnosis and the fitting of hearing aids for milder hearing losses due to the uncertainty on the part of both audiologists and parents.[1,2,3]

3. **What factors seem to have influenced the decision to consider amplification?**
   The impact of hearing loss of mild degree on language development and social functioning can be difficult to discern, particularly in the early years. Indeed, there are mixed findings regarding the effects of milder hearing losses on language acquisition. In this case, parents observed more difficulty hearing in noisy situations as Dylan became more independent and involved in group learning situations. In addition, his speech assessment at 3 years, 2 months showed difficulty with production of some speech sounds in words. These observations, coupled with comments from the LSL specialist and the classroom teacher, likely influenced their decision to finally proceed with hearing aids.

4. **Although this child's language development remains on par with his peers, the audiology clinic recommended the services of an LSL specialist. Why?**
   There is some debate about whether children whose spoken language is on par with peers with normal hearing should be eligible for services. In this case, there was some

concern about the child's speech development during the preschool period. Furthermore, an important role of the LSL specialist is to encourage and support parents in stimulating auditory and spoken language development. Parents were very hesitant about hearing aid use, and it was hoped that continued guidance from an LSL specialist in the preschool program would provide them with support to make the decision, while monitoring the child's spoken language development to identify/prevent delays in Dylan's language progress. For this child, hearing aid fitting occurred late in life, and he is particularly at risk of not using hearing aids. The services and encouragement of an LSL specialist in the school system can be expected to facilitate the adaptation to hearing aids for both the child and parents, which will hopefully lead to consistent use. The LSL specialist can also support the classroom teacher in using the remote microphone system and monitoring hearing aid use. Finally, the LSL specialist can work in close partnership with the family and the audiology clinic to ensure that any fine tuning of the hearing aids can be carried out in a timely manner as the child adapts to amplification.

9.5 Diagnosis and Recommended Treatment

Dylan presents with a bilateral, mild to moderate sensorineural hearing loss, which appears to be late onset. Since the initial diagnosis at age 2 years, 6 months, hearing loss has remained stable. The use of hearing aids has been recommended since the initial confirmation of ear-specific information. After his parents agreed to purchase hearing aids when Dylan reached age 6 years, bilateral hearing aids were prescribed, as well as a remote microphone system at school. The audiology clinic has also recommended monitoring of Dylan's language and academic development by an LSL specialist in his local school system to assist with adaptation to hearing aids and to ensure that Dylan's spoken language development and learning trajectory follow that of his hearing peers.

9.6 Outcome

Dylan's mild to moderate sensorineural hearing loss, which appears to be late onset, was confirmed at age 2 years, 6 months. He received consistent audiologic follow-up, and the parents received guidance in spoken language development. However, Dylan was not fitted with hearing aids until after age 6 years, due to parents' hesitation about the benefits of amplification and the impact of the hearing loss. At school, parents began observing more difficult listening situations and decided to proceed with hearing aids after about 18 months at school, especially after concern was expressed by the classroom teacher and the LSL specialist. Dylan's spoken language development, with his parents' rich input, seems to have progressed well, despite his hearing loss.

9.7 Acknowledgements

The author thanks Joanne Whittingham for assisting with extracting data for this case report as well as the clinical team at the Children's Hospital of Eastern Ontario Audiology Clinic. Financial support for the author's work is acknowledged from a grant from the Canadian Institutes of Health Research.

Suggested Readings

[1] Porter H, Bess FH, Tharpe AM. Minimal hearing loss in children. In: Tharpe AM, Seewald R, eds. Comprehensive Handbook of Pediatric Audiology. 2nd ed. San Diego, CA: Plural Publishing; 2016:887–914

References

[1] Fitzpatrick EM, Whittingham J, Durieux-Smith A. Mild bilateral and unilateral hearing loss in children: A 20 year view of characteristics and practices. Ear Hear. 2014; 35(1):10–18
[2] Fitzpatrick E, Grandpierre V, Durieux-Smith A, et al. Children with mild bilateral and unilateral hearing loss: Parents' reflections on experiences and outcomes. J Deaf Stud Deaf Educ. 2016; 21(1):34–43
[3] McKay S, Gravel JS, Tharpe AM. Amplification considerations for children with minimal or mild bilateral hearing loss and unilateral hearing loss. Trends Amplif. 2008; 12(1):43–54

10 Pfeiffer's Syndrome

Stacey R. Lim

10.1 Clinical History and Description

Julie is an 8-year-old girl with Pfeiffer's syndrome.

Julie was brought to the clinic to obtain additional opinions and suggestions about amplification. Julie was first identified with bilateral, moderately severe conductive hearing loss at 2 years of age and has received multiple audiologic evaluations at previous centers, confirming this hearing loss.

Her mother reported that Julie has received many reconstructive (cranial/facial) surgeries since infancy. Her last surgical procedure was approximately 6 months ago, and it is anticipated that Julie will continue to need surgeries throughout the rest of her childhood and adolescence. Julie also has a high palate and missing front teeth. Owing to the repeated surgeries and the tracheostomy that Julie has undergone, she has a nurse assisting her during school hours. Julie also has an ongoing history of ear infections and respiratory congestion. In addition, she has stenotic ear canals that are usually impacted with cerumen and for which she receives continuous medical management. Her mother reported feeling overwhelmed with the complexity of Julie's management needs.

At 2 years of age, when Julie was first identified with her bilateral, moderately severe conductive hearing loss, she was fitted with behind-the-ear (BTE) hearing aids coupled to full-shell earmolds. However, Julie's mother reports that Julie does not seem to hear much with them, and takes them off as soon as she arrives home from school. The earmolds are usually clogged with cerumen.

Because of the difficulty with the BTE hearing aids, Julie was also fitted with a bone conduction hearing device when she was a little over 2 years of age. However, Julie has been reluctant to wear the bone conduction hearing device because of its appearance and long-term physical discomfort; it is a body-worn instrument, coupled to a bone conduction stimulator that is worn on a metal headband. As a result, Julie's use of and benefit from both forms of amplification has been inconsistent.

Julie, now in the second grade, reportedly struggles in school. Her teachers have observed that Julie is a quiet, soft-spoken student who often sits by herself. She does not hold many conversations with others (including teachers, students, and support staff). At times, Julie's speech is difficult to understand.

10.2 Audiologic Testing

Otoscopy confirmed stenotic ear canals; the tympanic membranes could not be visualized and there appeared to be substantial cerumen blockage in both ear canals. Tympanometry could not be completed due to the stenotic ear canals and cerumen occlusion.

Insert earphones could not be used due to the stenotic ear canals and cerumen occlusion, and supra-aural earphones were painful for Julie; she would not tolerate them on her head during this test session, even with a sponge/foam padding. Therefore, even though binaural thresholds must be obtained as soon as possible to compare with previous results, sound-field testing, using warble tones, was implemented during this initial test session. Results indicated a moderately severe hearing loss, in at least the better ear (▶ Fig. 10.1), consistent with reports from previous clinics. A sound-field speech reception threshold (SRT) was obtained at 65 dB HL, also consistent with reports from previous clinics.

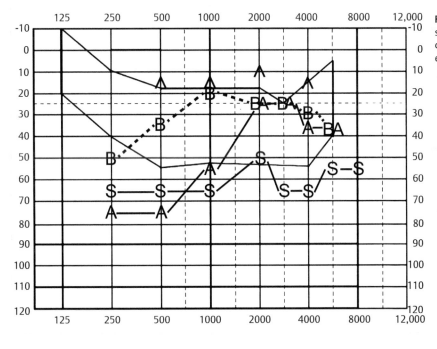

Fig. 10.1 Julie's audiogram at 8 years of age. S, soundfield air conduction; Λ, unspecified bone conduction; A, binaural hearing aids behind the ear; B, hearing aids with bone conduction device.

The PBK-50 was administered in the sound field at 95 dB HL (30 dB SL), and Julie's word recognition score was 68%. When target words were presented at a level of 50 dB HL, Julie's word recognition score was 0%, confirming that when she is not wearing hearing aids, conversational-level speech is not sufficiently audible or intelligible. The PBK-50 word lists were used due to Julie's delayed language level.

Bone conduction testing revealed thresholds in the normal hearing range for at least one ear (▶ Fig. 10.1), suggesting that Julie's hearing loss is conductive in nature—again, consistent with previous reports from other centers. As it was not possible to mask, it is not possible to confirm that hearing loss is conductive in both ears.

Aided sound-field testing was also completed with Julie's BTE hearing aids. Her aided binaural thresholds, obtained using warble tones in the sound field, revealed aided thresholds in the severe rising to mild hearing loss range when wearing her hearing aids (▶ Fig. 10.1). The aided SRT was obtained at 60 dB HL. When the PBK-50 was presented at a soft conversational level (35 dB HL), Julie's word recognition score was 0%. When the PKB-50 was presented at 50 dB HL, Julie's word recognition score was 12%. Julie's BTE hearing aids are providing virtually no benefit.

Next, aided sound-field testing was completed with Julie's bone conduction hearing device. Her aided thresholds with the bone conduction hearing device, obtained using warble tones in the sound field, were obtained in the moderate, rising to mild hearing loss range (▶ Fig. 10.1). An aided SRT was obtained at 35 dB HL. Her aided PBK-50 word recognition score was 84% at a presentation level of 50 dB HL. Julie's bone conduction hearing device is providing substantially more audibility than her BTE hearing aids, but not delivering full access of the entire speech spectrum to Julie's brain.

10.3 Questions for the Reader

1. What is Pfeiffer's syndrome, and what are some of the associated characteristics?
2. Was Julie's amplification an appropriate choice for her? Why or why not?
3. Given that Julie has had and will continue to have multiple surgeries over the coming years, what recommendations would you make in regard to Julie's amplification devices?
4. How could Julie's hearing loss affect academic and social development?

10.4 Discussion of Questions

1. **What is Pfeiffer's Syndrome and what are some of the associated characteristics?**

Pfeiffer's syndrome is an autosomal dominant genetic condition.[1] Children who have Pfeiffer's syndrome have premature fusion of the skull sutures, resulting in deformity of the skull. Other characteristics of Pfeiffer's syndrome can include bulging wide-set eyes, underdevelopment of the midface, and broad, short thumbs and big toes, with some possible webbing of the hands and feet. Other issues may include dental problems resulting from crowded teeth and often a high palate, poor vision, and hearing loss. Fifty percent of children with Pfeiffer's syndrome have either conductive and/or sensorineural hearing loss and may also have stenosis (narrowing) of the ear canals.[1]

2. **Was Julie's amplification an appropriate choice for her? Why or why not?**

Based on the history of stenosis with continued cerumen blockage of both her ear canals and earmolds, BTE hearing aids were not the most appropriate option for Julie. Moreover, aided sound-field testing revealed little benefit from her BTE hearing aids (▶ Fig. 10.1). In fact, when the aided and unaided audiologic assessments were compared, it was obvious that Julie was receiving little to no benefit from the BTE hearing aids. Thus, it is not surprising that Julie has been reluctant to wear her BTE hearing aids.

Julie's bone conduction hearing device offered better audibility than her BTE hearing aids, but it still provided insufficient amplification. In addition, Julie did not like the appearance of the bone conduction hearing device, and reportedly often took it off in school and at home.

3. **Given that Julie has had and will continue to have multiple cranial/facial surgeries over the coming years, what recommendations would you make in regard to Julie's amplification devices?**

As mentioned previously, Julie received little benefit from her BTE hearing aids. However, word recognition testing completed through bone conduction suggests that Julie has good speech recognition abilities in quiet, when her outer and middle ear systems are bypassed. Although Julie has been reluctant to wear her bone conduction hearing device due to aesthetics of the device and long-term discomfort (it was a body-worn instrument, coupled to a bone conduction stimulator that was worn on a metal headband), amplification provided through a bone conduction device would be a better option for auditory brain access.

Because Julie has multiple upcoming cranial/facial surgeries, an auditory osseointegrated implant system (AOIS) may not be one the family is able to consider at present. However, depending on the surgeon's evaluations and the family's interest, an AOIS may be a future option.

In the meantime, a strong recommendation is to replace the original, cumbersome, bone conduction hearing device with a softband application of an AOIS. The softband is a transcutaneous (across the skin) fitting of the AOIS, consisting of an adjustable band and a snap coupler that connects the sound processor to the band, holding the device to the skin.[2]

4. **How could Julie's hearing loss affect academic skills and social development?**

A brain of a child with hearing loss who does not have appropriate hearing technology does not have complete access to auditory information. Lack of good audibility of spoken communication will negatively impact all aspects of the child's life, including language, academic, and social development.[3,4] Due to her hearing loss and inappropriate amplification that caused reduced audibility, Julie is already behind in her linguistic, academic, and social knowledge, and will require extensive language and academic enrichment, and tutoring to catch up.

10.5 Recommended Treatment

Julie has a moderately severe conductive hearing loss, consistent with Pfeiffer's syndrome. When Julie wears her BTE hearing aids, she has limited access to intelligible speech, which negatively impacts her academic learning and social conversations with family members and classmates. This lack of access to intelligible speech also affects her ability to learn new information in school. However, when she has better brain access to auditory information through bone conduction amplification, she has enhanced speech understanding at conversational levels.

It was recommended that

- Bilateral testing must be completed to compare with results obtained at previous centers. The supra-aural earphones can be held to each ear, one at a time by a test assistant, to allow for ear-specific assessment.
- Julie should replace her old bone conduction hearing device with a new softband AOIS—beginning with a unilateral fitting. The goal, however, is a bilateral fitting of softband AOIS because research shows better speech recognition in noise and localization with the use of the two devices relative to monaural performance.[5] A remote microphone system should be used in all learning environments. Julie will require ongoing, attentive audiologic management of her hearing and amplification devices.
- When the family decides they are ready, they should contact Julie's otologist to investigate AOIS devices.
- The parents should schedule an Individualized Education Program (IEP) meeting to discuss Julie's auditory, speech/language, academic, and social needs, including more in-depth psychoeducational testing and intervention.
- The family would benefit from a support group with families who experience similar health and auditory challenges. The mother reported feeling isolated and overwhelmed with complex needs. This Web site about Pfeiffer's syndrome could be a place to start: http://www.faces-cranio.org/Disord/Pfeiffer.htm.

10.6 Outcome

With repeated, short, test sessions, thresholds were obtained for each ear, and results were consistent with those obtained at previous centers: stable, bilateral, moderately severe conductive hearing loss.

During counseling after audiologic assessments, the audiologist confirmed that Julie's reluctance to wear her bone conduction hearing device was due to discomfort and aesthetics. The audiologist then asked Julie whether she would be interested wearing a soft fabric headband instead of a metal headband. The audiologist also explained that fabric headbands come in a variety of colors that could be matched to Julie's outfits for the day. Julie appeared excited about this option, because even though she was reluctant to wear her original bone conduction hearing device, she admitted that she heard better when it was worn.

The audiology clinic did not do AOIS programming or fitting. Thus, the audiologist suggested that while Julie waited for an appointment at an area clinic specializing in AOIS fittings, Julie could wear the bone oscillator (removed from the metal headband) underneath a fabric headband purchased from an accessories store. The audiologist suggested that this could be an option while Julie and her family went through the decision-making and evaluation process to pursue AOIS. After wearing the bone conduction hearing device under a fabric headband for a month, Julie and her family decided to continue with a unilateral softband fitting of AOIS, because she found this to be a more comfortable and aesthetically pleasing option.

While the goal is a bilateral AOIS softband fitting, Julie and her family are currently very happy with a unilateral softband fitting. Her aided thresholds with the AOIS are in the normal to mild hearing loss range—much better than those obtained with her original bone conduction hearing device. The soft elastic bands are comfortable, and the color and pattern options for the band are very appealing to Julie. Therefore, she is amenable to wearing the device during all waking hours.

A wireless remote microphone is used at home and in school to provide enriched language environments for Julie.

Because the school district did not have an educational audiologist, the clinical audiologist met with Julie's IEP team and teachers to describe Julie's hearing loss and technologies, and also to discuss different strategies for creating optimal acoustic learning environments that support Julie's needs and desire for more social engagement. Although Julie still remains shy and withdrawn at times, her interactions with her peers reportedly have improved. The school has developed a "buddy system" where some of Julie's peers assist Julie if she appears confused during activities. Julie's speech-language therapy and tutoring sessions have been increased to twice weekly.

The teacher, classroom aide, nurse, and Julie's mother have reported that since her updated amplification changes, Julie's confidence, speech intelligibility, social skills, and awareness of the listening environment have improved.

References

[1] Katzen JT, McCarthy JG. Syndromes involving craniosynostosis and midface hypoplasia. Otolaryngol Clin North Am. 2000; 33(6):1257–1284, vi

[2] Christensen LV. Bone-anchored implants for children. In: Madell JR, Flexer C, eds. Pediatric Audiology: Diagnosis, Technology, and Management. 2nd ed. New York, NY: Thieme; 2014:228–237

[3] McCreery RW, Walker EA, Spratford M, et al. Longitudinal predictors of aided speech audibility in infants and children. Ear Hear. 2015; 36 Suppl 1:24S–37S

[4] Moeller MP, Tomblin JB, Yoshinaga-Itano C, Connor CM, Jerger S. Current state of knowledge: language and literacy of children with hearing impairment. Ear Hear. 2007; 28(6):740–753

[5] Dun CAJ, Agterberg MJH, Cremers CWRJ, Hol MKS, Snik AFM. Bilateral bone conduction devices: improved hearing ability in children with bilateral conductive hearing loss. Ear Hear. 2013; 34(6):806–808

11 Probable Ménière's Disease in a 10-Year-Old Child

Erin Schafer

11.1 Clinical History and Description

At the age of 10 years, Greg was diagnosed by another facility with a right unilateral, severe rising to normal sensorineural hearing loss. His pure-tone average (PTA) of 48 dB HL in the right ear and 7 dB HL in the left ear was within 5 dB of his speech reception threshold (SRT). Word recognition was 32% correct in his right ear and 100% correct in his left ear. Tympanograms were type A bilaterally, showing no evidence of middle ear pathology. Acoustic reflex thresholds were present ipsilaterally and contralaterally probe right at intensities ranging from 85 to 95 dB SPL and present ipsilaterally and contralaterally probe left at slightly elevated presentation levels (i.e., 100 dB SPL). Reflex decay was negative bilaterally at 500 and 1,000 Hz. Greg also presented with right ear tinnitus, migraines, intermittent dizziness, and one severe episode of vertigo. He was seen by an ear, nose, and throat doctor (ENT) for medical clearance before discussing amplification; the ENT ordered a magnetic resonance imaging (MRI). The MRI results showed no sign of retrocochlear pathology.

11.2 Audiologic Findings at Our Center

One month after the initial testing, Greg, at age 10 years, was referred to an audiologist at our clinic to rule out auditory neuropathy spectrum disorder (ANSD) or other possible causes of the hearing loss. On the date of this exam, case history revealed normal birth history and developmental milestones, including speech and language. His parents reported he passed his newborn hearing screening. There is a possible family history of Ménière's disease, through his paternal grandfather. The patient reported no fluctuations in hearing, aural fullness, or aural pressure associated with the dizziness. Greg still presents with dizziness that improves with allergy medications (i.e., Sudafed) and worsens with any head movement, migraines with nausea managed with ibuprofen, and no changes in known low-frequency hearing loss.

At this initial appointment at our center, Greg received a complete hearing evaluation and electrophysiological testing, including electrocochleography (ECochG) and auditory brainstem response (ABR) testing. Otoscopy revealed clear ear canals bilaterally. Tympanograms were type A bilaterally, showing no evidence of middle ear pathology. Acoustic reflex thresholds were measured ipsilaterally and contralaterally probe right at normal presentation levels (85–95 dB SPL), but present at elevated presentation levels or absent ipsilaterally and contralaterally probe left. This finding could not be explained, as the hearing loss was on the right. Pure-tone thresholds improved since his previous testing approximately 1 year before. Previous testing yielded severe (80 dB HL) rising to mild sensorineural hearing loss, and current testing is consistent with a moderately severe (55–60 dB HL) rising to normal sensorineural hearing loss (▶ Fig. 11.1, ▶ Fig. 11.2).

The testing at our center revealed that his SRTs were similar to his PTAs, with thresholds of 50 dB HL in the right ear and 0 dB HL in the left ear. Word recognition scores were obtained in the right ear at 90 dB HL (56% correct) and at 70 dB HL (68% correct) with masking (speech-weighted noise) in the left ear. Scores were slightly worse (by 12%) at the higher intensity. Word recognition performance was 100% correct in the left ear with a 40 dB HL presentation level. Distortion-product otoacoustic emissions (DPOAEs) were present at approximately 2.8 to 8.0 kHz in the right ear, and from approximately 1.4 to 8.0 kHz in the left. Transient-evoked OAEs were essentially absent in the right ear and present in the left ear.

ABR testing in the right ear revealed a well-defined wave I, III, and V to a click stimulus presented at 80 dB nHL. There was no evidence of a reversal in the waveform during a reversal in polarity of the click stimuli (rarefaction vs. condensation), indicating no evidence of ANSD. ECochG testing revealed a summating potential / actional potential (SP/AP) ratio of 0.54 (or 54%) in the right ear, which indicates abnormal hydromechanical function of the cochlea.

11.3 Question: What is the probable diagnosis? What findings led you to this conclusion?

Together, the change in his low-frequency hearing loss, symptoms of dizziness and tinnitus, and ECochG findings are suggestive of a Ménière's diagnosis. Normal ABR findings effectively ruled out ANSD. He was referred to an otologist for further medical evaluation and to confirm a Ménière's diagnosis.

11.4 Additional Testing

According to parent report regarding the medication evaluation following our testing, the otologist disagreed with the diagnosis of Ménière's disease. He referred the child for a repeat computed tomography (CT) scan to check for enlarged vestibular aqueduct syndrome (EVAS), and the CT scan showed no evidence of EVAS. Because of his recent audiological evaluation at our center, a repeat audiological exam was not performed. A hearing aid for Greg's right ear was recommended, and he has been using successfully a digital behind-the-ear hearing aid since that time. According to his audiologist, the hearing aid was fit to prescribed targets using real ear measures, but no aided thresholds were measured. Additionally, Greg began to use a frequency modulation (FM) system at school, and his mother reported benefit from the FM system when it was used. Upon speaking to the parent about the results, our audiologist, who initially performed ABR and ECochG testing, suggested that Greg's mother might seek a second opinion from an otologist who specializes in Ménière's disease in children.

A few months following the appointment with the otologist, Greg's family moved to another city. According to

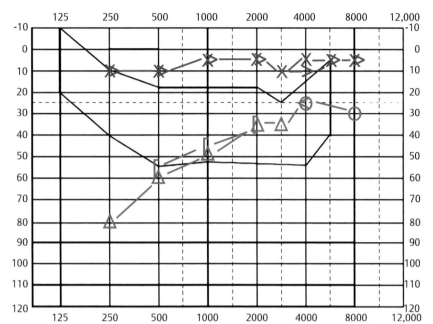

Fig. 11.1 Pure-tone test results at the initial appointment at another center (age: 10 years, 3 months). O, right ear air conduction; X, left ear air conduction; <, right ear bone conduction; >, left ear bone conduction; △, right ear air conduction masked; [, right ear bone conduction masked.

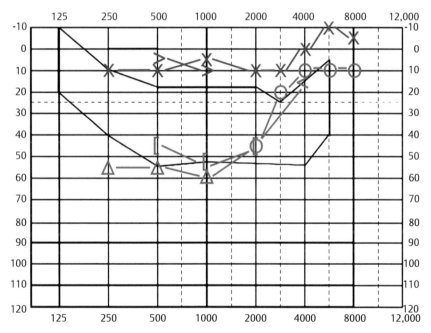

Fig. 11.2 Pure-tone test results at our center 1 year following the initial exam (age: 10 years, 4 months). O, right ear air conduction; X, left ear air conduction; <, right ear bone conduction; >, left ear bone conduction; △, right ear air conduction masked; [, right ear bone conduction masked.

Greg's mother, they followed up with a new otologist who also questioned the "Ménière's disease" diagnosis. The otologist stated that he just "had not heard of this in kids." Audiological testing at this appointment revealed similar audiological results as those obtained a few months prior. Right aided thresholds, with the left ear plugged, revealed good benefit from his hearing aid, and his aided SRT was 25 dB HL. Immittance was not performed at this appointment. The otologist asked Greg's parents to return when he was experiencing another dizzy spell so that videonystagmography (VNG) could be performed. Greg's mother reported that he had several dizzy spells following their appointment with the otologist, but when she called the office, she was unable to get an appointment for the VNG.

It has been 2 years since the recommendation for the VNG. Although he has received two follow-up audiological exams, Greg has not been able to get an appointment during a dizzy spell. His results suggest stable results relative to his previous exam 1 year prior (▶ Fig. 11.3). Word recognition (left: 100%; right: 60%) were consistent with his pure-tone hearing thresholds, and his SRTs were not tested. His results suggest better hearing thresholds in his right ear. However, Greg's mother reports that his hearing fluctuates fairly often; the family can tell a difference in his good-hearing days and bad-hearing days even when he does not seem to be dizzy. At this final appointment, Greg's word recognition score (left: 100%; right: 96%) as well as his SRT improved substantially in the right ear (left: 5 dB HL; right: 25 dB HL) (▶ Fig. 11.4, ▶ Fig. 11.5).

At present, Greg, age 12 years, continues to use the hearing aid in his right ear but does not use an FM system at his new school. Greg's mother reports that he does not need the FM system because he receives more attention at the new school. The school is smaller, and the teachers are a lot more helpful and understanding. He has preferential seating in the classroom, receives a printed copy of class notes, and is given extra test time when needed.

11.5 Questions for the Reader

1. What are the diagnostic criteria for Ménière's disease in children?

2. How prevalent is Ménière's disease in children?
3. Would you recommend amplification in this case? If so, what would you recommend?
4. Do you think he should resume using the FM system at his new school?
5. What other recommendations would you suggest for this family?

11.6 Discussion of Questions

1. **What are the diagnostic criteria for Ménière's disease in children?**

The criteria for diagnosis in children are the same as for

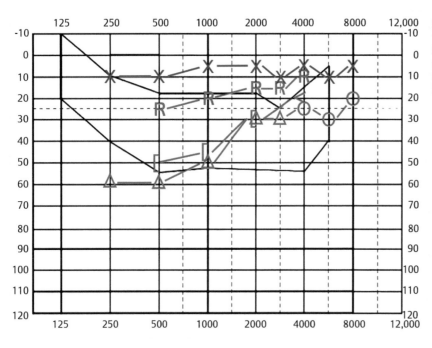

Fig. 11.3 Pure-tone test results in new city (age: 10 years, 7 months). O, right ear air conduction; X, left ear air conduction; <, right ear bone conduction; △, right ear air conduction masked; [, right ear bone conduction masked; R, right ear hearing aid.

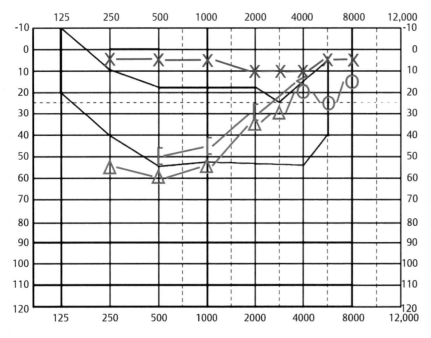

Fig. 11.4 Pure-tone test results 1 year following previous exam (age: 11 years, 4 months). O, right ear air conduction; X, left ear air conduction; <, right ear bone conduction; △, right ear air conduction masked; [, right ear bone conduction masked.

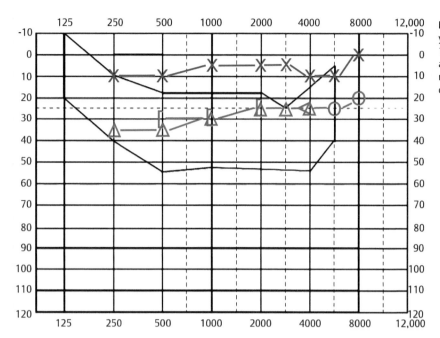

Fig. 11.5 Most recent pure-tone test results 1 year following previous exam (age: 11 years, 10 months). O, right ear air conduction; X, left ear air conduction; <, right ear bone conduction; △, right ear air conduction masked; [, right ear bone conduction masked.

adults, regardless of age. There are four levels of Ménière's disease defined by the American Academy of Otolaryngology: possible, probable, definite, and certain. A possible diagnosis requires either episodic, Ménière's-like vertigo without documented hearing loss or "sensorineural hearing loss, fluctuating or fixed, with disequilibrium but without definitive episodes," with other causes being ruled out.[1] A probable diagnosis requires one episode of vertigo, a documented hearing loss (occurring at least one time), and tinnitus and/or aural fullness in the affected ear, to the exclusion of other diagnoses. A definite diagnosis of Ménière's disease requires the same criteria as above, but with two definite episodes of vertigo. Lastly, a certain diagnosis requires all of the above, along with histopathological confirmation.

2. **How prevalent is Ménière's disease in children?**
Ménière's disease is exceedingly rare in the pediatric population. There have been very few studies that examined the exact frequency of occurrence, but Choung et al reported that, of the 114 people with Ménière's disease who visited their clinic over 9 years, only 2.6% were children.[2] In addition, of the children who presented with vertigo, only 2.0% would be diagnosed with Ménière's disease. Similarly, Hausler et al reported that, of the 598 dizzy children examined, only 9 were diagnosed with Ménière's disease was evaluated.[3] In another study, Brantberg et al reported on four pediatric cases in which the diagnostic criteria for Ménière's disease.[4] Initially, the four children did not meet the criteria for Ménière's disease, and the authors believe that the delay in diagnosis to 8 years of age was related to the children's inability to communicate their auditory symptoms. Based on these studies, it is clear that a low proportion of people diagnosed with Ménière's disease are children and also that it is a rare diagnosis even among children exhibiting dizziness. However, at the same time, this research

suggests that it is possible for a pediatric patient to be diagnosed with Ménière's disease.

3. **Would you recommend amplification and/or hearing assistance technology in this case? If so, what would you recommend?**
Yes, we would strongly recommend the use of a behind-the-ear hearing aid on his right ear, pending medical clearance, which was obtained in the present case. He had fairly stable hearing thresholds for most of the hearing tests, with the exception of the most recent test. This unilateral loss would certainly result in difficulty localizing sound, hearing at a distance, and hearing in a noisy environment, such as a classroom. He would experience the most difficulty when the signal of interest is on his right side, which is likely to occur at school during group discussions, in project-based learning activities, or when the teacher moves around the classroom. In addition to amplification for his right ear, we would recommend that Greg use digital, wireless remote-microphone technology during instruction at school to combat the difficulties he is likely to encounter. In addition to technology considerations, Greg should have several accommodations listed in his Individualized Education Plan (IEP) or 504 services, some of which may include preferential seating, class notes, printed announcement made over the public address system, and frequent checks for understanding by his teacher.

4. **What other recommendations would you suggest for this family?**
If Greg returned to our center, we would perform a repeat ECochG as well as a VNG as recommended by his current otologist. It is certainly possible that Greg has some other type of vestibular disorder, and further testing will be necessary to explore this possibility. The family should be encouraged to arrange for a VNG during a dizziness episode.

References

[1] Committee on hearing and equilibrium guidelines for the diagnosis and evaluation of therapy in Ménière's disease. American Academy of Otolaryngology-Head and Neck Foundation, Inc. Otolaryngol Head Neck Surg. 1995; 113(3):181–185

[2] Choung YH, Park K, Kim CH, Kim HJ, Kim K. Rare cases of Ménière's disease in children. J Laryngol Otol. 2006; 120(4):343–352

[3] Hausler R, Toupet M, Guidetti G, Basseres F, Montandon P. Ménière's disease in children. Am J Otolaryngol. 1987; 8(4):187–193

[4] Brantberg K, Duan M, Falahat B. Ménière's disease in children aged 4–7 years. Acta Otolaryngol. 2012; 132(5):505–509

12 Transient Auditory Neuropathy Spectrum Disorder or Delayed Auditory Maturation in a Well Baby

Andi Seibold

12.1 Clinical History

Jacob was born a healthy, full-term, 9-pound baby. The pregnancy and birth were unremarkable with no complications warranting neonatal intensive care. Before discharge from the hospital, Jacob referred on his newborn hearing screening in the left ear four times.

Jacob was seen at 4 weeks of age for diagnostic auditory brainstem response (ABR) testing at an outpatient pediatric audiology clinic. After obtaining a full case history, no family history of hearing loss was reported, and his mother believed he startled to sounds. Upon testing, there were no synchronous responses to click or toneburst stimuli in either ear under insert earphones. A low-amplitude wave V with poor morphology was identified but did not follow a normal latency-intensity function with a decrease in intensity to clicks, 4,000-Hz or 500-Hz toneburst stimuli (▶ Fig. 12.1). It was also noted that wave III had a larger amplitude in relation to waves I and V. Responses were recorded down to approximately 65 to 75 dB eHL in both ears, although this was not an estimate of hearing sensitivity in light of the abnormal ABR.

A large cochlear microphonic was noted to click stimuli at 95 dB nHL in both ears to both rarefaction and condensation stimuli. The mirror image of the preneural response was noted out to 2.6 ms in the right ear and 2.9 ms in the left ear. An alternating run showed a smoothing and near-cancellation of the cochlear microphonic, which was to be expected.

Transient-evoked otoacoustic emissions (TEOAEs) with normal amplitudes were recorded at four frequencies in the left ear and three frequencies in the right ear, indicating normal cochlear function at least through the level of the outer hair cells. Tympanometry was performed using a 1,000-Hz probe tone and showed mobile tympanic membranes. Knowing this, acoustic reflexes were performed and were found to be elevated (100–105 dB HL) at 500, 1,000, and 2,000 Hz and absent at 4,000 Hz, bilaterally. A confirmation ABR was done at 8 weeks and yielded the same results.

12.1.1 Question: What is the probable diagnosis? What diagnostic findings led you to this diagnosis?

Following the testing, a diagnosis of auditory neuropathy spectrum disorder (ANSD) was given. This diagnosis was made in the presence of the following: poor morphology/near-absence of wave V at high intensities to click; abnormal latency-intensity shift to tonebursts on the auditory evoked test; a large cochlear microphonic to rarefaction and condensation clicks; present OAEs bilaterally; and elevated to absent acoustic reflexes.

12.2 Diagnosis and Treatment

A referral was made to a pediatric otologist who also specialized in cochlear implantation. To determine how Jacob was using his hearing, behavioral observation audiometry (BOA) was performed, specifically using an approach to watch suckling reflexes during a feeding.[1] Two pediatric audiologists trained in this technique performed the test.

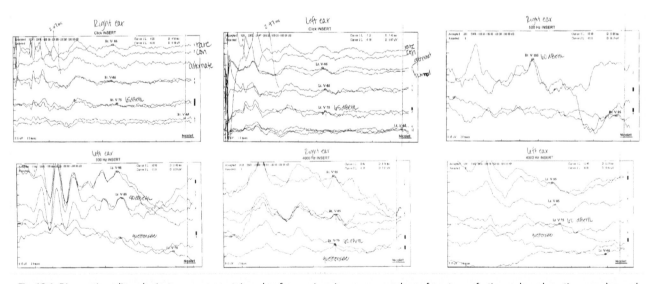

Fig. 12.1 Diagnostic auditory brainstem response at 4 weeks of age; mirror-image preneural waveform to rarefaction and condensation was observed well beyond 2 ms bilaterally, with poor wave V morphology. Questionable waveforms were marked as a note to the audiologist and otologist, and were not used as a means of estimating threshold.

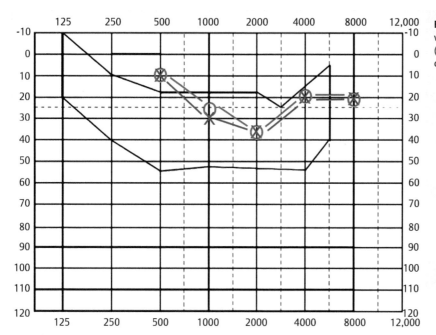

Fig. 12.2 Behavioral hearing thresholds at 12 weeks using BOA. Speech awareness threshold (dB HL): right, 10; left, 20. O, right ear air conduction; X, left ear air conduction.

Table 12.1 Aided speech awareness threshold to warbled pure tones

	500 Hz	1,000 Hz	2,000 Hz	4,000 Hz
Binaural aided (dB HL)	10	15	15	20

Jacob was 12 weeks old at the time of his first booth test; 1,000-Hz tympanometry revealed mobile tympanic membranes, bilaterally, and elevated acoustic reflexes. Warbled pure tones and narrowband noise were used as test stimuli. Responses to 500, 1,000, 2,000, 4,000, and 8,000 Hz were obtained in both ears using insert earphones in a mild cookie-bite configuration (▶ Fig. 12.2). A speech awareness threshold (SAT) by BOA was also obtained at 10 dB in the right and 20 dB in the left.

Due to a mild hearing impairment, amplification was recommended as a first step in treatment to the family, and this recommendation was supported by his otologist. Jacob was fitted with low-gain hearing aids at 13 weeks, according to Desired Sensation Level 5.0 targets and a real-ear-to-coupler difference (RECD) measure obtained in the right ear; due to inability to obtain RECD on the left ear, the right ear values were also applied to his left ear. He was then scheduled for an initial evaluation by an auditory-verbal therapist who would help monitor his progress over time.

12.3 Outcome

Jacob was seen every 2 to 3 months for the first year of his life and had both aided and unaided testing using BOA and insert earphones to track his progress. His first aided testing showed responses to warbled tones in the normal range, with an SAT obtained binaurally at 15 dB HL (▶ Table 12.1). Ling sounds were not tested due to rapid patient fatigue.

A magnetic resonance imaging of the internal auditory canals at 3 months of age yielded no abnormal findings.

Jacob had a sedated ABR at 6 months to reevaluate the neural integrity of his auditory system (▶ Fig. 12.3). This test confirmed poor wave morphology, but showed slight improvements since his first diagnostic ABR. Additionally, a present cochlear microphonic with reversal noted out to 2.4 ms was still noted with a large wave III in relation to waves I and V in both ears. Thresholds to alternating click stimuli were obtained down to 15 dB eHL, bilaterally, which was an improvement from the 65 dB eHL thresholds previously obtained. Toneburst testing was recorded down to thresholds with better morphology than his previous ABR at 4 weeks. In light of the polarity reversals and poor morphology, behavioral test results were still used to estimate Jacob's hearing.

To evaluate auditory maturation in the presence of abnormal ABRs, behavioral hearing loss, and hearing aid use, evoked P1 cortical testing was performed within a week of his 6-month ABR in the aided condition. Results were in the normal range, indicating adequate stimulation for auditory maturation (▶ Fig. 12.4).[2]

At 7 months, visual reinforcement audiometry (VRA) was attempted but Jacob could not reliably be conditioned. BOA still showed a mild hearing loss with Type A tympanograms, but acoustic reflexes were present at 90 dB at all frequencies, which was an improvement over his testing at 2 months of age (▶ Table 12.2). It is important to note that present acoustic reflexes at 90 dB are fairly uncommon for children with ANSD.[3]

At 9 months, Jacob responded to speech and tones reliably in the normal hearing range in both ears using VRA (▶ Fig. 12.5). A sedated ABR was scheduled at 1 year of age.

ABR responses showed synchronous, neural responses with waves I, III, and V at normal latencies down to 15 to 20 dB eHL in both ears for click and toneburst stimuli (▶ Fig. 12.6). His latency-intensity shift was normal, and no inversion of waveforms to a change in polarity was noted at all. It was also noted that peak amplitudes were normal for waves I, III, and V. His auditory-verbal therapist reported that he was on target for his speech and language. At this point, discontinued use of the hearing aids was recommended.

Jacob returned at 15 months for confirmation testing, which also revealed responses to speech and tones in the normal hearing range, bilaterally (▶ Table 12.3).

One last ABR was performed at 18 months of age to document consistent neural responses, with present OAEs. Since this time, Jacob has had normal behavioral audiograms, normal

speech development, and no known auditory side effects from his use of hearing aids or ANSD.

12.4 Questions for the Reader

1. What is the prevalence of ANSD in children?
2. What diagnostic manifestations are present in ANSD, and is it primarily a pediatric disorder?
3. What challenges are present when managing infants with ANSD?
4. Could there be another approach to managing this case?

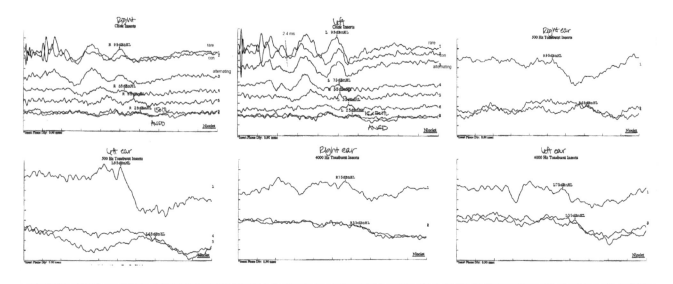

Fig. 12.3 Sedated ABR results at 6 months of age. Note large wave III responses to click stimuli in comparison to wave V.

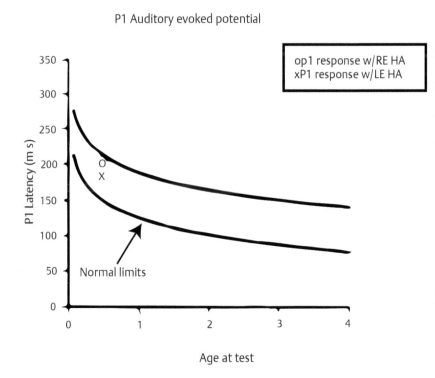

P1 Auditory evoked potential

op1 response w/RE HA
xP1 response w/LE HA

Fig. 12.4 Aided P1 latency responses at 6 months of age (o = right ear; x = left ear).

12.5 Discussion of Questions

1. **What is the prevalence of ANSD in children?**

In a recent small-scale literature review, the prevalence of ANSD in well babies undergoing hearing screening is low, estimated to be less than 1%, while the false-negative rate (passing babies who do have ANSD) was between 4 and 17%.[4] Of infants who are diagnosed with sensorineural hearing loss, approximately 5 to 10% will have ANSD.[5] There are some known contributing risk factors that make an infant more susceptible to the impairment, including prematurity, low birth weight, stay of greater than 5 days in the neonatal intensive care unit, mechanical ventilation, and hyperbilirubinemia, often with a blood transfusion.[5]

2. **What diagnostic manifestations are present in ANSD? Is it primarily a pediatric disorder?**

In this case, initially, Jacob presented with classic ANSD symptoms: abnormal or absent ABR including inversion of responses to rarefaction and condensation stimuli, abnormal latency-intensity function, present cochlear microphonic, and present otoacoustic emissions.[6] These findings indicate evidence of normal outer hair cell function but an impaired neurological or transmission pathway to the brain.[7,8] It is important to include imaging studies in the diagnosis to determine if there is another underlying anatomical retrocochlear

Table 12.2 Behavioral hearing thresholds at 7 months using BOA

Ear	500 Hz	1,000 Hz	2,000 Hz	4,000 Hz
Right (dB HL)	DNT	25	35	25
Left (dB HL)	DNT	25	30	25
Unmasked BC		20		

Abbreviations: BC, bone conduction; DNT, did not test.
Note: **V**isual reinforcement audiometry attempted, but patient could not be conditioned.

pathology, such as cochlear nerve agenesis or aplasia, that may be contributory to the ANSD.[9] In severe cases where implantation may be a recommendation, this imaging is an important consideration in the initial phase of the diagnostic process.

Universal newborn hearing screenings have been paramount in helping to identify babies with ANSD. It should be considered that, in this case, as well as others, an automated ABR was essential as part of his diagnosis; had OAEs alone been performed at birth, he would have passed the test in the presence of the disorder. Perhaps, it seems that more children than adults have the disorder, but this is likely due in part to newborn hearing screenings, which have identified far more newborns than those identified prior to the inception of mandated hearing screenings.[10] Many adults or older children with ANSD report difficulty hearing in noise and have lower-than-expected word recognition in relation to their audiometric thresholds.[6] More attention has been given to pediatric cases due to increased identification through newborn hearing screenings, the difficulty and challenges of infant diagnosis, and the time-sensitive nature of speech development and variety of management techniques. As children diagnosed with ANSD grow into adults, it is likely that more research will be forthcoming about how these children progress with regard to hearing, speech, and language, as well as what ongoing management techniques are necessary and beneficial.

3. **What challenges are present when managing infants with ANSD?**

As with any hearing loss diagnosis in infants, obtaining reliable and repeatable results is one of the biggest challenges when managing ANSD. However, evidence-based practices coupled with professionals of various backgrounds and expertise on the team are the best way to successfully manage infantile ANSD.

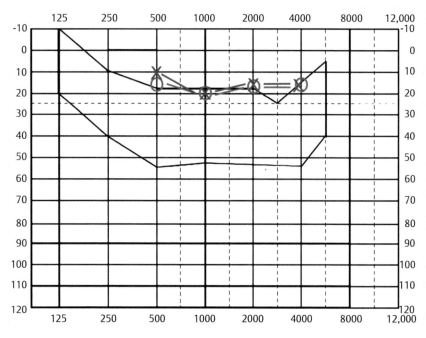

Fig. 12.5 Behavioral responses at 9 months of age using VRA under insert earphones. Speech awareness threshold (dB HL): right, 15; left, 10. O, right ear air conduction; X, left ear air conduction.

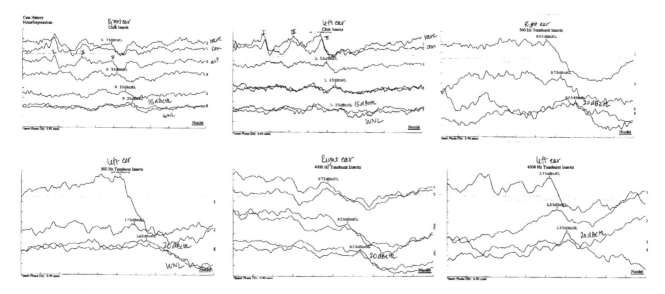

Fig. 12.6 ABR showing synchronous neural responses, normal thresholds with appropriate latency-intensity shift, and absence of waveform reversal to changing stimulus polarity.

Table 12.3 Behavioral hearing thresholds at 15 months using VRA, exactly 1 year after first behavioral test

Ear	500 Hz	1,000 Hz	2,000 Hz	4,000 Hz
Right (dB HL)	15	20	15	15
Left (dB HL)	10	20	15	15

As a spectrum disorder, not all markers are present in every case. Some children may fluctuate, some may progressively worsen, some spontaneously resolve, some receive benefit from management, and others receive little benefit from management and are recommended for cochlear implantation.[1]

In Jacob's case, transient ANSD was observed becaparause, according to the audiological testing, his disorder resolved.[11] The commitment to short- and long-term management of transient ANSD should not be underestimated. These children may require more frequent follow-up visits and frequent serial electrophysiological testing. The diagnostic test battery may be quite broad. For example, acoustic reflexes and OAEs may not be a standard procedure for every child at every pediatric audiology appointment. However, with ANSD, this type of data should be monitored at every visit. Continued management is necessary, even if the ANSD appears to resolve, because the long-term ramifications of transient ANSD are unknown, and could include auditory delay or dysfunction later in life. Additionally, children with transient ANSD should receive annual speech-language evaluations to monitor progress over time.

These cases often require referrals to other specialists. In this case, we required assistance from an auditory-verbal therapist, otologist, audiologists equipped for cortical evoked-potential evaluation, and dedicated parents to ensure Jacob's success. Having a multidisciplinary network of skilled professionals will make the experience as seamless as it can be.

ABR should be the primary method for estimating hearing sensitivity in most children from birth to 6 months. However, ABR does not provide valid information regarding hearing sensitivity for children with ANSD. BOA testing can provide insight into an infant's responsiveness to sound. BOA assessment should be coupled with other cross-check measures, such as SAT, tympanometry, and parent report, as well. It is especially valuable in monitoring hearing with technology. Lastly, management with amplification versus cochlear implantation remains a controversial topic. The use of behavioral hearing thresholds as well as ongoing speech and language evaluation becomes paramount in guiding this decision. While too encompassing a topic for this discussion, it can be summarized to say that each child must be monitored closely, frequently, and individually, as the criteria for each case will be as unique as the diagnosis itself. However, the primary factors for determining cochlear implant candidacy should be the child's auditory, speech, and language development relative to norms for standardized assessments.

The future course of ANSD is unknown at the time of diagnosis, which is often shortly after birth. Parents are saddened with the news of a hearing impairment, and unfortunately, professionals often cannot provide a clear prognosis compared with other types of hearing loss.

4. **Could there be another approach to managing this case? This is a difficult case that resulted in the unexpected resolution of ANSD. Thus, the classic symptoms of ANSD may have been representative of delayed auditory maturation, which is fairly uncommon in full-term, healthy infants.**

As stated previously, many audiologists are uncomfortable or untrained in obtaining BOA responses using the sucking-response paradigm, and do not see BOA as a means of determining threshold. The Joint Committee on Infant Hearing (2007) supports the use of BOA as a cross-check in combination with electrophysiological data; however, the Committee does not support the use of BOA responses in isolation to fit hearing aids. This recommendation may relate to published data showing the presence of minimal response levels rather than thresholds obtained in some infants by using BOA.[12,13] As a result, to validate and solidify the value of BOA in the ascertainment of hearing sensitivity as well as in the hearing aid fitting process, more peer-reviewed, published research is needed to validate the sucking protocol for BOA.

For audiologists who do not use BOA, a "wait-and-see" approach for hearing aids might have been utilized in this case of a possible mild hearing loss, until VRA responses could be obtained. VRA thresholds were attempted at 7 months, but the child was unable to condition to the task at that time. However, VRA at 9 months showed normal-hearing sensitivity. Therefore, the audiologist would not have fitted hearing aids, but rather would have coached the family to keep the baby physically close while providing an enriched auditory/linguistic environment (talking, reading, singing, etc.). In addition, vigilant audiologic assessments and management every 4 to 6 weeks would be optimal to monitor the baby's auditory development.

References

[1] Madell J. Using behavioral observation audiometry to evaluate hearing in infants from birth to 6 months. In:Madell J, Flexer C, eds. Pediatric Audiology, Diagnosis, Technology and Management. New York, NY: Thieme Medical Publishers: 2014:68–78

[2] Sharma A, Martin K, Roland P, et al. P1 latency as a biomarker for central auditory development in children with hearing impairment. J Am Acad Audiol. 2005; 16(8):564–573

[3] Berlin CI, Hood LJ, Morlet T, et al. Multi-site diagnosis and management of 260 patients with auditory neuropathy/dys-synchrony (auditory neuropathy spectrum disorder). Int J Audiol. 2010; 49(1):30–43

[4] Korver AM, van Zanten GA, Meuwese-Jongejeugd A, van Straaten HL, Oudesluys-Murphy AM. Auditory neuropathy in a low-risk population: a review of the literature. Int J Pediatr Otorhinolaryngol. 2012; 76 (12):1708–1711

[5] Bielecki I, Horbulewicz A, Wolan T. Prevalence and risk factors for auditory neuropathy spectrum disorder in a screened newborn population at risk for hearing loss. Int J Pediatr Otorhinolaryngol. 2012; 76(11):1668–1670

[6] Starr A, Picton TW, Sininger Y, Hood LJ, Berlin CI. Auditory neuropathy. Brain. 1996; 119(Pt 3):741–753

[7] Rance G. Auditory neuropathy/dys-synchrony and its perceptual consequences. Trends Amplif. 2005; 9(1):1–43

[8] Roush PA. Children with auditory neuropathy spectrum disorder. In: Seewald R, Tharpe AM, eds. Comprehensive Handbook of Pediatric Audiology. San Diego, CA: Plural Publishing; 2011:734–750

[9] Buchman CA, Roush PA, Teagle HF, Brown CJ, Zdanski CJ, Grose JH. Auditory neuropathy characteristics in children with cochlear nerve deficiency. Ear Hear. 2006; 27(4):399–408

[10] Ngo RY, Tan HK, Balakrishnan A, Lim SB, Lazaroo DT. Auditory neuropathy/ auditory dys-synchrony detected by universal newborn hearing screening. Int J Pediatr Otorhinolaryngol. 2006; 70(7):1299–1306

[11] Madden C, Rutter M, Hilbert L, Greinwald JH, Jr, Choo DI. Clinical and audiological features in auditory neuropathy. Arch Otolaryngol Head Neck Surg. 2002; 128(9):1026–1030

[12] Norrix LW. Hearing thresholds, minimum response levels, and cross-check measures in pediatric audiology. Am J Audiol. 2015; 24(2):137–144

[13] Parry G, Hacking C, Bamford J, Day J. Minimal response levels for visual reinforcement audiometry in infants. Int J Audiol. 2003; 42(7):413–417

13 Auditory Neuropathy Spectrum Disorder: Delayed Diagnosis

Shelley Moats

13.1 Clinical History and Description

David, a 21-month-old boy, was referred to our center for a sedated auditory brainstem response (ABR) evaluation following an abnormal hearing evaluation by another audiologist. This evaluation was initiated by the family due to concerns regarding "inconsistent" hearing and a significant speech and language delay. These concerns also were reported by the referring audiologist. His mother reported that David had little to no spoken language and that he appeared to hear better on some days than others. He was in good general health at the time of the appointment.

Review of medical history indicated that David was delivered at 35 weeks of gestation due to maternal preeclampsia. He spent 2 weeks in the neonatal intensive care unit (NICU) and received 5 days of mechanical ventilation; intravenous (IV) antibiotics were administered per mechanical ventilation protocol.

David was jaundiced and his peak bilirubin level was reported to be 19 mg/dL; he received phototherapy for approximately 1 week. He failed the automated ABR newborn hearing screening in both ears prior to discharge per his mother's report, but had a normal follow-up screening at 7 months of age, at a facility that provides only otoacoustic emissions (OAEs) screenings. Review of state Early Hearing Detection and Intervention (EHDI) records indicates a refer result in the right ear only, with none of the above-mentioned medical history reported. David was enrolled in early intervention at approximately 20 months of age due to parental concern regarding communication delays.

David had a reported history of chronic otitis media and had bilateral pressure equalization (PE) tubes placed at 16 months of age. No preoperative or postoperative hearing evaluations were completed at the otolaryngologist's office per his mother's report. She and other family members did not notice any improvement in hearing following surgery.

Audiologic evaluation completed by the referring clinic, using sound field visual reinforcement audiometry, indicated a severe hearing loss in at least the better ear. PE tubes were patent bilaterally. A sedated ABR was requested for thorough, ear-specific assessment of David's auditory status.

13.2 Audiologic Testing

David had been without food/drink prior to sedation and was upset on the day of testing; therefore, otoscopy was completed after he was sedated. External ear canals were clear of cerumen, and PE tubes were visualized in both ears. Tympanometry revealed large ear canal volumes bilaterally, indicating that both PE tubes were patent.

Distortion product otoacoustic emissions (DPOAEs) were present at normal to slightly reduced amplitudes bilaterally for the 2,000- to 8,000-Hz range based on Vanderbilt 65/55 normative data (▶ Fig. 13.1).

High-level click-evoked ABR was completed using rarefaction and condensation polarities. A cochlear microphonic was observed, which reversed with change in stimulus polarity, in both ears. There were no other identifiable waveforms in either ear. This finding is consistent with auditory neuropathy spectrum disorder (ANSD; ▶ Fig. 13.2).

13.3 Questions for the Reader

1. Based on Joint Committee on Infant Hearing (JCIH) 2007 guidelines, what risk factors for hearing loss are present in David's history?
2. Is a bilirubin level of 19 mg/dL significant?
3. Discuss the rationale for repeat ABR screening versus OAEs screening based on David's history and JCIH guidelines for newborn hearing screening.

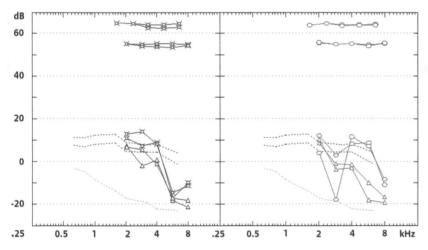

Fig. 13.1 Distortion product otoacoustic emissions (DPOAEs) obtained during initial sedated evaluation.

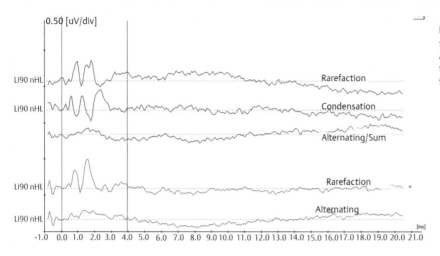

Fig. 13.2 Click-evoked auditory brainstem response (ABR) waveforms obtained during sedated ABR evaluation. Please note that condensation tracing for right ear was missing from file, but findings are recorded in all clinic documentation.

4. JCIH 2007 indicates that a team approach is necessary in diagnosis and management of pediatric hearing loss. Where did the system break down for David?
5. What other testing could be completed as part of a recommended battery for ANSD?
6. Based on the obtained results, what additional referrals should be recommended for David?

13.4 Discussion of Questions

1. **Based on JCIH 2007,[1] what risk factors for hearing loss are present in David's history?**
   David's risk factors for hearing loss include premature birth, NICU stay > 5 days, IV antibiotics, peak bilirubin level > 18 mg/dL, and prolonged mechanical ventilation.

2. **Is a bilirubin level of 19 mg/dL significant?**
   Ninety-seven percent of term infants are born with peak bilirubin levels of < 13 mg/dL; and exchange transfusion is generally discussed at levels of 20 mg/dL on the first day of life. While David's peak bilirubin level was 19 mg/dL, and he was considered a preterm birth, this could still be a significant medical issue. Previous JCIH recommendations indicate further evaluation when peak bilirubin levels are ≥ 18 mg/dL.

3. **Discuss the rationale for repeat ABR screening versus OAEs screening based on David's history.**
   Based on the risk of ANSD with elevated peak bilirubin, as well as the fact that David was an NICU graduate and was originally screened with ABR, JCIH protocol indicates that he should have been rescreened with ABR. If this had occurred, David may have received a more timely diagnosis.

4. **JCIH 2007 indicates that a team approach is necessary in diagnosis and management of pediatric hearing loss.[1] Where did the system break down for David?**
   - The birthing hospital did not provide accurate information about risk factors for hearing loss to the EHDI program, which could have resulted in a more aggressive monitoring plan appropriate for David's history.
   - EHDI did not receive information about a lower level of screening being completed for the follow-up screening; if they had, the family could have been contacted by the EHDI program to recommend further testing.

   - The managing ENT physician did not complete, or refer for, a comprehensive evaluation of David's hearing status despite expressed parental concerns.

5. **What other testing could be completed as part of a recommended battery for ANSD?**
   If PE tubes were not in place, acoustic reflex testing could have been performed to obtain additional support for the ANSD diagnosis. It would also be useful to complete a "tubing-clamped" run of click-evoked ABR, to ensure that polarity reversal is actually related to the cochlear microphonic and not stimulus artifact.

6. **Based on the obtained results, what additional referrals should be recommended for David?**
   - Otology consultation with imaging studies.
   - Genetic testing, specifically for the otoferlin gene (OTOF), based on the diagnosis of ANSD.
   - Neurologic evaluation to assess for other peripheral neuropathies due to elevated bilirubin.
   - Eye health and vision examination in accordance with JCIH 2007 recommendations.
   - Ongoing audiologic evaluation and monitoring of speech-language status using standardized measures.

13.5 Additional Testing

Prior to fitting David with amplification, behavioral thresholds were requested to be obtained by the referring audiologist in David's hometown; this prevented the need to travel several hours prior to behavioral testing, so he would be ready to participate. Per referring audiologist's report, David conditioned reliably to visual reinforcers while wearing insert earphones. Speech awareness thresholds were obtained at 75 dB HL in each ear. Frequency-specific thresholds were consistent with severe to profound hearing loss in each ear for the 500- to 4,000-Hz range (▶ Fig. 13.3).

13.6 Additional Questions for the Reader

1. Why is it necessary to obtain behavioral thresholds prior to fitting hearing aids for all children, and particularly in cases of ANSD?

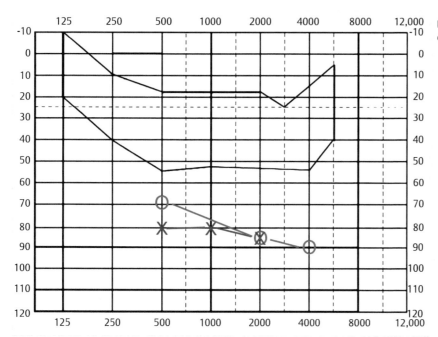

Fig. 13.3 Frequency-specific thresholds. O, right ear air conduction; X, left ear air conduction.

13.7 Discussion of Additional Questions

1. **Why is it necessary to obtain behavioral thresholds prior to fitting hearing aids for all children, and particularly in cases of ANSD?**

   In cases of ANSD, since the ABR is absent or highly abnormal, it cannot be used to predict behavioral thresholds. Moreover, in ANSD patients, behavioral responses can range from within normal limits to profound hearing loss. The audiologist must also consider the variability in using ABR to predict behavioral thresholds for all children with hearing loss regardless of etiology. We must know exactly what the child is hearing before fitting with hearing devices, or benefit cannot be determined and appropriate follow-up recommendations cannot be made. In addition, hearing thresholds can fluctuate in ANSD and must be monitored regularly.

13.8 Recommended Treatment

David was diagnosed with ANSD. Once accurate behavioral thresholds were obtained, David was fitted with bilateral hearing aids. After a 3-month trial with properly programmed hearing aids, David was not making significant progress in his communication development based on speech-language pathologist (SLP) report and administration of the LittlEARS Auditory Questionnaire. LittlEARS scores were consistent with a delay in auditory skill development compared to his chronological age (score of 18). ABR was repeated at that time to reevaluate auditory status, and results were again consistent with ANSD. A cochlear implant evaluation was completed, and David received bilateral sequential cochlear implants approximately 5 months apart.

13.9 Outcome

Neural response telemetry was completed to achieve initial mappings for both ears; responses were noted on all electrodes in both ears which suggest that the cochlear implants have been successful at restoring neural synchrony. He readily conditioned to behavioral mappings once listening skills were better established. At David's most recent cochlear implant follow-up appointment, he was able to detect calibrated Ling 6 sounds with each individual speech processor between 15 and 25 dB HL. He scored 80% correct on a picture-based Northwestern University-Children's Perception of Speech (NU-CHIPS) when using both processors at 50 dB HL in the auditory-only condition. David would not participate for ear-specific testing or for speech in noise testing on this date, and tends to strongly indicate preference for listening with both processors versus one at a time. Ear-specific testing is recommended for follow-up appointments.

In addition to the ANSD, David has been diagnosed with significant sensory issues and remains somewhat delayed in his speech and language development. The family had originally pursued an auditory-verbal approach, but noted that David's performance and behavior improved significantly when sign support was added. He now uses a total communication approach. David is now enrolled in kindergarten at a public school. He receives school-based services from an occupational therapist, a Teacher of the Deaf, and a sign language interpreter. Additionally, he has access to an ear-level remote microphone system in the classroom. He also receives private occupational and speech-language therapy services.

Reference

[1] American Academy of Pediatrics, Joint Committee on Infant Hearing. Year 2007 position statement: principles and guidelines for early hearing detection and intervention programs. Pediatrics. 2007; 120(4):898–921

Suggested Readings

[1] American Academy of Audiology. Guidelines for the Assessment of Hearing in Infants and Young Children. August 2012

[2] American Academy of Audiology. Clinical Practice Guidelines for Pediatric Amplification. June 2013. Available at: http://galster.net/wp-content/uploads/2013/07/AAA-2013-Pediatric-Amp-Guidelines.pdf

[3] Berlin CI, Bordelon J, St John P, et al. Reversing click polarity may uncover auditory neuropathy in infants. Ear Hear. 1998; 19(1):37–47

[4] Berlin CI, Hood LJ, Morlet T, et al. Absent or elevated middle ear muscle reflexes in the presence of normal otoacoustic emissions: a universal finding in 136 cases of auditory neuropathy/dys-synchrony. J Am Acad Audiol. 2005; 16(8):546–553

[5] Coninx F, Weichbold V, Tsiakpini L. LittlEARS® Auditory Questionnaire, MED-EL. 2003

[6] Hood LJ, Berlin CI, Morlet T, Brashears S, Rose K, Tedesco S. Considerations in the clinical evaluation of auditory neuropathy/dys-synchrony. Semin Hear. 2002; 23:201–208

[7] Madell JR, Flexer C. Pediatric Audiology: Diagnosis, Technology and Management. 2nd ed. New York, NY: Thieme Medical Publishers; 2014

14 Child with Progressive Hearing Loss

Elizabeth M. Fitzpatrick

14.1 Clinical History and Description

Baby Simon was referred to the audiology clinic in a pediatric hospital, the local diagnostic center for the region's screening program, after receiving a "refer" result from the universal newborn hearing screening program. Two screens, one in hospital before discharge and one a month later in a follow-up community clinic, showed a pass for the right ear and a refer for the left ear. Case history information indicated that Simon's birth history was unremarkable, and there were no risk indicators for hearing loss. A first diagnostic assessment was completed just before 3 months of age.

14.2 Audiologic Testing

The initial assessment involved auditory brainstem response (ABR) testing using tone pips and distortion product otoacoustic emissions (DPOAEs). ABR responses were consistent with normal hearing in the right ear and a mild to moderate hearing loss in the left ear (tone pip responses recorded at 0.5, 1, and 2 kHz in each ear). ABR thresholds, converted to estimated behavioral thresholds, are shown in the audiogram (▶ Fig. 14.1). DPOAEs were present and normal in the right ear and absent in the left ear. Immittance results suggested normal middle ear function in each ear. Parents were counselled regarding the results, and they indicated that they would prefer to wait a few months before further testing. Audiologic reassessment and referral to an Ear, Nose and Throat (ENT) specialist was scheduled at age 9 months.

Simon was reassessed in the audiology clinic at age 9 months. Ear-specific information could not be obtained as he would not tolerate earphones, but behavioral testing in sound field using visual reinforcement audiometry (VRA) suggested a mild to moderate loss in the 30 to 60 dB HL range in the better ear. DPOAEs were absent in each ear. Given this apparent deterioration in hearing, he was immediately seen in ENT, and a comprehensive medical evaluation was initiated which included genetics consultation, magnetic resonance imaging (MRI), and electrocardiogram. He returned to audiology a few days later for further assessment, and this time ear-specific information obtained using VRA showed bilateral hearing loss of mild to moderate degree in the right ear and mild to severe in the left ear as presented in the audiogram (▶ Fig. 14.2). Based on the MRI results, the ENT also concluded that the child had enlarged vestibular aqueduct syndrome (EVAS). Amplification options were discussed with parents, and they made an informed decision to proceed with a binaural hearing aid fitting. Simon was referred to a Family Support Worker in the Infant Hearing Program, who guides the family in discussing intervention options and accessing resources, when needed. Hearing aids were fitted at 9.5 months of age, and the family enrolled in weekly family-centered intervention sessions with a Listening and Spoken Language Specialist in the same audiology clinic.

In conjunction with his therapy program, Simon was seen regularly for audiologic reassessment to monitor hearing and development of auditory function with his hearing aids. Follow-up evaluation at 12 months showed essentially no clinically important change in hearing thresholds. Simon was interactive, and developmental milestones seemed to be on track. At age 14 months, based on therapy observation and assessment, receptive and expressive language were found to be progressing

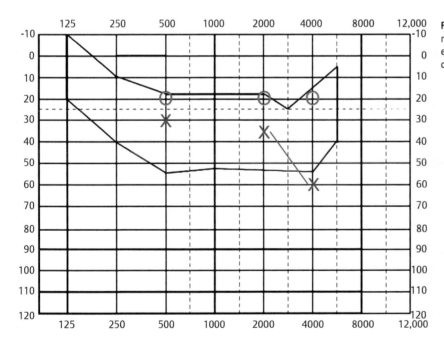

Fig. 14.1 Thresholds obtained at initial assessment with ABR tone pip testing, and converted to estimated audiometric thresholds. O, right ear air conduction; X, left ear air conduction.

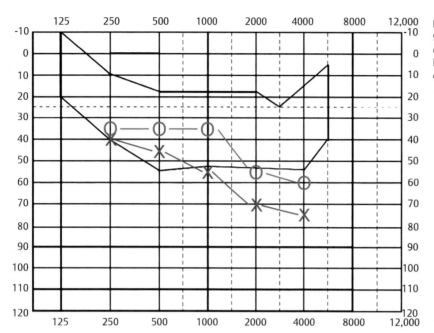

Fig. 14.2 Audiometric information obtained at 9 months showing bilateral mild-moderate right ear (O) and mild to severe left ear (X) hearing loss. Results obtained using VRA. O, right ear air conduction; X, left ear air conduction.

according to expectations for his age. However, by age 16 months, as shown in the audiogram later, further decrease in hearing thresholds was noted, and Simon presented with a moderate to severe loss in each ear (▶ Fig. 14.3). Tympanometry suggested abnormal middle ear function in the right ear (Type B). Bone conduction thresholds suggested a mixed hearing loss with an air–bone gap at 0.5 and 1 kHz. Reassessment within 1 month at 17 months of age showed further deterioration in some thresholds in the right ear (25 dB decrease at 2 and 4 K in the right ear) and no clinical difference in thresholds in the left ear. Based on tympanometry results and ENT evaluation, bilateral myringotomy and placement of ventilation tubes were carried out. Retesting shortly after this treatment showed thresholds in the 60 to 105 dB range for the right ear and 45 to 85 dB range for the left ear.

Given the changes in hearing levels, the clinical team and family started to discuss the potential benefits of cochlear implantation. However, subsequently, within a month, hearing thresholds in the right ear returned to previous levels, ranging from 35 to 65 dB, but testing could not be completed for the left ear. At this assessment, bone conduction thresholds were consistent with a sensorineural hearing loss. However, about a month later, reassessment showed that, while hearing remained similar in the right ear, there was now a marked deterioration in the left ear with levels of 100, 115, and 120 dB recorded at 1, 2, and 4 kHz. Within 2 months, with patent tubes in place, there was considerable improvement in the left ear, but hearing remained in the moderate to profound range, with the worse threshold being 95 dB at 2 kHz. Careful audiologic monitoring at approximately monthly intervals and observation through therapy continued from age 18 to 24 months. Hearing loss continued to show some fluctuation and was complicated by middle ear pathology including otorrhea and impacted cerumen. During this period, a comprehensive cochlear implant evaluation was conducted, as the family continued to consider the possibility of a cochlear implant.

Simon continued to be monitored through therapy and maintained good progress in language development. Results on the Pre-

school-Language Scale test, which evaluates auditory expression and expressive communication again showed age-appropriate skills at 22 months of age (standard score total language of 104). By 24 months, a complete audiogram was obtained using play audiometry (▶ Fig. 14.4) and showed borderline profound hearing loss at 2 kHz in the left ear. Subsequent testing the next month was less conclusive in terms of the child's responses but suggested further deterioration at 0.5 and 2 kHz in the left ear, with no change in the right ear. By this time, the family and team had decided to proceed with cochlear implantation.

Simon received a cochlear implant in the left ear at age 27 months. He was seen for regular programming of his speech processor; he adapted well, and thresholds obtained with his implant were within the expected range of 20 to 25 dB HL across the speech frequency range. He also continued to use his hearing aid on the right ear. Speech perception testing at 8 months with his implant only showed 92% on the monosyllabic subtest of the Early Speech Perception (ESP) test. At 1 year postimplant, scores were 100% on both ESP spondees and monosyllabic subtest when wearing the cochlear implant and hearing aid. Speech and language assessment 8 months postcochlear implant (age, 35 months) showed age-appropriate scores for the Goldman-Fristoe Test of Articulation and the Peabody Picture Vocabulary Test. Assessment of the right ear (nonimplanted) shortly after cochlear implantation, and in subsequent test sessions, showed no further deterioration with thresholds remaining in the moderate to severe range. The family was then transferred to an intervention program closer to their home, where they continue to receive support for language development.

14.3 Questions for the Reader

1. Why was reassessment not carried out immediately after the first assessment to confirm hearing loss and proceed with intervention?
2. How might the rapid deterioration in hearing from the first to the second assessment be explained?

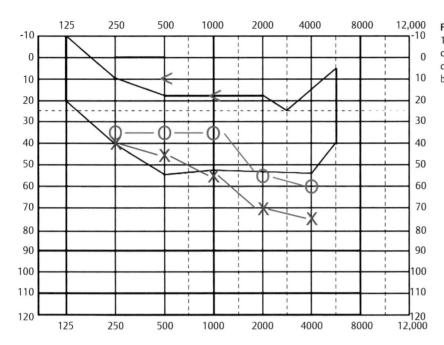

Fig. 14.3 Audiometric information obtained at 16 months showing further decrease in air conduction thresholds in each ear. O, right ear air conduction; X, left ear air conduction; <, right ear bone conduction.

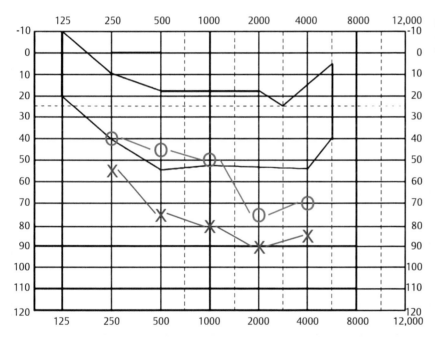

Fig. 14.4 Complete audiogram obtained with play audiometry at 24 months of age. O, right ear air conduction; X, left ear air conduction.

3. What factors besides audiometric hearing levels may have influenced the decision to consider a cochlear implant, despite the moderate to severe hearing loss in one ear?
4. What is the appropriate postimplant audiological management for this child?

14.4 Discussion of Questions

1. **Why was reassessment not carried out immediately after the first assessment to confirm hearing loss and proceed with intervention?**
   Parents were provided with information about the assessment results, which pointed to a unilateral sensorineural hearing loss of mild to moderate degree. They also were counselled about the importance of talking to their 3-month-old baby on the side of the ear with normal hearing. The option for earlier reassessment in audiology was provided. However, given normal hearing in one ear, and the milder degree of hearing loss in the left ear, parents felt they would prefer to wait until their baby was a little older so that behavioral responses could more likely be obtained. The audiologist encouraged the parents to contact the audiology clinic with any questions or concerns during the waiting period. Previous research has shown that there is often a gap in the fitting of amplification for unilateral and mild hearing losses in young children due to the lack of evidence for benefit and therefore uncertainty on the part of audiologists and parents.[1,2]

2. **How might the rapid deterioration in hearing from the first to the second assessment be explained?**

The MRI after the second assessment revealed that the child had enlarged vestibular aqueducts, known to be associated with sensorineural or in some cases mixed hearing loss in the low frequencies.[3] EVAS is also associated with sudden changes in hearing and progressive and/or fluctuating hearing loss, all of which were characteristic of this child's hearing loss.[4,5]

3. **What factors besides audiometric hearing levels may have influenced the decision to consider a cochlear implant, despite the moderate to severe hearing loss in one ear?**

Given the fluctuating nature of the child's hearing in both ears, as documented at various assessments, he was likely receiving inconsistent auditory input/information to his brain. Despite that language acquisition was progressing well at the point that cochlear implantation was discussed, high-frequency thresholds had dipped into the borderline profound range in the implanted (left) ear. These levels coupled with constant changes in hearing made auditory brain access with a conventional hearing aid increasingly difficult, particularly binaural access to high-frequency speech sounds.

4. **What is the appropriate postimplant audiological management for this child?**

Consistent with best practices for any child, regular follow-up is required to ensure optimal programming of both the cochlear implant and hearing aid. Of particular importance in this case is the additional requirement for close attention to hearing in the right ear. The right ear has remained "stable" for about 2 years and the child is receiving adequate brain access to the speech spectrum with his hearing aid. However, it is essential to continue close audiological monitoring of hearing levels so that hearing aid adjustments can be made or a decision can be made about cochlear implantation if there is a decrease in thresholds. Since the parents no longer attend weekly sessions in the audiology clinic, it is important that the child's therapist and parents carefully observe the child's functioning with the right ear and communicate with audiology if any difference in auditory function is noted.

14.5 Final Diagnosis and Recommended Treatment

Frequency-specific ABR testing was completed at age 2 months and indicated a unilateral mild to moderate hearing loss. The hearing progressed to bilateral loss, which fluctuated in both ears for the first 2 years. By age 2 years, hearing loss had progressed from a severe to a profound degree in the left ear and the right ear continued to show a moderate to severe hearing loss. The family wished to provide Simon with every opportunity to maintain age-appropriate auditory and spoken communication skills and proceeded with a cochlear implant in the left ear combined with the continued use of a hearing aid in the right ear. They continued to receive careful audiological monitoring and family-focused support from a Listening and Spoken Language Specialist to facilitate the development of spoken communication.

14.6 Outcome

Simon was identified at an early age and had consistent and frequent audiological follow-up, resulting in good awareness of the status of his progressive and fluctuating hearing throughout early childhood. When hearing deteriorated to severe to borderline profound levels, in the left ear, he received a cochlear implant. He and his family were enrolled in a Listening and Spoken Language intervention program from age 10 months, when hearing first progressed from a unilateral to a bilateral loss. His development suggests good auditory brain access, first from hearing aids and then a cochlear implant combined with a hearing aid. He also received optimal auditory and language input from his family, and therefore made excellent progress in spoken language acquisition. He continues to use bimodal hearing and has developed spoken language similarly to typically developing children.

14.7 Acknowledgements

The author thanks Joanne Whittingham for collecting data for this case report, Eunjung Na for assistance with figures, and the clinicians at the Children's Hospital of Eastern Ontario Audiology Clinic for their input. Financial support for the author's work is gratefully acknowledged from the Canadian Institutes of Health Research and the Canadian Child Health Clinician Scientist Program.

References

[1] Fitzpatrick EM, Whittingham J, Durieux-Smith A. Mild bilateral and unilateral hearing loss in childhood: a 20-year view of hearing characteristics, and audiologic practices before and after newborn hearing screening. Ear Hear. 2014; 35(1):10–18

[2] McKay S, Gravel JS, Tharpe AM. Amplification considerations for children with minimal or mild bilateral hearing loss and unilateral hearing loss. Trends Amplif. 2008; 12(1):43–54

[3] Seo YJ, Kim JM, Choi JY. Correlation of vestibular aqueduct size with air-bone gap in enlarged vestibular aqueduct syndrome. Laryngoscope. 2016; 126 (7):1633–1638

[4] Boston M, Halsted M, Meinzen-Derr J, et al. The large vestibular aqueduct: a new definition based on audiologic and computed tomography correlation. Otolaryngol Head Neck Surg. 2007; 136(6):972–977

[5] Papsin BC. Cochlear implantation in children with anomalous cochleovestibular anatomy. Laryngoscope. 2005; 115(1, Pt 2) Suppl 106:1–26

Suggested Readings

[1] American Speech-Language Hearing Association. Large vestibular aqueduct (LVA) disorders. Available at: http://www.asha.org/aud/articles/LVADisorders/. Accessed on February 20, 2016

[2] Dewan K, Wippold FJ, II, Lieu JE. Enlarged vestibular aqueduct in pediatric sensorineural hearing loss. Otolaryngol Head Neck Surg. 2009; 140(4):552–558

15 School-Aged, Unidentified Minimal/Mild Hearing Loss

Lori A. Pakulski

15.1 Clinical History and Description

Tom, 8 years old, is a second grade student, who has been struggling with comprehension and other academic skills. Kate, a speech-language pathology (SLP) undergraduate student, who was volunteering at the school, was assigned to tutor him. Kate first noticed that Tom was misunderstanding what she said. For example, when she said, "The boy skipped down the driveway," Tom thought she said, "slipped." Upon further investigation, Kate realized that Tom also was making other unusual sound confusions. For example, when she asked him about a *sled* in a picture, he replied, "I don't see a *flag*."

After getting permission to review his records, Kate found that there was no information about speech-language or hearing concerns. Later, Tom's mother reported that he had failed his infant hearing screenings. She further explained that the pediatrician recommended a "wait-and-see approach," rather than return for a complete evaluation. Because Tom was developing spoken language and meeting other developmental milestones, a follow-up had not been conducted. In fact, Tom's mother stated that she had been told that "failing the infant hearing screening wasn't a big deal and many children with normal hearing failed the infant screening."

During a tutoring session, Kate performed a basic "Ling Six Sound Test" at conversational level while sitting next to Tom in order to investigate whether Tom could hear the components of speech. He correctly identified four of the sounds (oo, ah, m, and sh), but missed /s/ and confused /ee/ for /oo/. Kate later analyzed Tom's listening errors utilizing the Tools for Schools "The SOUNDS of Speech" reference card from Advanced Bionics (available online: http://www.advancedbionics.com/content/dam/ab/Global/en_ce/documents/libraries/TFS%20Learning%20About%20Hearing%20Loss/3–01066-B-6_Sounds%20of%20Speech-FNL.pdf). Kate realized that the Ling Six Sound Test errors were actually similar to the errors Tom had made in his schoolwork for words such as "flag" and "sled." It appeared to her that Tom was hearing low- and mid-frequency sounds (250–2,000 Hz), which allowed him to correctly identify most sounds of speech. However, he did not consistently respond to speech sounds that required hearing higher frequency formants[1] ($\geq$ 3,000 Hz), as shown in ▶ Fig. 15.1.

With this information, Kate was able to convince the staff that a hearing screening was warranted. The educational audiologist scheduled the screening and found that, although Tom had normal middle ear function, and was able to respond to 20 dB HL tones at 1,000 and 2,000 Hz, he did not respond to the 4,000 Hz tones in either ear. As a result, a full audiometric evaluation was scheduled.

15.2 Audiologic Testing

An otoscopic examination was unremarkable. Acoustic immittance testing revealed normal middle ear functioning. Results of the audiometric evaluation (▶ Fig. 15.2) showed hearing sensitivity well within the normal limits between 250 and 2,000 Hz, decreasing to a slight sensorineural loss at 4,000 Hz and a mild loss at 8,000 Hz, bilaterally. Tom's word recognition ability, in a quiet background, was good at 92% in the right ear and 96% in the left ear. However, when the words were presented in background noise that was equal in intensity to the speech signal, his word recognition ability decreased to 76% in the right ear and 80% in the left ear. These results support the findings of the Ling Six Sound Test.

15.3 Diagnosis and Recommended Treatment

Tom's hearing sensitivity is well within normal limits between 250 and 2,000 Hz, decreasing to a slight sensorineural loss at 4,000 Hz and to a mild sensorineural hearing loss at 8,000 Hz, bilaterally (▶ Fig. 15.2). Mild-gain behind-the-ear hearing aids were recommended for both ears, which were coupled to a wireless remote microphone system at school. The hearing aids provide high frequency amplification, with open earmolds, to reduce the amount of noise amplified. The wireless remote microphone system is also in place to mitigate classroom noise and distance issues, thus allowing Tom to have full auditory brain access to all the sounds of speech. While Tom was somewhat hesitant at first, he quickly realized the benefit of hearing technology, and now he uses it most waking hours. His teacher reported an improvement in his academic and social skills, and noted a remarkable increase in his confidence.

15.4 Questions for the Reader

1. Why might professionals tell parents that a failed hearing screening is not something that should alarm them?
2. What are some of the potential challenges or ways in which minimal hearing loss can impact a school-aged child?
3. What is the impact of highly sensitive (better than average) low-frequency hearing?
4. Why might Tom not qualify for school services given his hearing level?
5. What are some other important recommendations for a school-aged child with hearing loss?
6. What is the impact of classroom acoustics on a child with minimal hearing loss?
7. What differences can a savvy SLP make in the life of a child with hearing loss?

15.5 Discussion of Questions

1. **Why might professionals tell parents that a failed hearing screening is not something that should alarm them?**
Some pediatricians are not comfortable with infant hearing screening testing and do not believe that the results are reliable. Additionally, they may not believe that a mild hearing loss will have a significant effect on a child's development.

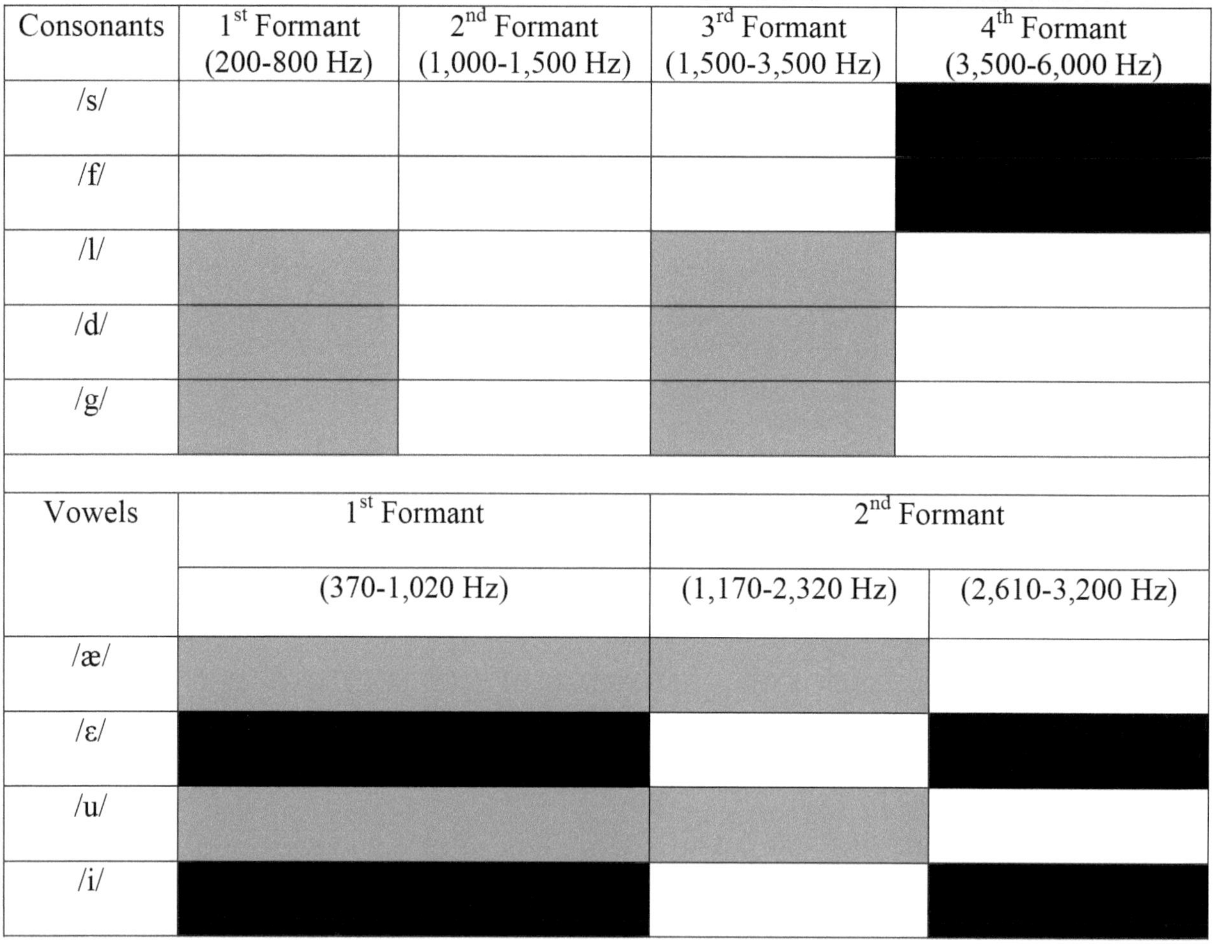

Consonants	1st Formant (200-800 Hz)	2nd Formant (1,000-1,500 Hz)	3rd Formant (1,500-3,500 Hz)	4th Formant (3,500-6,000 Hz)
/s/				██████████
/f/				██████████
/l/	███████		███████	
/d/	███████		███████	
/g/	███████		███████	

Vowels	1st Formant	2nd Formant	
	(370-1,020 Hz)	(1,170-2,320 Hz)	(2,610-3,200 Hz)
/æ/	███████	███████	
/ɛ/	███████		███████
/u/	███████	███████	
/i/	███████		███████

Fig. 15.1 Frequency range of selected English speech sounds. Gray box indicates Tom correctly identified the formant frequencies of the sound; black box indicates incorrect response.

It is important for parents to understand that a failed hearing screening indicates there may be a hearing problem but does not confirm a hearing loss. Some professionals underestimate the value of hearing screenings and may not encourage parents to follow through with a full evaluation. Instead, they take a "wait-and-see" approach. If a child is developing speech and language, as often is the case for someone with a minimal/mild hearing loss, there may not appear to be a problem. The signs of a minimal or mild hearing loss can be rather subtle, and may be mistaken for other issues (such as behavior, inattention, cognitive, etc.). As a result, the hearing loss may go unrecognized for many years, as is the case for Tom, and not be identified until the child develops language or learning problems.

2. **What are some of the potential challenges or ways in which minimal hearing loss can impact a school-aged child?**
Minimal/mild hearing loss can impact a child in nearly every aspect of life from general well-being, to socialization and human relationships, to academic performance. It may appear as though a child is not interested, not paying attention, or trying to get attention, and/or it may look as though he or she has a language learning problem. Missing the subtleties of spoken language may lead to surface-level errors, such as

missing plurals, possessives, and past tense sounds. However, a mild hearing loss can also cause a child to misunderstand nuances of language that help the learning of idioms, understanding jokes, and so forth. Confidence and general well-being may also be impacted as a child may struggle to understand what everyone else seems to be learning without effort.

3. **What is the impact of highly sensitive (better than average) low-frequency hearing?**
The loudness of speech originates from the low-frequency sounds, making it difficult for people with a high-frequency hearing loss to realize that they are not hearing well. In other words, Tom will hear the loudness of speech, but will miss important soft or moderate intensity sounds that are critical to understanding. As a result, it is common for people with this configuration of hearing loss to report that they have very sensitive hearing, if only other people would speak more clearly. A second concern is that noise, which tends to be low frequency in nature, can be overwhelming to someone with better than average low-frequency hearing sensitivity. Consequently, Tom is likely to exhibit greater listening fatigue than his peers, and become overwhelmed in noisy environments.

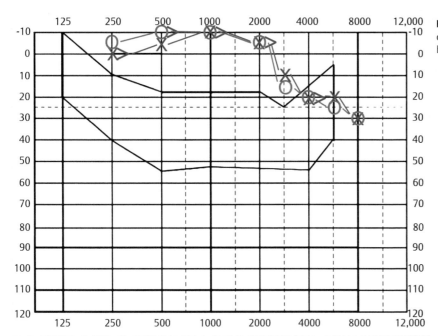

Fig. 15.2 Audiometric evaluation. O, right ear air conduction; X, left ear air conduction; >, left ear bone conduction.

4. **Why might Tom not qualify for school services given his hearing level?**

Despite the fact that without hearing technology Tom does not have auditory brain access to all the sounds of speech, it is possible that his hearing loss will not qualify him for an Individualized Education Plan (IEP), and all of the supports, modifications, and accommodations that go with it. States have varying definitions on what qualifies a child, and if Tom is a fairly successful student (despite his struggles), he may not meet the qualifications. However, under Section 504 of the Rehabilitation Act, he would qualify for accommodations that provide equal access to instruction.

5. **What are some other important recommendations for a school-aged child with hearing loss?**

Once a person has hearing loss, other forms of hearing damage create a cumulative effect that may contribute to many of the problems associated with hearing loss. For example, Tom should be taught hearing conservation, and should be monitored for noise exposure among other hearing-related concerns. He should also be provided social and academic supports both in and out of school.

A second recommendation pertains to Tom's speech testing, which was conducted in a quiet background as well as in noise. Generally, testing in noise is useful because children, especially those with hearing loss, perform more poorly as the intensity level of the desired speech approximates the intensity level of the background noise (referred to as signal-to-noise ratio or SNR). Thus, measuring a child's speech-in-noise abilities provides information about how that child may perform in a noisy classroom and may indicate the need for a particular hearing technology. However, in Tom's case, the audiologist may not have had access to the best speech-in-noise test protocol. Rather than adding noise to the NU6 words, the audiologist should use a published test that has high sensitivity, validity, and reliability.[2]

6. **What is the impact of classroom acoustics on a child with minimal hearing loss?**

According to the Acoustical Society of America, the speech intelligibility rating of many U.S. classrooms is 75% or less, meaning that even listeners with normal hearing can understand only three of four words read.[3] The impact of poor acoustics is worse for students with hearing loss. The acoustics of a classroom can be difficult for a school to measure and track, and may be related to architectural design, classroom and extraneous noise, and reverberation. There are some fairly simple improvements that can be made, such as covering hard surfaces with area rugs or window treatments; other concerns such as the heating, ventilation, and air conditioning (HVAC) system and traffic noise may be more difficult to address.

7. **What differences can a savvy SLP make in the life of a child with hearing loss?**

Kate, a preservice SLP, was able to identify a hearing concern that had otherwise gone unidentified for many years. While this might seem like an unusual case, hearing loss goes undetected far too often. Even when hearing loss has been identified, hearing technology may be malfunctioning without anyone realizing. This can be attributed, at least in part, to the fact that majority of preservice education and health care students (in programs other than speech-language or audiology) do not receive coursework or experience related to hearing loss prevention, identification, or management.[4] Although audiologists see patients periodically, SLPs most often see clients on a weekly basis. Thus, SLPs who are knowledgeable about hearing loss can identify concerns early. Another example of the importance of a savvy SLP was presented in Case 29 in the first edition of the *Pediatric Audiology Casebook*.

References

[1] Ling D. Speech and the Hearing-Impaired Child: Theory and Practice. 2nd ed. Washington, DC: AG Bell; 2002

[2] Schafer EC. Speech perception in noise measures for children: a critical review and case studies. J Educ Audiol. 2010; 16:4–15

[3] Seep B, Glosemeyer R, Hulce E, Linn M, Aytar P. Classroom Acoustics: A Resource for Creating Learning Environments with Desirable Listening Conditions. Melville, NY: Acoustical Society of America; 2000

[4] Squires E, Pakulski LA, Glassman J, Diehm E. Knowledge of hearing loss among university students pursuing careers in health care [In review]

Suggested Readings

[1] Khairi Md Daud M, Noor RM, Rahman NA, Sidek DS, Mohamad A. The effect of mild hearing loss on academic performance in primary school children. Int J Pediatr Otorhinolaryngol. 2010; 74(1):67–70

[2] Goldberg L, McCormick Richburg C. Minimal hearing impairment major myths with more than minimal implications. Commun Disord Q. 2004; 25(3):152–160

[3] Klatte M, Hellbruck J, Seidel J, Leistner P. Effects of classroom acoustics on performance and well-being in elementary school children: a field study. Environ Behav. 2010; 42(5):659–692

[4] McCormick Richburg C, Goldberg LR. Teachers' perceptions about minimal hearing loss: a role for educational audiologists. Commun Disord Q. 2005; 27(1):4–19

[5] McFadden B, Pittman A. Effect of minimal hearing loss on children's ability to multitask in quiet and in noise. Lang Speech Hear Serv Sch. 2008; 39 (3):342–351

[6] Pakulski LA, Kaderavek JN. Children with minimal hearing loss: interventions in the classroom. Interv Sch Clin. 2002; 38(2):96–103

[7] Tharpe AM. Unilateral and mild bilateral hearing loss in children: past and current perspectives. Trends Amplif. 2008; 12(1):7–15

[8] Tharpe AM, Sladen D, Dodd-Murphy J, Boney S. Minimal hearing loss in children: minimal but not inconsequential. Semin Hear. 2009; 30(2):80–93

16 What Was Missed?

Christi Barbee and Andrew B. John

16.1 Clinical History and Description

George presented to our clinic as a 7.5-year-old boy with a history of speech delay, dysarthria, severe allergies, and parental concerns about hearing. Newborn hearing screening results, as reported by parent, were that he passed for both ears. George was noted to have a large skull but no cranial abnormality as well as a history of asthma, eczema, and poor diction. His family history was positive for heart disease, hypertension, diabetes, reactive airway disease, and thyroid disease. He was being treated with Claritin, Nasonex, Singulair, grapefruit seed extract, and an albuterol inhaler for severe allergies.

Review of George's chart revealed several previous appointments with an ENT practice specializing in allergy care. These records are summarized here.

16.1.1 At Age 2

George received pressure equalization (PE) tubes as a result of middle ear effusion and concerns about hearing. However, the mother's concerns about George's hearing were not resolved by the PE tubes, and George was referred for an auditory brainstem response (ABR) test. Per mother's report, the ABR results were "completely normal." These test results were not provided to our clinic.

16.1.2 At Age 5

George was evaluated for allergies. The ENT reported removing cerumen and noted that PE tubes were extruded and also removed at this appointment. George's tympanic membranes appeared retracted with mild tympanosclerosis. An audiogram at four frequencies in the right ear revealed minimal response levels in the mild hearing loss range for both ears (▶ Fig. 16.1). Notes on the audiogram indicated that only one response was obtained at the intensities marked as threshold. Tympanograms were noted as normal. Acoustic reflexes and word recognition testing were not attempted. Distortion-product otoacoustic emissions (DPOAE) were attempted but unsuccessful due to "congested breathing." The report of this appointment described George's hearing as "within normal limits" but noted that the parents still had concerns about George's hearing.

16.1.3 At Age 5.5

George was seen on three dates for allergy-related evaluations. An adenoidectomy and nasal endoscopy were performed, and allergen testing of George's home and school environments were conducted, revealing very high levels of mold in both locations. Reports also noted the presence of a dog (to which George is allergic) in the home, but parents indicated that the dog was kept out of George's room. The ENT recommended air filtration systems for home and school.

16.1.4 First Audiologic Appointment (at ENT Clinic) at Age 7

George was evaluated due to continued parental concern of hearing problems. An audiological evaluation was conducted revealing responses in the slight hearing loss range (▶ Fig. 16.2). Notes on the audiogram indicated that some thresholds are marked based on one response (as in the age-5 evaluation) and

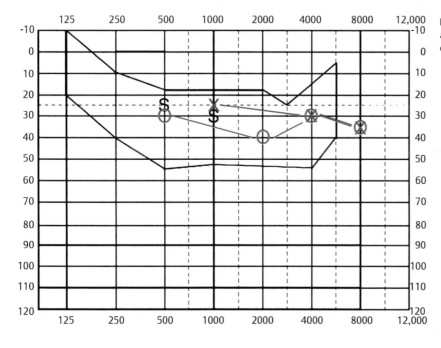

Fig. 16.1 Results of first available audiogram at age 5. O, right ear air conduction; X, left ear air conduction; S, sound field air conduction.

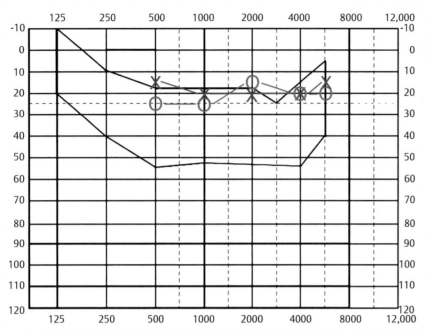

Fig. 16.2 Results of second available audiogram at age 5. O, right ear air conduction; X, left ear air conduction.

that reliability was "fair to poor." Word-recognition responses were noted as difficult to understand with need for frequent reinstruction. Tympanograms were noted as normal, and acoustic reflexes were not tested. A DPOAE screening found no evidence of OAE bilaterally (▶ Fig. 16.3). Results were characterized as "abnormal inner ear function with questionable hearing detection thresholds," and the audiologist recommended an ABR and testing for auditory processing disorder (APD).

16.1.5 Second Audiologic Appointment (at ENT Clinic) at Age 7

Three weeks later, George was evaluated by the audiologist again. Results of the *previous* appointment are described here as "behavioral thresholds ... normal, with SRT of 20 and excellent discrimination; however ... some difficulty understanding in the left ear for speech discrimination ... DPOAE appeared to be relatively normal." A new audiologic evaluation was conducted revealing responses in the slight to mild hearing loss range (▶ Fig. 16.4). Tympanograms were normal. Acoustic reflex and word recognition testing were not attempted. Both DPOAE and transient evoked otoacoustic emissions (TEOAE) were tested and reported as absent bilaterally. A click ABR was conducted, revealing present responses to click stimuli at 45 dB nHL. Waveforms and latencies are noted in ▶ Fig. 16.5. The audiologist noted that frequency-specific ABR testing could not be conducted due to myogenic artifact. Results were characterized as "normal auditory thresholds on behavioral testing ... abnormal inner ear testing ... testing discrepancies ... cannot rule out central auditory processing abnormality." George was then referred to our clinic for an APD evaluation.

16.2 Audiologic Testing

George was seen in our clinic, for the first time, at age 7.5, approximately 5 months after his last appointment, for an APD evaluation. However, following an audiologic examination, the APD evaluation was deferred.

Audiometric test results revealed a mild sloping to severe sensorineural hearing loss (SNHL) bilaterally (▶ Fig. 16.5). George was cooperative during testing and compliant when tones were presented at an elevated intensity (60 dB HL at 1,000 Hz). Speech reception thresholds were consistent with the audiogram. Otoscopy revealed no visible abnormality. Tympanometry suggested normal middle ear pressure and peak compensated static acoustic admittance bilaterally. Evaluation of DPOAE revealed absent emissions (▶ Fig. 16.6). Acoustic reflex and word recognition testing were not attempted at this visit.

George's mother was counseled regarding the results of the evaluation. She expressed relief, noting that she believed George had been having difficulty hearing for a few years and that these problems had not been resolved after PE tube placement. We recommended that George be fitted with bilateral behind-the-ear hearing aids, use a wireless remote microphone system at school, and receive speech and language therapy.

16.3 Questions for the Reader

1. Review the test results and interpretation for the audiologic evaluations at age 5 (▶ Fig. 16.1) and age 7 (▶ Fig. 16.2; ▶ Fig. 16.4). Do you agree or disagree with the report's characterization of hearing test results provided here? Why? Are

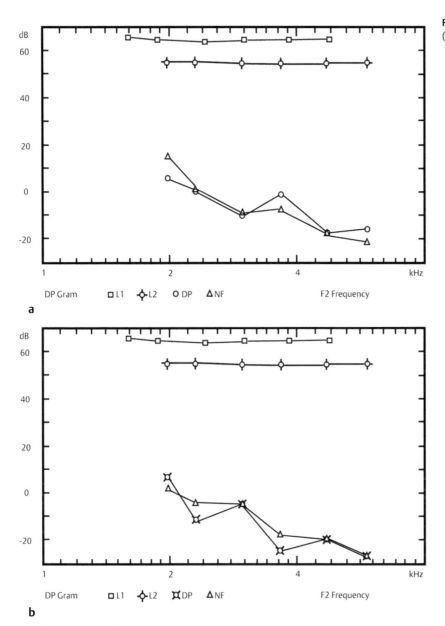

Fig. 16.3 Results of DPOAE screening at age 7. (**a**) right ear and (**b**) left ear.

there any other tests you would like to have seen performed?

2. Why do you think that the audiologic evaluation at age 7.5 (▶ Fig. 16.7) revealed SNHL that was not reported in the previous evaluations?

3. What elements of the child's case history and comorbid conditions may have made diagnosis of SNHL difficult?

4. Do you think that George may be faking or exaggerating his hearing loss? Why or why not?

16.4 Discussion of Questions

1. **Review the test results and interpretation for the audiologic evaluations at age 5** (▶ Fig. 16.1) **and age 7** (▶ Fig. 16.2; ▶ Fig. 16.4). **Do you agree or disagree with the report's characterization of hearing test results provided here? Why? Are there any other tests you would like to have seen performed?**

Results at age 5 (▶ Fig. 16.1) suggested elevated pure-tone thresholds. Monitored live voice was used to obtain a speech reception threshold in the sound field, which did seem to be in agreement with the sound field thresholds for 500 and 1,000 Hz. We would not consider the thresholds to be within normal limits for a 5-year-old child. These results suggested to us the possibility of a significant hearing loss, which would affect George's ability to develop appropriate speech and language. At age 7 (▶ Fig. 16.2), word recognition scores were lower than we expected given that the presentation level was 35 dB HL above the speech reception threshold. One might consider that George was not hearing as well as the audiogram indicated. At the second age-7 appointment (▶ Fig. 16.4), the speech reception threshold is elevated when compared to the

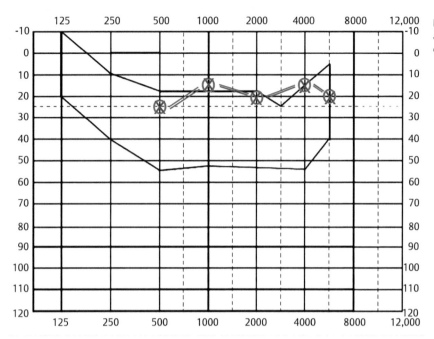

Fig. 16.4 Results of second available audiogram at age 7. O, right ear air conduction; X, left ear air conduction.

pure-tone average. The absence of DPOAE and TEOAE at these appointments is concerning, but hearing was characterized as "within normal limits" or "questionable" without further investigation of test discrepancies. Also the results of the ABR conducted at age 7 (▶ Fig. 16.5) were not normal. Peaks marked as wave V demonstrate prolonged absolute latencies. Ideally, acoustic reflex threshold assessment would have been completed at this appointment, because the patient presumably was diagnosed with otitis media (OM), requiring the placement of PE tubes at age 2. It would be helpful to know whether middle ear function was within normal limits, but only tympanometry results were available.

2. **Why do you think that the audiologic evaluation at age 7.5 (▶ Fig. 16.7) revealed SNHL that was not reported in the previous evaluations?**
It is hard to know for sure. It is possible that the patient's hearing loss fluctuated, but there is no evidence from the provided test results to suggest a disorder that would cause such a loss. It is possible that the tester interpretations of the patient's test results were over-reliant on pure-tone thresholds which suggested normal hearing but (1) were often marked after only one response, which is inconsistent with recommended threshold procedure, and (2) were not always consistent with other tests.

3. **What elements of the child's case history and comorbid conditions may have made diagnosis of SNHL difficult?**
Given the patient's history of PE tube placement, severe allergies, and upper respiratory disease, it would be reasonable to expect that hearing difficulties reported by the parent were a result of negative middle ear pressure and/or OM. This case is a good example of a child whose hearing loss was *not* attributable to the most likely explanation.

4. **Do you think that George may be faking or exaggerating his hearing loss? Why or why not?**
We do not think George was faking hearing difficulties. His test results at age 7.5 were consistent (note air and bone thresholds and speech reception threshold [SRT] and pure tone average [PTA]). Malingerers often provide a better-than-expected speech reception threshold. In this case where the speech reception threshold is elevated and notes on the audiogram indicate frequent repetition of instructions with one-time responses taken for some pure-tone thresholds, we tend to doubt the pure-tone thresholds.

16.5 Final Diagnosis and Recommended Treatment

George was reevaluated 1 month later. Hearing thresholds were rechecked and were unchanged from the previous appointment. He was fitted with hearing aids shortly thereafter, following medical clearance from his pediatric otolaryngologist physician. We recommended that George be evaluated by a pediatric otologist to rule out a large vestibular aqueduct (via magnetic resonance imaging) and to investigate other possible causes for George's sensorineural hearing loss.

16.6 Outcome

Hearing aid outputs were matched to generic prescriptive fitting targets, and aided thresholds were obtained between 20 and 25 dB HL for each aided ear. At subsequent appointments, George's mother noted that George is making significant improvement in his speech therapy appointments and that she has noticed an immediate difference in his hearing. He also asks for "his ears" as soon as he wakes up in the morning.

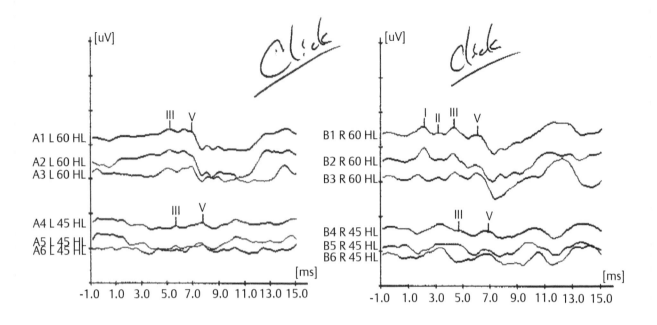

Fig. 16.5 Results of click ABR testing at age 7.

Collection Parameters						Latencies (ms)					Interlatencies (ms)		
Wave	Transducer	Ear	Intensity	Type	Frequency	I	II	III	IV	V	I-III	III-V	I-V
A1	Insert Earphone	Left	60dB HL	Click	N/A			5.20		6.89		1.69	
A2	Insert Earphone	Left	60dB HL	Click	N/A								
A3	Insert Earphone	Left	60dB HL	Click	N/A								
A4	Insert Earphone	Left	45dB HL	Click	N/A			5.64		7.76		2.13	
A5	Insert Earphone	Left	45dB HL	Click	N/A								
A6	Insert Earphone	Left	45dB HL	Click	N/A								
B1	Insert Earphone	Right	60dB HL	Click	N/A	2.14	3.20	4.32		6.07	2.19	1.75	3.94
B2	Insert Earphone	Right	60dB HL	Click	N/A								
B3	Insert Earphone	Right	60dB HL	Click	N/A								
B4	Insert Earphone	Right	45dB HL	Click	N/A			4.70		6.89		2.19	
B5	Insert Earphone	Right	45dB HL	Click	N/A								
B6	Insert Earphone	Right	45dB HL	Click	N/A								

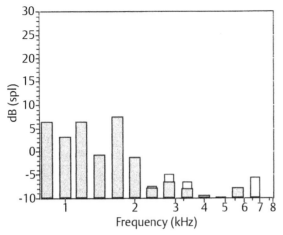

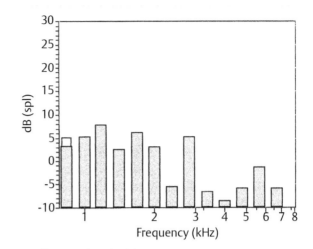

Half octave band OAE power

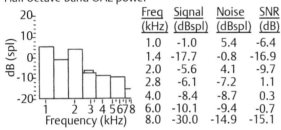

Freq (kHz)	Signal (dBspl)	Noise (dBspl)	SNR (dB)
1.0	-1.0	5.4	-6.4
1.4	-17.7	-0.8	-16.9
2.0	-5.6	4.1	-9.7
2.8	-6.1	-7.2	1.1
4.0	-8.4	-8.7	0.3
6.0	-10.1	-9.4	-0.7
8.0	-30.0	-14.9	-15.1

Test Summary
Sum all 1/2 octave= -4.1dBspl Ave DP 1/2oct (1-6)= -11.9dBspl

Half octave band OAE power

Freq (kHz)	Signal (dBspl)	Noise (dBspl)	SNR (dB)
1.0	1.5	5.6	-4.1
1.4	-9.1	2.6	-11.7
2.0	-4.5	4.7	-9.2
2.8	-12.0	1.4	-13.4
4.0	-10.6	-7.5	-3.1
6.0	-19.4	-4.0	-15.4
8.0	-19.8	-10.7	-9.1

Test Summary
Sum all 1/2 octave = ----dBspl Ave DP 1/2oct (1-6)= ----dBspl

Fig. 16.6 Results of DPOAE testing at age 7.5.

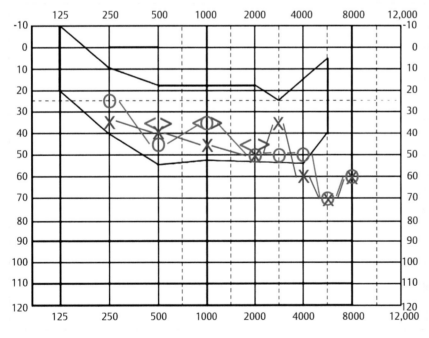

Fig. 16.7 Results of audiogram obtained at our clinic at age 7.5 prior to scheduled central auditory processing disorder evaluation. O, right ear air conduction; X, left ear air conduction; <, right ear bone conduction; >, left ear bone conduction.

Suggested Readings

[1] Jerger JF, Hayes D. The cross-check principle in pediatric audiometry. Arch Otolaryngol. 1976; 102(10):614–620

[2] Norrix LW. Hearing thresholds, minimum response levels, and cross-check measures in pediatric audiology. Am J Audiol. 2015; 24(2):137–144

17 A Case of Progressive Vestibular Impairment

Kelsey Hatton, Devin McCaslin, and Marc Bennett

17.1 Clinical History and Description

A 9-year-old girl presents with report of long-standing dizziness. She has unilateral hearing loss and a history of multiple head injuries in the setting of chronic headaches/migraines.

According to the family, from age 7, the patient began to experience episodes of nausea and dizziness lasting for minutes to hours at a time. The case history revealed multiple falls with significant injuries warranting a visit to the emergency room, including

- Age 2: the patient fell off a couch at home and had a bruise on her neck.
- Age 3: the patient fell and hit her head (occiput) on a rock with no imaging follow-up at the time.
- Age 4: the patient fell off a swing onto the back of her head and had bleeding from her injury. There was no loss of consciousness.
- Age 7: the patient ran into a parked car and fell to the ground, hitting her head and yielding abrasions on her forehead and around her eye.

Documentation notes the patient to be happy, cheerful, and interacting at an age-appropriate level with family and providers. No signs of abuse, domestic violence, or neglect were noted when the patient was seen in various departments. Her previous medical history is notable for a normal full-term birth without complications, passing her newborn hearing screening, and no history of ear infections. She reportedly performed well in school. The family history revealed her mother had a history of migraine headaches and hearing loss.

17.1.1 Initial Audiometric, Vestibular, and Imaging Results

The patient's hearing was tested using conventional pure tone audiometry. Audiometry revealed normal hearing sensitivity for the left ear. For the right ear results showed a mild conductive hearing loss at 250 Hz, rising to normal hearing through 4,000 Hz, and then precipitously sloping to moderately severe to severe sensorineural loss from 6,000 to 8,000 Hz. Tympanometry and acoustic reflex testing from 500 to 2,000 Hz were considered normal, bilaterally. Word recognition was excellent for both ears (▶ Fig. 17.1).

Vestibular function testing consisted of videonystagmography, sinusoidal harmonic acceleration, cervical and ocular vestibular-evoked myogenic potentials (i.e., cVEMP and oVEMPs), and electrocochleography (ECochG). ECochG was normal on the left side, and no repeatable response could be obtained for the right side. Both cVEMP and oVEMP responses were normal on the left side and absent on the right. Remaining testing was significant for a compensated right peripheral vestibular impairment with a right posterior semicircular canal benign paroxysmal positional vertigo (pSCC BPPV). Referral to neurotology was recommended due to asymmetrical nature of hearing loss, family history of hearing loss, family history of headache, and documented vestibular impairment.

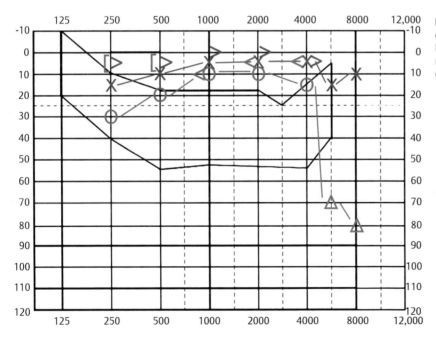

Fig. 17.1 Audiometric data. O, right ear air conduction; X, left ear air conduction; <, right ear bone conduction; >, left ear bone conduction; △, right ear air conduction masked; [, right ear bone conduction masked.

A computed tomography (CT) scan report from another facility indicated "normal appearance of temporal bones." Internal review of this CT scan demonstrated "a previous right occipital skull fracture."

17.2 Questions for the Reader

1. Do the case history and test results support an etiology for this patient's hearing and balance function?
2. Is any other audiological testing needed for workup?
3. How often would you recommend evaluating the patient's hearing or balance?
4. What would you discuss in counseling this family and child?

17.3 Discussion of Questions

1. **Do the case history and test results support an etiology for this patient's hearing and balance function?**
   Key components of the case history are a primary complaint of dizziness, report of episodic vertigo, recurrent patient head injuries, and family history of migraine headaches. The most common forms of childhood vertigo are migraine precursors or migraine variants.[1] Taken with a family history of migraine headache, benign paroxysmal vertigo of childhood (BPVC) or vestibular migraine could be possible contributors to the patient's reports of episodic vertigo.

   Significant test results are BPPV, a right-sided peripheral vestibular impairment, and asymmetrical right-sided hearing loss. The unilateral nature of both the vestibular and hearing impairment would be concerning for some type of physical difference between ears. Peripheral vestibular dysfunction is not commonly documented in children; however, up to 45% of patients with enlarged vestibular aqueduct (EVA) have vestibular signs and symptoms.[2] With a CT scan revealing a history of previous head trauma, a third-window disorder such as EVA would be a strong candidate disorder correlated to both hearing and balance impairments. Progressive loss of cochlear function secondary to head trauma is commonly seen in EVA.[3,4] A history of head injury among EVA patients has also been seen to significantly increase the number of vestibular signs and symptoms.[2]

2. **Is any other audiological testing needed for workup?**
   This patient was able to participate in a complete diagnostic vestibular test battery. Audiometric workup was also relatively complete. Distortion product otoacoustic emissions (DPOAEs) might have been tested to further evaluate right ear function. However, with present acoustic reflexes, good performance on word recognition, and no complaint of hearing difficulty, the added value of DPOAE testing might be limited for this case.

3. **How often would you recommend evaluating the patient's hearing or balance?**
   Due to the sensorineural nature of the hearing loss and stability demonstrated across external and internal audiograms over a 6-month interval, repeat hearing evaluation within 6 months to 1 year was recommended, or sooner should the family feel there was a change in hearing. Repeat vestibular testing was recommended within 6 months to 1 year if the severity of dizziness worsened or the quality of

dizziness symptoms changed. Continued follow-up with neurotology and audiology to further assess the source of the patient's dizziness is important. In this case, if the vestibular symptoms are associated with a migraine variant, there is a potential for dizziness to resolve over time.[1] Research also supports the potential for progressive hearing loss or balance impairment in patients with EVA.[2,3]

4. **What would you discuss in counseling this family and child?**
   Counseling should cover the patient's vestibular impairment and expected limitations. Exercises to increase stability and central vestibular compensation with physical therapy would likely be beneficial. While the cause of vestibular loss may be unclear, the fact that the patient has incurred multiple head injuries is concerning. Avoiding future head injuries may be important for preventing a recurrence of her BPPV or a worsening of her overall vestibular function. Counseling could also introduce the potential for migrainous influence on vestibular disorders of childhood. If migraine contributes to vestibular symptoms in this case, the patient's symptoms are likely to change or improve over time.

17.4 Diagnosis and Recommended Treatment

A canalith repositioning procedure was performed to address positional vertigo symptoms. After vestibular function testing and treatment for BPPV, the patient was seen by neurotology and diagnosed with resolved posterior semicircular canal BPPV and possible BPVC. Possible BPVC is a disorder that is a strong predictor of a child acquiring migraines. A migraine diet was recommended.

17.5 Outcome

Canalith repositioning treatment yielded successful resolution of right pSCC BPPV following two maneuvers. After a migraine diet was initiated, the family reported a reduction in frequency and severity of the patient's symptoms. Additional workup was pursued, including an order for a magnetic resonance imaging (MRI) to rule out retrocochlear pathology.

17.6 Progressive Vestibular Impairment

17.6.1 Subsequent Audiometric, Vestibular, and Imaging Results

Following the initial appointments, the family returned for a follow-up with neurotology due to patient's continued and frequent vertiginous episodes which reportedly lasted for 7 to 8 hours at a time. She also reported concurrent headache with sensitivity to light and sound. The frequency of symptoms began to affect her performance in school. Additional audiograms were performed using pure tone audiometry at ages 9, 11, 12, and 13 years. On all occasions, thresholds have remained clinically stable. When tympanometry and acoustic reflex testing from 500 to 2,000 Hz were completed, responses remained normal. Word recognition remained excellent at all visits with all materials (PBK and NU-6).

Subsequent vestibular examinations were performed at ages 10 years 2 months, 12 years 4 months, and 12 years 9 months. On all occasions, the patient had absent right-sided cVEMP and oVEMP responses, with a right peripheral vestibular impairment. However, there was decompensation for her peripheral vestibular impairment over subsequent visits with a reduction in total caloric response (▶ Table 17.1). She also had notable reduction of left VEMP responses over time (▶ Table 17.2). Additional imaging was performed with an MRI at ages 10 and 11, and a repeat CT scan was performed at age 12. MRI results show "enlargement of right endolymphatic sac without appreciable cochlear dysplasia," which was stable at the second MRI (▶ Fig. 17.2). The repeat CT scan revealed "enlarged right vestibular aqueduct (2.5 mm in diameter) with the left vestibular aqueduct within upper limits of normal" (▶ Fig. 17.3). An EVA is defined as greater than or equal to 2.0 mm at the operculum and/or greater than or equal to 1.0 mm at the midpoint.[5]

17.7 Additional Questions for the Reader

1. Are there further recommendations you would make?
2. What are some of the complicating factors in this case?

17.8 Discussion of Additional Questions

1. **Are there further recommendations you would make?**
   The patient experienced some improvement in her migraines and unsteadiness symptoms via diet. Further medical management may be beneficial if headache symptoms continue. Continued unsteadiness may be helped with vestibular rehabilitative therapy (VRT). An added benefit of therapy is that the patient can help to set mobility/steadiness goals that are relevant to her daily activities.

2. **What are some of the complicating factors in this case?**
   For this patient, the presence of initial BPPV and vestibular migraines prolonged the final diagnosis of EVA. There is also the potential for migraine-induced nystagmus to mimic BPPV. When a patient is experiencing a migraine, he or she is more likely to have positive vestibular findings, such as spontaneous nystagmus or nystagmus characteristic of central vestibular disorder (i.e., strong vertical component). The high-frequency nature of her hearing loss is an additional complicating factor in determining appropriate diagnosis because third-window disorders most typically result in low-frequency hearing losses with air–bone gaps.

Table 17.1 Caloric and rotational chair data

Patient age	Right warm	Left warm	Right cool	Left cool	Asymmetry (%)	Total SPV	SHA
9 y 3 mo	6	27	6	36	68	75	Normal
10 y 11 mo	4	27	4	31	76	66	Low gain, 0.01–0.04 Hz
12 y 4 mo	1	7	4	10	55	22	Phase leads with low gain, 0.01–0.04 Hz
12 y 9 mo	1	17	4	14	72	36	Normal

Abbreviation: SHA, sinusoidal harmonic acceleration; SPV, slow phase velocity.

Table 17.2 VEMP data

Patient age	cVEMP P1 latency		cVEMP amplitude		oVEMP N1 latency		oVEMP amplitude	
	Right	Left	Right	Left	Right	Left	Right	Left
9 y 3 mo	NR	13.58	NR	471.19	NR	11.19	NR	5.18
10 y 11 mo	NR	14.55	NR	63.97	NR	13.26	NR	2.94
12 y 4 mo	NR	15.72	NR	37.60	NR	12.18	NR	7.01
12 y 9 mo	NR	NR	NR	NR	NR	NR	NR	NR

Abbreviations: cVEMP, cervical vestibular-evoked myogenic potential; NR, no response; oVEMP, ocular vestibular-evoked myogenic potential.

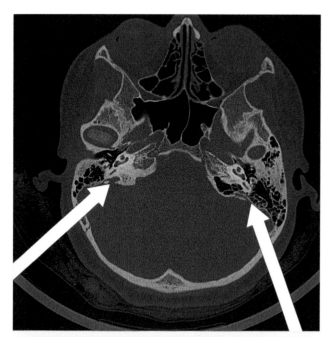

Fig. 17.2 Magnetic resonance imaging. An axial cut viewed from below the patient. The white arrows indicate an enlarged right vestibular aqueduct.

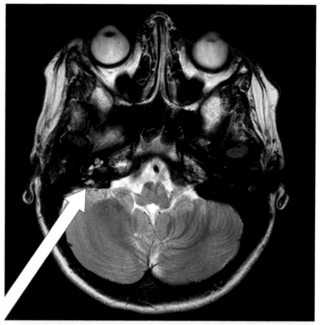

Fig. 17.3 Computed tomographic scan. An axial cut viewed from below the patient. The white arrow indicates the location of the vestibular aqueduct.

17.9 Subsequent Diagnoses and Recommended Treatments

Upon return visits during age 9, migraine diet and a repeated repositioning were reported to reduce the frequency of patient symptoms. Preferential seating was recommended as the family was not interested in amplification. With continued symptoms at age 10, an MRI was ordered, and results supported right EVA. VRT and neurological consult were recommended. Minimization and avoidance of head trauma were discussed. At age 11, further medical treatment for migraines was recommended should dizziness worsen. Monitoring of right-sided EVA revealed no change. The patient had not participated in or scheduled to enroll in VRT up to this point. At age 12, repeat imaging to investigate possible left EVA was ordered. Due to increased dizziness with stress, counseling was recommended to alleviate tension. The family initiated VRT at this time, and the patient was discharged as she met all assigned goals at age 12 years 11 months. Specific goals met included

- Normal age-matched scores for gaze stabilization and dynamic visual acuity.
- Standing independently on foam surface with eyes closed > 30 seconds.
- Independent ambulation over community distances (> 1,000 feet) on various surfaces with head turns.
- Composite score on the sensory organization test was above age-matched normative data. There were no deficits in the

use of vestibular, somatosensory, or visual cues for the maintenance of upright posture. Her center of gravity was determined to be well aligned.

17.10 Outcome

Continued migraine diet helped to partially manage patient symptoms. Enrollment in and completion of a 10-week course of VRT yielded "an increase in stability and ability to participate in age-appropriate mobility tasks without loss of balance or report of dizziness." The patient has not contacted clinic with further complaints of imbalance to date.

References

[1] Lagman-Bartolome AM, Lay C. Pediatric migraine variants: a review of epidemiology, diagnosis, treatment, and outcome. Curr Neurol Neurosci Rep. 2015; 15(6):34

[2] Zalewski CK, Chien WW, King KA, et al. Vestibular dysfunction in patients with enlarged vestibular aqueduct. Otolaryngol Head Neck Surg. 2015; 153 (2):257–262

[3] Alemi AS, Chan DK. Progressive hearing loss and head trauma in enlarged vestibular aqueduct: a systematic review and meta-analysis. Otolaryngol Head Neck Surg. 2015; 153(4):512–517

[4] Noordman B, van Beeck Calkoen E, Witte B, Goverts T, Hensen E, Merkus P. Prognostic factors for sudden drops in hearing level after minor head injury in patients with an enlarged vestibular aqueduct: a meta-analysis. Otol Neurotol. 2015; 36(1):4–11

[5] Valvassori GE, Clemis JD. The large vestibular aqueduct syndrome. Laryngoscope. 1978; 88(5):723–728

18 Auditory Processing Evaluation: 12-Year-Old Male

Erin C. Schafer and Shelby Landes

18.1 Clinical History and Description

GF, a 12-year-old sixth-grade male homeschool student, was seen for a complete auditory processing evaluation. His medical history includes an unremarkable pregnancy with minor complications during birth. He was diagnosed with verbal and motor tics, high anxiety, and some traits reminiscent of autism spectrum disorder (ASD). The results of a full individual evaluation (FIE) completed at GF's school indicated that he qualified for special education services under emotional disturbance. His mother decided to homeschool GF after poor experiences with school personnel, and she reports that he seems to be regressing and not performing at the level expected for his age. She is concerned about his ability to understand verbal instructions, academic performance (especially math, reading, and writing), and frequent misinterpretation and/or overgeneralization of conversations. He often asks for repetition or states that he did not understand what was said. According to his mother, GF exhibits high levels of anxiety, particularly when trying new things for fear of making a mistake or not understanding directions. He enjoys computer games and game design, something he feels relieves stress and anxiety.

18.2 Diagnostic Auditory Processing Evaluation Results

18.2.1 Audiologic Evaluation

Otoscopy revealed clear ear canals with good visualization of a healthy tympanic membrane bilaterally. Immittance results yielded a type A tympanogram in both ears, and ipsilateral acoustic reflex thresholds were present and within normal limits bilaterally. Responses to pure-tone stimuli were within normal limits bilaterally, and speech reception thresholds were obtained at 10 dB hearing level (HL) in both ears. Word recognition scores were 100% bilaterally.

18.2.2 Speech Perception in Noise

The Bamford–Kowal–Bench speech-in-noise (BKB-SIN) test was used to estimate GF's speech recognition in noise at the 50% correct level. In other words, the test determines the signal-to-noise ratio (SNR) that is required by the listener to understand 50% of key words in the presence of background noise. Sentences were presented at 0-degree azimuth (directly in front of the listener), and noise was presented from two locations: 0 and 180 degrees. GF's thresholds in noise were +2-dB SNR with noise at 0-degree azimuth and +1-dB SNR with noise at 180-degree azimuth. These results are outside the normal limits provided in the test manual in the 0-degree noise condition, with the average SNR needed for peers of the same age being –0.9-dB SNR. The 180-degree noise condition

suggests that his performance will improve slightly when background noise is spatially separated from the sentences. During the test, GF made several comments that suggested difficulties with auditory working memory skills. For example, he would say "I heard that one, but I don't remember what it said" or "I heard it, but it was too long." GF became anxious and continued to struggle with this, especially at more difficult SNRs, despite being reinstructed that he can say as many or as few words as he can remember.

18.2.3 Binaural Integration

GF's binaural integration skills were tested to determine his ability to process different stimuli when they were presented to each ear at the same time. Deficits in binaural integration often demonstrate a large right ear advantage and can result in increased difficulty understanding speech in the presence of background noise or when there are multiple talkers.

The dichotic digits test (DDT) is a method of assessing binaural integration by presenting four digits dichotically (two different digits per ear) and asking the child to repeat each number heard using free recall. GF's scores for 50 stimuli sets in the right and left ears were 84% (norm = 96.2 ± 4.1%) and 60% (norm = 90.7 ±- 5.7%), respectively, suggesting performance that was two standard deviations below the mean for his age. There was an atypical difference between scores in the right and left ears (24%), suggesting a strong right ear advantage.

The competing words—directed ear (CW-DE) subtest of the SCAN-3 was also used to assess binaural integration. This test involves presenting words dichotically and asking the child to repeat both words. The directed ear component asks the child to repeat the words in a specific order based on which ear heard each word. This is a means of identifying the large right ear advantage common to the auditory processing disorder (APD) diagnosis. GF's total scaled score of 4 places him in the 2nd percentile, which is in the borderline disordered range. A large atypical right ear advantage (cumulative preference = 5%) was seen in the directed right ear task, and a typical right ear advantage was seen in the directed left ear task. Cumulative preference can range from 2 to 15%, with lower scores associated with a greater likelihood of an auditory-based disorder.

GF's performance on both tests suggests a deficit in binaural integration. This is evident in his borderline to abnormal overall performance on the dichotic listening tasks as well as the large right ear advantage identified on both the DDT and the CW-DE.

18.2.4 Binaural Separation

The competing sentences (CS) subtest of the SCAN-3 was used to evaluate his binaural separation abilities. Binaural separation is the ability to ignore a stimulus in one ear and focus on a different stimulus in the other ear when both stimuli are presented simultaneously. Abnormal results in this domain typically are associated with increased difficulty understanding speech in background noise or when there are multiple talkers.

GF's scaled score on the CS subtest was 7. This falls in the lower range of normal limits in the 16th percentile. A large atypical right ear advantage (cumulative preference = 5%) was observed for this measure. These results are consistent with abnormal binaural separation abilities due to the right ear advantage.

18.2.5 Temporal Processing

The random gap detection test (RGDT) was used to determine GF's temporal processing abilities by asking him to identify whether two stimuli are perceived as one sound or two. Abnormality in the ability to detect small fluctuations in the timing of speech cues is consistent with temporal processing deficits and can increase difficulty with speech perception. The composite gap detection threshold is calculated by averaging the lowest identifiable gap for pure tones of 500 to 4,000 Hz. Results of the RGDT indicated a threshold of 2 ms, which falls within normal limits on this measure.

18.2.6 Temporal Patterning

The pitch pattern sequence (PPS) test was used to examine GF's temporal-patterning abilities, which are the recognition of presentation patterns of nonlinguistic auditory stimuli. The PPS requires children to discriminate between high and low pitches in sets of three tones (e.g., high–high–low, high–low–high, low–low–high) that are presented monaurally. A percentage of the pitch patterns correctly identified is calculated. GF correctly identified 100% of the PPSs in the right ear and 100% of the sequences in the left ear. This is consistent with normal temporal-patterning abilities.

Table 18.1 Summary of GF's performance on speech perception in noise, binaural listening, and temporal processing/patterning tasks

Speech perception in noise			
BKB-SIN	+2 dB SNR (0-degree azimuth)	+1 dB SNR (180-degree azimuth)	Outside normal limits
Binaural integration			
DDT	84%: right ear (RE) 60%: left ear	24% difference	Outside normal limits Strong RE advantage
CW-DE	4 (2nd percentile)	Directed RE = 5% cumulative preference	Outside normal limits Strong RE advantage
Binaural separation			
CS	7 (16th percentile)	5% cumulative preference, RE	WNL Strong RE advantage
Temporal processing/patterning			
RGDT	Gap detection threshold = 2 ms		WNL
PPS	100%: RE	100%: LE	WNL

Abbreviations: BKB-SIN, Bamford–Kowal–Bench speech-in-noise test; CS, competing sentences; CW-DE, competing words–directed ear; DDT, dichotic digits test; PPS, pitch pattern sequence; RGDT, random gap detection test; SNR, signal-to-noise ratio; WNL, within normal limits.

18.3 Summary of Test Results

18.3.1 Spatial Stream Segregation

Auditory stream segregation is the listener's ability to separate simultaneous incoming auditory signals and attach meaningful representations to those signals (▶ Table 18.1). The Listening in Spatialized Noise—Sentences Test (LiSN-S) evaluates these skills by varying the spatial and pitch characteristics of incoming stimuli and by calculating speech recognition thresholds (SRT) in noise as well as advantage scores for each of the test conditions. Sentences are presented in the presence of distracter stories, with the intensity level of the phrase adjusted to find the patient's SRT in noise at the 50% correct level. The distracter stories are varied in regard to their position in space (± 0- vs. ± 90-degree azimuth) and the vocal quality of the speakers (same voice vs. different voices). The low-cue SRT represents listening skills when no spatial or vocal cues are available, while the total advantage and high-cue SRT represent listening skills when both vocal and spatial cues are available. Talker advantage indicates the listener's ability to use differences in vocal quality to distinguish the signal of interest, and spatial advantage reflects a listener's ability to use differences in the physical location of incoming stimuli to perceive the signal of interest amidst competing signals. GF's results are summarized in ▶ Table 18.2.

18.3.2 Informal Evaluation

The Children's Auditory Performance Scale (C.H.A.P.S.) is a teacher questionnaire designed to examine the listening difficulties of a child compared with age-matched, typically functioning peers. Six listening conditions are evaluated, including noise, quiet, ideal, multiple inputs (i.e., auditory, visual, tactile), auditory memory (i.e., recalling spoken information), and auditory attention span. Because GF is homeschooled, his mother completed the survey. Her responses indicate that GF is in the at-risk range for all listening conditions except for the ideal and multiple-input conditions. These responses suggest that GF has substantially greater difficulties listening in classroom-type environments than his peers.

The Children's Communication Checklist-2 (CCC-2) is a comprehensive parent/caregiver survey of a child's communication skills across language and pragmatic domains. Based

Table 18.2 GF's average test scores and normal test scores on the Listening in Spatialized Noise—Sentences Test (LiSN-S)

Measure	Average score for age	GF's score (dB)	Normal limits	Standard deviation
Low-cue SRT	−1.1	−0.9	Within	−0.2
High-cue SRT	−12.4	−11.2	Within	−0.6
Talker advantage	6.9	7.6	Within	0.3
Spatial advantage	10.5	8.3	Within	−1.3
Total advantage	11.3	10.3	Within	−0.5

Abbreviation: SRT, speech recognition threshold.

on responses from GF's mother, the General Communication Composite score was 27, indicating an overall communicative competence in the 0.3 percentile (one-third of the 1st percentile). Typical scores of other children are around 100 (standard deviation = 15), which places GF well below normal limits. The Social Interaction Difference Index (SIDI) was −2, suggesting a communicative profile within the normal range (not characteristic of a specific language disorder or ASD).

Fisher's Auditory Problems Checklist collects information from the parent/caregiver about the perceived auditory problems experienced by the child and is often used as an informal screening tool for APD. Responses from GF's mother were converted into a score of 48%. This suggests that he has a range of auditory difficulties 2 SDs below the mean for peers of the same age, with the average score for sixth graders being 80%.

18.4 Questions for the Reader

1. What were the strengths and deficit areas identified in the auditory processing evaluation?
2. Would you diagnose GF with an APD? Why or why not?
3. Would you recommend any additional testing for GF?
4. What would you recommend for GF to address his listening issues?

18.5 Discussion of Questions

1. **What were the strengths and deficit areas identified in the auditory processing evaluation?**

   The comprehensive test results are indicative of normal auditory processing abilities for temporal processing, temporal patterning, and spatial stream segregation. Deficits were seen in GF's speech perception in noise, binaural integration, and binaural separation. This profile suggests asymmetry between the function of the right and left auditory cortices. In fact, a comment from GF during the test session highlighted the asymmetry he experiences. He stated, "I can do this thing where I turn off my left side and only listen to the right ear, but I can't do it the other way around." This interaural asymmetry may lead to increased difficulty listening in noisy environments and greater difficulty attending to auditory information.[1] During testing GF also demonstrated difficulty with auditory working memory, and according to informal evaluations completed by GF's mother, he has substantial listening difficulties both at home and in noisy environments.

2. **Would you diagnose GF with an APD? Why or why not?**

   Yes. We diagnosed GF with APD given his deficits in speech perception in noise, binaural integration, and binaural separation. Although his FIE at school indicated emotional disturbance, there were no other formal evaluations obtained to confirm a diagnoses of ASD or other disorders that may confound results.[2] Although it is not relevant in the present case, it is important to note that a diagnosis of ASD or other disorders, such as attention deficit hyperactivity disorder, cognitive disabilities, or language disorders, may negatively influence results on behavioral auditory processing tests.

3. **Would you recommend any additional testing for GF?**

   Given the fact that GF had a recent FIE, comprehensive speech-language, educational, and physical, and testing has already been conducted, it is likely that no outside referrals are necessary. However, we would confirm that he is receiving professional counseling services for his anxiety and emotional issues. In addition, we may recommend additional speech-language or psychological testing focused on auditory memory, which appeared to be a difficult task for GF. There are also several other auditory processing test measures that were not utilized in our test protocol; however, we attempted to address each domain of auditory processing with one to two measures.[2,3] In an ideal world, our protocol would also include electrophysiological measures from the level of the brainstem to the cortex in response to speech stimuli, which could corroborate behavioral measures by shedding some additional light on the functional integrity of the auditory system relative to age-matched, typically functioning peers.[2]

4. **What would you recommend for GF to address his listening issues?**

   The following recommendations were provided to attempt to improve GF's ability to attend to auditory stimuli:
   - Consider a dichotic training treatment program with Auditory Rehabilitation for Interaural Asymmetry (ARIA)[4,5] or CAPDOTS. Note that there is emerging evidence to support dichotic training in children with processing deficits. For example, one study (N = 21) showed significant improvements in dichotic left ear performance, which was initially weak, after dichotic training in the soundfield.[4,5] Additionally, a single-subject research study (N = 3) yielded positive results with dichotic training under earphones.[6]
   - Engage in the following at-home activities[7]:
     o Practice following verbal instructions of increasing difficulty. For example, "Draw a dot. Next, draw a dot connected by a line to another dot. Now, draw a dot connected by a line to another dot and then draw another line underneath."
     o Play "Simon Says" with verbal commands specifically targeting actions on the left side of the body (e.g., hop to your left foot, raise your left arm, use your left pointer finger to touch your nose, etc.).
     o Play games to strengthen processing abilities in multiple modalities and auditory memory such as Bop-It, Simon, charades, and Pictionary.
   - Consider a comprehensive receptive language evaluation or psychological evaluation to evaluate potential auditory memory deficits.
   - If he returns to a school environment, consider the use of remote-microphone technology (e.g., ear-level digital system) in the classroom and possibly at home.
   - If he returns to a school environment, use strategic seating in the classroom (close to the teacher, away from distracting outside noises such as hallways, projectors, fans, etc.).
   - Allow extra time for processing information.
   - Reduce visual distractions.
   - Check for understanding during verbal instruction.
   - Repeat or rephrase information when necessary.
   - Use hearing protection whenever in the presence of loud sounds.

References

[1] Moncrieff D, Keith W, Abramson M, Swann A. Diagnosis of amblyaudia in children referred for auditory processing assessment. Int J Audiol. 2016; 55 (6):333–345

[2] Jerger J, Musiek F. Report of the consensus conference on the diagnosis of auditory processing disorders in school-aged children. J Am Acad Audiol. 2000; 11(9):467–474

[3] Cameron S, Dillon H. Auditory processing disorder. —from screening to diagnosis and management:. a-step-by-step guide. Audiology Now. 2005; 21:47–55

[4] Moncrieff DW, Wertz D. Auditory rehabilitation for interaural asymmetry: preliminary evidence of improved dichotic listening performance following intensive training. Int J Audiol. 2008; 47(2):84–97

[5] Moncrieff D. Audia Dichotic and Auditory Rehabilitation for Interaural Asymmetry Software [computer software]. Version 1.4.4.0. Dichotics Inc.; 2016

[6] Denman I, Banajee M, Hurley A. Dichotic listening training in children with autism spectrum disorder:. a single subject design. Int J Audiol. 2015; 54 (12):991–996

[7] Cokely C, Wilson PL. Remediation of auditory processing disorders in children: an overview. In: Roeser R, Downs M, eds. Auditory Disorders in School Children. 4th ed. New York, NY: Thieme Medical Publishers; 2004:365–393

Suggested Readings

[1] American Speech-Language-Hearing Association. Central auditory processing disorders [technical report]. American Speech-Language-Hearing Association. http://www.asha.org/policy/TR2005–00043/. Published 2005. Accessed June 27, 2016

[2] Bellis TJ, Anzalone AM. Intervention approaches for individuals with (central) auditory processing disorder. Contemp Issues Commun Sci Disord. 2008; 35:143–153

[3] Loo JH, Rosen S, Bamiou DE. Auditory training effects on the listening skills of children with auditory processing disorder. Ear Hear. 2016; 37(1):38–47

19 Hearing and Vestibular Loss in a 9-Month-Old Child

Kristen Janky

19.1 Clinical History and Description

The patient is a 9-month, 3-week-old female patient who is currently being followed for unilateral, profound, sensorineural hearing loss in the right ear. The patient's family wanted to determine the underlying etiology of the hearing loss; therefore, she was seen for interdisciplinary assessment including audiologic, vestibular, ophthalmology, ear, nose, and throat (ENT), and genetics evaluations.

The patient was born full-term without any complications. At age 9 months, she is reportedly meeting all gross motor milestones in that she is sitting independently and demonstrates good head control. She has history of middle ear effusion.

19.2 Audiologic Findings

The patient did not pass her newborn hearing screen in either ear. At her rescreen, age 8 days, she passed in her left ear, but not in her right ear. Confirmatory auditory brainstem response (ABR) and distortion product otoacoustic emission (DPOAE) testing were completed at age 2 months. Tympanometry with use of a 1,000-Hz probe tone was normal in both ears prior to ABR and DPOAE testing. Responses to tone-burst ABR suggested normal hearing sensitivity in the left ear with DPOAEs present at normal absolute amplitudes from 1 to 8 kHz and profound hearing loss in the right ear with absent DPOAEs from 1 to 8 kHz. Interpeak latencies were normal, which ruled out neuropathy affecting the auditory brainstem pathways for the left ear, but it could not be ruled out for the right ear due to the degree of hearing loss. The normal tympanograms ruled out any conductive component to the hearing loss. Use of an auditory osseointegrated device (AOD) on a soft band as well as interdisciplinary evaluation, including audiologic, vestibular, ophthalmology, ENT, and genetics evaluations, was recommended, which were all completed at age 9 months.

Conventional audiometric assessment using visual reinforcement techniques was attempted at age 9 months, albeit with poor reliability. Tympanograms were consistent with middle ear effusion bilaterally. Use of an AOD on a soft band was again recommended; however, the child's mother declined to follow up on this recommendation.

19.3 Vestibular Findings

Rotary chair testing was completed at age 9 months to assess for vestibular loss as part of the interdisciplinary evaluation. The vestibulo-ocular reflex was monitored during rotation using electrodes with the patient seated on her parent's lap. Rotary chair findings are shown in ▶ Fig. 19.1. Given the abnormal phase lead at 0.01 and borderline phase lead at 0.02 Hz, these findings do not rule out unilateral peripheral vestibular system involvement. Because rotary chair is a test of overall responsiveness of the vestibular system, it does not localize to the right or left ear. However, due to the profound hearing loss in the right ear, vestibular function would most likely be affected in the right ear.

Additional testing to confirm a unilateral vestibular weakness could not be completed for this patient. Typically, in addition to rotary chair testing, the cervical vestibular evoked myogenic potential (VEMP) is evaluated in children. The cervical VEMP is an assessment of the inferior portion of the vestibular nerve and saccule and, therefore, complements the rotary chair test, which is an assessment of the horizontal semicircular canals and superior branch of the vestibular nerve. Cervical VEMP testing with air-conducted stimuli can be completed in the presence of sensorineural hearing loss as it is strictly a test of vestibular function; however, cervical VEMP testing requires normal middle ear function as conductive hearing loss attenuates the intensity of sound getting to the vestibular system. Therefore, due to the presence of abnormal tympanograms, and subsequent conductive hearing loss, cervical VEMP testing could not be completed for this patient.

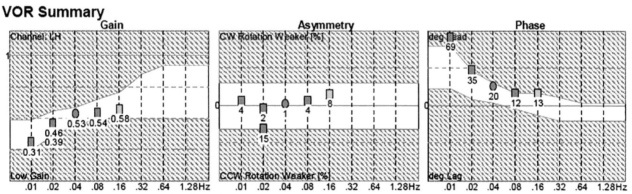

Fig. 19.1 Rotary chair findings demonstrate a phase lead, clockwise (rightward) asymmetry at 0.01 Hz and borderline phase lead at 0.02 Hz.

19.4 Other Findings

19.4.1 Genetics

Physical exam was not suggestive of any type of syndromic hearing loss; therefore, genetic testing was not recommended.

19.4.2 ENT

Physical exam was normal with the exception of possible bilateral effusion. In children with unilateral sensorineural hearing loss, the most common cause of hearing loss is a form of inner ear anomaly; therefore, magnetic resonance imaging (MRI), including the brainstem, with and without contrast was recommended after the patient's first birthday.

19.4.3 MRI

At age 12 months, MRI of the brain and internal auditory canals with and without contrast under sedation was completed (▶ Fig. 19.2). On the right, the eighth cranial nerve and superior portion of the vestibular nerve were visualized; however, the cochlear nerve and inferior division of the vestibular nerve were markedly hypoplastic or absent (▶ Fig. 19.2b,c). The MRI was otherwise unremarkable for the left ear (▶ Fig. 19.2a–c).

The rotary chair phase lead in the present patient would suggest that the superior portion of the vestibular nerve, while visualized on MRI, may still be affected and that cervical VEMP would likely have been absent.

19.4.4 Ophthalmology

The patient was noted to have a moderate amount of far-sightedness with astigmatism. Prescription lenses were recommended.

19.5 Questions for the Reader

1. In children with hearing loss, who is at risk for also having vestibular loss?
2. Which tests of vestibular function are typically completed in children?
3. When should a child be referred for vestibular testing?

4. What are the functional consequences of vestibular loss in children?
5. If a child with hearing loss is diagnosed with vestibular loss, what are some additional recommendations?

19.6 Discussion of Questions

1. **In children with hearing loss, who is at risk for also having vestibular loss?**
The presence of hearing loss puts children at risk for also having vestibular loss[1]; however, not all children with hearing loss will have vestibular loss. Vestibular loss is more likely to occur in children with greater severity of hearing loss,[2,3] which is why it is not surprising that in children who receive a cochlear implant, approximately 50% demonstrate some degree of vestibular loss, with 30% having bilateral vestibular loss.[4,5]

Vestibular loss is also more likely to occur with specific etiologies of hearing loss. Etiologies of hearing loss that are associated with vestibular loss include cytomegalovirus, meningitis, Usher's syndrome, Pendred's syndrome, enlarged vestibular aqueduct syndrome and other inner ear malformations, Waardenburg's syndrome, auditory neuropathy, connexin mutations (GJB2), measles, mumps, and ototoxicity, among others.[6,7,8,9,10,11,12]

2. **Which tests of vestibular function are typically completed in children?**
Vestibular testing includes traditional videonystagmography with caloric testing, video head impulse testing (vHIT), ocular and cervical VEMPs, rotary chair, and computerized dynamic posturography (CDP). Each of these exams provides complementary information regarding vestibular function; however, not all exams are appropriate for children, particularly children younger than 5 years. Therefore, the age and ability of the child are important considerations when choosing which tests of vestibular function are appropriate.

Additionally, it is important to consider the information provided by each vestibular test when choosing which tests of vestibular function are appropriate. The vestibular system is made up of five rate sensors: three semicircular canals (horizontal, posterior, and anterior canals) and two otolith organs

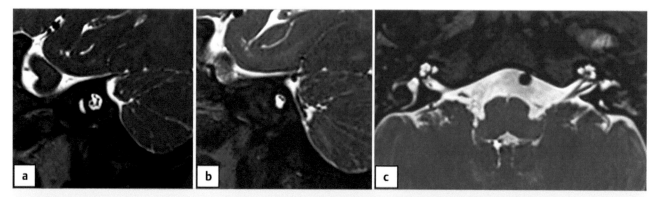

Fig. 19.2 (a) MRI, *left* sagittal cut of the internal auditory canal showing normal facial and vestibulocochlear nerve branches; **(b)** MRI, *right* sagittal cut of the internal auditory canal, showing facial and probable superior branch of the vestibular nerve with no visualization of the cochlear and inferior vestibular nerve branches; and **(c)** MRI, axial cut, showing the internal auditory canal. Two nerve branches (darker lines) can be seen on the left (one going to the cochlea, the other going to the vestibular system) and almost no evidence of innervation on the right.

(utricle and saccule). The vestibular portion of the eighth cranial nerve is divided into two branches, superior and inferior. The superior branch of the nerve innervates the horizontal canal, superior canal, and utricle, while the inferior branch of the nerve innervates the posterior canal and saccule. Vestibular testing has the ability to assess each of the rate sensors and both portions of the vestibular nerve (▶ Table 19.1).

Taking into account the age and ability of the child and the information provided by each vestibular test, we generally use the following recommendations at our institution. Rotary chair, cervical VEMPs, and a parent case history (outlining whether the child exhibits signs and symptoms of a vestibular disorder, including gross motor milestone delay) are recommended as part of the vestibular evaluation for children younger than 4 to 5 years. For children older than 4 to 5 years, ocular VEMP and vHIT would be included. Based on the preference and ability of the child, caloric testing would eventually be substituted for rotary chair testing. Either CDP, starting at age 3 years, or an appointment with vestibular rehabilitation, for children of any age, would additionally be recommended for an assessment of functional balance and treatment plan regarding gross motor skill attainment, if needed.

3. **When should a child be referred for vestibular testing?**
Vestibular testing is typically recommended in children who exhibit symptoms of dizziness and in children with hearing loss, particularly in children with hearing loss who also exhibit gross motor delay or whose etiology of hearing loss is known to have concomitant vestibular loss. Because vestibular loss is more likely to occur in children with greater severity of hearing loss, vestibular testing would be recommended in all children prior to cochlear implantation.

Table 19.1 Tests of vestibular function, the rate sensor, and portion of the vestibular nerve assessed

Test of vestibular function	Rate sensor assessed	Portion of vestibular nerve assessed
Caloric testing	Horizontal canal	Superior
vHIT	Horizontal canal	Superior
vHIT	Superior canal	Superior
vHIT	Posterior canal	Inferior
Cervical VEMP	Saccule	Inferior
Ocular VEMP	Utricle	Superior
Rotary chair	Horizontal canal	Superior
Computerized dynamic posturography	Does not assess a specific rate sensor; however, it is a functional assessment of overall balance function	

Abbreviations: VEMP, vestibular evoked myogenic potential; vHIT, video head impulse test.

4. **What are the functional consequences of vestibular loss in children?**
Compared to adults, relatively little is known about the functional consequences of vestibular loss in children; however, the presence of vestibular loss in children has been associated with the following functional deficits. First, children with significant vestibular loss are delayed in their acquisition of gross motor skills, including head control, sitting, standing, walking, and maintaining balance.[9,13,14] The degree of gross motor developmental delay and imbalance has been linked to the degree of vestibular loss, where children with greater severity of vestibular loss exhibit greater delay in gross motor development in early childhood and greater imbalance as an older child.[5,9,13,15] Children with vestibular loss also demonstrate reduced dynamic visual acuity (i.e., the ability to see while their head is in motion).[5,16,17] The functional implications of having reduced visual acuity with head motion are not fully understood; however, preliminary evidence suggests this may affect reading acuity.[18] Additionally, children with hearing and vestibular loss demonstrate reduced quality of life.[19] There is also speculation that vestibular loss can result in deficits of specific domains of cognitive function.[20]

Several additional outcome measures have been noted in children with vestibular loss who have also received a cochlear implant. As noted earlier, approximately 50% of children with cochlear implants have some degree of vestibular loss.[4,21] While children with cochlear implants perform many of the same activities as children with normal hearing, parents report that some children have a difficult time sustaining certain activities, such as riding a bike.[21] Overall, balance is reportedly better with the device turned on, likely because the vestibular nerve is receiving some degree of electrical stimulation[21]; however, in spite of this, children with cochlear implants and vestibular loss have increased falls and balance impairment, which has been shown to result in a higher rate of internal device failure.[22]

For these reasons, questioning parents regarding the attainment of gross motor milestones, their current balance abilities, and the patterns of their child's play, which can be important indicators of the potential for vestibular loss in children, is essential.

5. **If a child is diagnosed with vestibular loss, what are some additional recommendations?**
Regardless of the degree of vestibular loss, referral to a physical therapist in vestibular rehabilitation is recommended when vestibular loss is diagnosed. The purpose of physical therapy is to assess for functional consequences of vestibular loss, such as delays in gross motor acquisition and reduced dynamic visual acuity, as discussed earlier, and to provide treatment for any realized deficits or delays. While there is the notion that children will overcome these delays without intervention and learn to adapt due to brain plasticity, there is evidence that gross motor delays can be progressive over

time and that children who participate in vestibular rehabilitation evidence improved postural control,[23,24,25] further compounding the importance of incorporating vestibular rehabilitation into treatment recommendations. Because maintenance of stance is dependent on vestibular, vision, and somatosensation, when children are diagnosed with hearing and/or vestibular loss, an eye exam is also recommended, as children with hearing loss have a greater number of refractive errors compared to children with normal hearing.[26] Additional recommendations include counseling parents on specific activities where having a vestibular loss might affect performance, such as swimming, riding a bike, seeing in the dark, scuba diving, and playing sports.

19.7 Summary

In stepping through each of these questions relative to the current case, this child would be considered to be at risk for having vestibular loss due to both the severity of the hearing loss (profound in the right ear) and the presence of an inner ear abnormality. Because the child was 9 months of age, rotary chair, cervical VEMP, and parent case history were recommended. Rotary chair was consistent with possible vestibular involvement, localizing most likely to the right ear given the presence of hearing loss in the right ear; parent case history was suggestive of normal gross motor skill attainment; and cervical VEMP testing was contraindicated due to the presence of middle ear effusion. With regard to functional consequences of vestibular loss, little is known about the functional consequences of vestibular loss in children with severe vestibular involvement (i.e., bilateral vestibular loss) and even less is known about the functional consequences of less severe vestibular involvement, as noted in the current case with unilateral vestibular loss. Although parent report was not consistent with gross motor delay, an evaluation with vestibular rehabilitation to assess gross motor function and visual acuity would be recommended due to the presence of vestibular loss, regardless of severity. Additionally, an evaluation by ophthalmology was also recommended. In this case, far-sightedness with astigmatism was diagnosed, and prescription lenses were recommended.

References

[1] O'Reilly RC, Morlet T, Nicholas BD, et al. Prevalence of vestibular and balance disorders in children. Otol Neurotol. 2010; 31(9):1441–1444

[2] Brookhouser PE, Cyr DG, Beauchaine KA. Vestibular findings in the deaf and hard of hearing. Otolaryngol Head Neck Surg. 1982; 90(6):773–777

[3] Tribukait A, Brantberg K, Bergenius J. Function of semicircular canals, utricles and saccules in deaf children. Acta Otolaryngol. 2004; 124(1):41–48

[4] Cushing SL, Gordon KA, Rutka JA, James AL, Papsin BC. Vestibular end-organ dysfunction in children with sensorineural hearing loss and cochlear implants: an expanded cohort and etiologic assessment. Otol Neurotol. 2013; 34(3):422–428

[5] Janky KL, Givens D. Vestibular, visual acuity, and balance outcomes in children with cochlear implants: a preliminary report. Ear Hear. 2015; 36(6):e364–e372

[6] Yetiser S, Kertmen M, Ozkaptan Y. Vestibular disturbance in patients with large vestibular aqueduct syndrome (LVAS). Acta Otolaryngol. 1999; 119(6):641–646

[7] Zagólski O. Vestibular-evoked myogenic potentials and caloric stimulation in infants with congenital cytomegalovirus infection. J Laryngol Otol. 2008; 122(6):574–579

[8] Cushing SL, Papsin BC, Rutka JA, James AL, Gordon KA. Evidence of vestibular and balance dysfunction in children with profound sensorineural hearing loss using cochlear implants. Laryngoscope. 2008; 118(10):1814–1823

[9] Inoue A, Iwasaki S, Ushio M, et al. Effect of vestibular dysfunction on the development of gross motor function in children with profound hearing loss. Audiol Neurootol. 2013; 18(3):143–151

[10] Zagólski O. Vestibular-evoked myogenic potentials and caloric tests in infants with congenital rubella. B-ENT. 2009; 5(1):7–12

[11] Black FO, Pesznecker SC, Allen K, Gianna C. A vestibular phenotype for Waardenburg syndrome? Otol Neurotol. 2001; 22(2):188–194

[12] Jackler RK, De La Cruz A. The large vestibular aqueduct syndrome. Laryngoscope. 1989; 99(12):1238–1242, discussion 1242–1243

[13] Shall MS. The importance of saccular function to motor development in children with hearing impairments. Int J Otolaryngol. 2009; 2009(3):972565

[14] Kaga K. Vestibular compensation in infants and children with congenital and acquired vestibular loss in both ears. Int J Pediatr Otorhinolaryngol. 1999; 49(3):215–224

[15] Abadie V, Wiener-Vacher S, Morisseau-Durand MP, et al. Vestibular anomalies in CHARGE syndrome: investigations on and consequences for postural development. Eur J Pediatr. 2000; 159(8):569–574

[16] Rine RM, Braswell J. A clinical test of dynamic visual acuity for children. Int J Pediatr Otorhinolaryngol. 2003; 67(11):1195–1201

[17] Martin W, Jelsma J, Rogers C. Motor proficiency and dynamic visual acuity in children with bilateral sensorineural hearing loss. Int J Pediatr Otorhinolaryngol. 2012; 76(10):1520–1525

[18] Braswell J, Rine RM. Evidence that vestibular hypofunction affects reading acuity in children. Int J Pediatr Otorhinolaryngol. 2006a; 70(11):1957–1965

[19] Rajendran V, Roy FG, Jeevanantham D. Postural control, motor skills, and health-related quality of life in children with hearing impairment: a systematic review. Eur Arch Otorhinolaryngol. 2012; 269(4):1063–1071

[20] Wiener-Vacher SR, Hamilton DA, Wiener SI. Vestibular activity and cognitive development in children: perspectives. Front Integr Nuerosci. 2013; 7:92

[21] Cushing SL, Chia R, James AL, Papsin BC, Gordon KA. A test of static and dynamic balance function in children with cochlear implants: the vestibular olympics. Arch Otolaryngol Head Neck Surg. 2008; 134(1):34–38

[22] Wolter NE, Gordon KA, Papsin BC, Cushing SL. Vestibular and balance impairment contributes to cochlear implant failure in children. Otol Neurotol. 2015; 36(6):1029–1034

[23] Braswell J, Rine RM. Preliminary evidence of improved gaze stability following exercise in two children with vestibular hypofunction. Int J Pediatr Otorhinolaryngol. 2006b; 70(11):1967–1973

[24] Rine RM, Cornwall G, Gan K, et al. Evidence of progressive delay of motor development in children with sensorineural hearing loss and concurrent vestibular dysfunction. Percept Mot Skills. 2000; 90(3, Pt 2):1101–1112

[25] Rine RM, Braswell J, Fisher D, Joyce K, Kalar K, Shaffer M. Improvement of motor development and postural control following intervention in children with sensorineural hearing loss and vestibular impairment. Int J Pediatr Otorhinolaryngol. 2004; 68(9):1141–1148

[26] Sharma A, Ruscetta MN, Chi DH. Ophthalmologic findings in children with sensorineural hearing loss. Arch Otolaryngol Head Neck Surg. 2009; 135(2):119–123

20 Magnetic Bone Conduction Hearing Implant System

Lisa Vaughan Christensen and Lindi Berry

20.1 Clinical History and Description

AW was born with bilateral atresia and microtia at 33 weeks of gestation, weighing 4 lb and 6 ounces. His family history was unremarkable for similar anomalies and no other medical history was significant. This condition was unknown prior to his birth. A newborn hearing screening was bypassed and an unsedated auditory brainstem response (ABR) shortly after birth revealed a moderate conductive hearing loss, for clicks, 500 and 4,000 Hz, in both ears. Masked bone conduction ABR testing for a click yielded a response within normal limits. A bone conduction hearing device was recommended.

At approximately 6 months of age, AW was fit with a traditional bone conduction device. Aided testing for AW utilizing the unilaterally fit bone conduction device revealed thresholds within the slight hearing loss to normal hearing range in Soundfield (▶ Fig. 20.1).

20.2 Audiologic Testing

AW wore the traditional bone conduction device until he was 9 years of age. During those first 9 years of age, the traditional bone conduction device provided good benefit. Aided testing continued to be in the near normal range of hearing. Areas of difficulty, as noted through the Children's Home Inventory for Listening Difficulties (CHILD), were listening in noisy situations and listening at a distance. A discussion regarding the benefits of a bone-anchored device was held during a routine audiological evaluation when AW was 9 years of age. AW had some speech and language delays as a younger child, but at the time of implantation, speech and language skills were noted as age appropriate.

At the age of 9 years, AW was implanted, bilaterally, with the Baha Attract implantable, transcutaneous bone conduction system utilizing Baha 4 processors. Three months after implantation, AW had improvements in low-frequency aided thresholds as compared to the traditional bone conduction device, but the Baha Attract system showed decreased results for the higher frequencies. Aided speech recognition testing conducted at 50 dB HL utilizing live monitored voice was excellent (▶ Fig. 20.2). At AW's 6-month follow-up, his aided thresholds were improved, with the exception of 4,000 Hz (▶ Fig. 20.3). Initial magnet strength at the 3-month follow-up was 2, and two pads were used for comfort. At the 6-month follow-up, magnet strength remained at 2, but one of the two pads was able to be removed. Magnet selection for the Attract should provide retention but still ensure comfort to the patient during wear time. Magnets have strength ratings from 1 to 5. A magnet strength of 1 represents the weakest magnet, while a strength of 5 represents the strongest magnet strength. If the magnet is too weak, the sound processor may have a tendency to fall off and if it is too strong, the patient may feel discomfort or experience skin soreness and irritation. To help ensure this delicate balance, soft stickable pads are available to stick to the magnets. These help the audiologist use a stronger magnet and ensure comfort.

20.3 Questions for the Reader

1. For what kind of hearing losses would you consider a Baha Attract over a traditional hearing aid?
2. What makes the Baha Attract system more "attractive" to families and patients?
3. Are there additional surgical considerations for the Baha Attract?

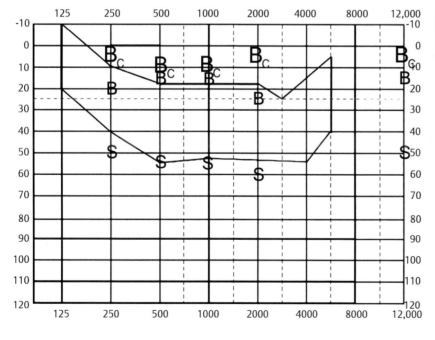

Fig. 20.1 Test results at 6 months of age. B, hearing aids with bone conduction device BC, binaural cochlear implant; S, soundfield air conduction.

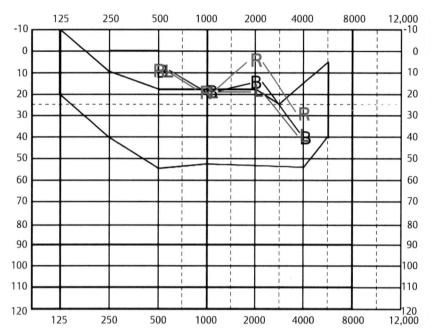

Fig. 20.2 Aided testing 3 months after Baha Attract implantation, at the age of 9 years. B, hearing aids with bone conduction device; L, left ear hearing aid; R, right ear hearing aid.

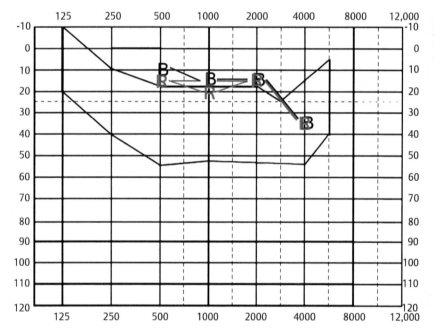

Fig. 20.3 Aided testing 6 months after Baha Attract implantation. B, hearing aids with bone conduction device; L, left ear hearing aid; R, right ear hearing aid.

4. Does the Baha Attract system help reduce the infection rates often seen with the Baha Connect system?

5. Because of the limitations of skin/hair, would a Baha Connect be better for patients?

6. What acoustic issues could you expect with an Attract fitting versus a Connect fitting, and how could you adjust for this in fitting and programming?

7. What extra precautions could you recommend and consider for an active pediatric patient using an Attract system?

8. With slightly poorer aided results at 4,000 Hz, what would be the impact on the child's speech and language development? How can this be addressed audiologically?

20.4 Discussion of Questions

1. **For what kind of hearing losses would you consider a Baha Attract over a traditional hearing aid?**
The Baha Attract should be considered an option in the same typical ways the Baha Connect is selected for any patient with conductive hearing loss. Cases of permanent unilateral or bilateral conductive hearing loss, especially those with abnormal outer ear anatomy and chronic infections of the middle or outer ear, can be considered good options for the Baha Attract. Cases of mixed unilateral or bilateral hearing loss with bone conduction thresholds of 40 dB HL or better should be considered as options for the Baha Attract but need to utilize a power processor.

2. **What makes the Baha Attract system more "attractive" to families and patients?**

Many times families and patients reject the idea of an external abutment of percutaneous, implantable bone conduction systems, such as the Connect system. This percutaneous coupling of the sound processor lends itself to risk of infection.[1] The Attract system utilizes a magnet coupling without a percutaneous abutment. This coupling is often more appealing to patients and families.

3. **Are there additional surgical considerations for the Baha Attract?**

The surgical time associated with implantation of the Attract has not differed greatly from the time required to implant the Baha Connect at our facility. Some considerations for the surgeon are the possibility of removing fatty tissue from the area near the magnet coupling, and because of the bone conduction component with both Baha systems, having a lesser amount of fatty tissue around the site helps with the utilization of bone conduction. The audiologists should also have an array of magnet strengths to trial, especially during the first few months after implantation, to help with the issues of fatty tissue and hair around the magnet site.

4. **Does the Baha Attract system help reduce the infection rates often seen with the Baha Connect system?**

A relatively high rate of skin infections was associated with the Baha Connect percutaneous system.[1] Preliminary data from the Cook Children's Medical Center has shown no infections outside of the initial surgical follow-up. We are hopeful that the lack of a percutaneous coupling will lead to no external infection rates.

5. **Because of the limitations of skin/hair, would a Baha Connect be a better option for patients?**

Preliminary raw data obtained from Baha Attract recipients at the Cook Children's Medical Center and the Texas Ear Clinic in Fort Worth, Texas, suggest similar results to Softband data with slight differences in aided thresholds at 4,000 Hz among patients. It is important to test aided thresholds and speech recognition at each appointment and to make corrections to get the best auditory information for each individual child.[2] Changing magnet strengths, increasing gain for high frequencies when necessary, and testing often after the initial fitting will all increase appropriate fittings and success with the Baha Attract. Also, to note is a lesser rate of infection when using the Attract over the Connect.

6. **What acoustic effects could you expect with an Attract fitting versus a Connect and how could you adjust for this in fitting and programming?**

Relative to a percutaneous implantable system, high-frequency attenuation is probable with use of a transcutaneous implantable device. It is helpful to measure with direct bone conduction within the Cochlear Baha programming software, which will potentially account for the high-frequency attenuation associated with transcutaneous bone conduction stimulation and provide an increase in high-frequency gain to increase access to high-frequency inputs. This can be done utilizing a laptop programming setup inside your booth to utilize visual reinforcement audiometry (VRA) methods with smaller children utilizing Softbands or with children with developmental delays. Also, because direct bone conduction is an in situ audiogram, Conditioned Play Audiometry (CPA) can be utilized to elicit these responses. It is also important to remember that high-frequency gain can be increased during the fitting when aided thresholds are not optimal.

7. **What extra precautions could you recommend and consider for an active pediatric patient using an Attract system?**

Working with pediatric patients can be challenging, especially busy toddlers and active children. As with any amplification device, pediatric audiologists must often come up with a plan of action to keep their patients wearing their devices during all waking hours. The Baha Attract system is no different in this aspect. The use of a retention line, provided by Cochlear in the care kit, is the best way to keep the device from being lost during busy play times or sports activities. Audiologists should keep in mind that a strong magnet could also help with retention of the device.

8. **With slightly poorer aided results at 4,000 Hz, what would be the impact on the child's speech and language development? How can this be addressed audiologically?**

Aided Soundfield thresholds are used in verification of the audibility of the speech spectrum when working with Osseo devices. Per the AAA Pediatric Amplification Guidelines, children who use hearing devices require more high-frequency audibility. This need for more high-frequency audibility occurs as children typically spend a majority of their time listening to other children and women. Both of these speech sources are typically greater in high-frequency content. These children who do not have full access to high-frequency sounds also miss subtle differences in language like plurals. Therefore, it is best to give a child with hearing loss the most high-frequency access possible. If, when using the Baha Attract, high frequencies are not optimal, it is critical that the audiologist make programming changes to increase high-frequency gain. It is also important to assess magnet strength, contact to the skin by the processor, and limit use of magnet pads to determine the maximum high-frequency audibility.

20.5 Outcome

- AW is described as an active boy, and his teachers report he has trouble sitting still during the day.
- After his implantation, his teachers reported that he is less "antsy" at school and more focused during the school day. He is currently using a frequency modulation (FM) system. No other outcome measures were used by the school.
- Aided testing continues to improve with routine testing and adjustments by his audiologist.

References

[1] Lee CE, Christensen L, Richter GT, Dornhoffer JL. Arkansas BAHA experience: transcalvarial fixture placement using osseointegration surgical hardware. Otol Neurotol. 2011; 32(3):444–447

Suggested Readings

[1] American Academy of Audiology. 2013 Pediatric Amplification Protocol. Available at: http://www.audiology.org. Accessed August 2016.

[2] Nicholson N, Christensen L, Dornhoffer J, Martin P, Smith-Olinde L. Verification of speech spectrum audibility for pediatric Baha Softband users with craniofacial anomalies. Cleft Palate Craniofac J. 2011; 48(1):56–65

[3] Christensen L, Smith-Olinde L, Kimberlain J, Richter GT, Dornhoffer JL. Comparison of traditional bone-conduction hearing AIDS with the Baha system. J Am Acad Audiol. 2010; 21(4):267–273

21 Startle Epilepsy and Tinnitus Masking

Lisa Vaughan Christensen

21.1 Clinical History and Description

LR is a 9-year-old girl with a history of epilepsy. Specifically, LR has a type of seizure that is evoked by loud or startling sounds. These seizures are known as startle-provoked epileptic seizures (SPES). Although she exhibited normal development prior to age 3, LR's mother reports a multiple-hour seizure at age 3, and LR now has global developmental delays and is nonverbal. She can follow some simple commands from her mother (finds some body parts); answers some yes/no questions with head shakes or nods; and loves to dance though her mobility is slightly impaired and restricted because of seizure activity.

For most patients, the occurrence of epileptic seizures is unforeseeable and, most of the time, sporadic. Manford et al[1] estimated that, in about 5% of patients, there are specific triggers for epilepsy. The most common being photosensitivity. With SPES, the trigger/stimuli can be sensory stimuli of various modalities, but most commonly this stimulus is noise. Manford et al also reported that same "noise" stimuli, if the patient is forewarned, will have no effect. Cases of SPES are considered rare.

Klinkenberg et al[2] reported that most children with SPES are known to have a congenital brain condition or an acquired brain injury early in life. Unexpected sounds are the most common trigger for these children. Somatosensory and visual stimuli have also been reported with these patients. Klinkenberg et al also noted that background sounds have been known to reduce the responses. They published their experiences of four children fit with tinnitus maskers to provide a consistent background sound. The children were aged 8 to 4 years old. They were all male and all suffered from epilepsy precipitated by sudden sounds. Two patients were noted to have triggers to visual stimuli as well as auditory stimuli. All four patients had multiple seizures each day. Some common triggers were a pencil falling in the classroom and a school bell ringing. All of the patients were fit with the Beltone TBR 62D utilizing a nonoccluding open fit style. A reduction in seizure frequency of 50% or more was reported in two of the four children. It is noted that one patient repeatedly removed the devices, and wear time was poor. It is also noted that the children with positive responses were able to be counseled and understood the treatment. The continuous sound masked sudden onset of sounds; however, it was also noted that the patient felt that the sound was a reassuring effect that helps with fear as well.

During her first audiology visit, LR's parents reported approximately 10 to 15 seizures each day. When questioned about typical sound triggers to her seizures, her parents reported loud sudden sounds and also sneezing, coughing, or dogs barking. They also noted specific places where her seizures were always minimal. One particular place was the mall, where her mother noted "there is always a loud roar of background noise." The other place noted was LR's room at home which always has a "white noise machine" on when she is in that room. Her parents also reported numerous emergency room visits yearly due to falls and other injuries related to these "drop" seizures. LR has the ability to walk but is not typically allowed to walk unaccompanied due to the risk of a seizure. She was not currently in a typical school placement due to unpredictable seizure activity in the noisy environment of her typical school day. LR does receive home-based school services from her local school district. The family's main concern was not having the ability to leave home and take LR places where they could not keep her safe.

21.2 Audiologic Testing

Owing to LR's specific noise-induced seizures, the family had no concerns about hearing. However, hearing was tested during her first audiological appointment. Because of her developmental delays, LR was evaluated utilizing visual reinforcement audiometry (VRA) with insert earphones. The evaluation was conducted using an ascending method to not startle LR in the quiet booth and, therefore, elicit a seizure during the evaluation. LR's hearing was normal in both ears (▸ Fig. 21.1).

21.3 Questions for the Reader

1. How do hearing aids for normal hearing get funded?
2. Is there a better option than hearing aids for this particular case?
3. How do you determine the "appropriate" level of masking?
4. Will the current hearing aid settings remain appropriate forever?
5. Should any additional therapies be considered for LR?

21.4 Discussion of Questions

1. **Is there a better option than hearing aids for this particular case?**
   For this particular child, audiology and neurology were both in agreement on the course of treatment. Because noise generators worked at home to reduce seizures, ear level tinnitus maskers seemed to make the most sense. Open fit hearing aids with a tinnitus feature allow tinnitus masking, and they do not occlude LR's ears so that she can still hear all sound surrounding her. Having a wearable device allows the family to go anywhere they desire with the comfort of their home set up with noise generators.

2. **How do hearing aids for normal hearing children get funded?**
   Funding for LR was expected to be difficult due to her normal hearing and the rarity of her condition. When the authorization was sent to her insurance company, the Klinkenberg article, a letter from the audiologist explaining the situation, and a letter from the neurologist were all included with the typical authorization paperwork. Luckily, LR's hearing aids were approved by her insurance company on the first request for reimbursement.

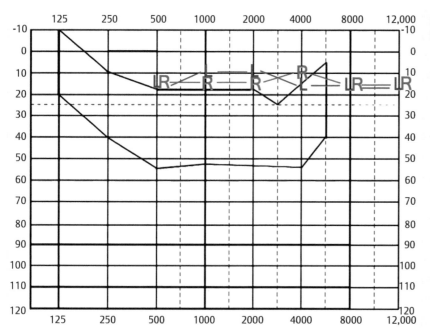

Fig. 21.1 Test results at the age of 9. L, left ear hearing aid; R, right ear hearing aid.

3. **How do you determine the "appropriate" level of masking?**

The type of masking was discussed with the family and white noise was chosen because they felt it would sound familiar to LR. The noise generator in her room at home was also white noise. The levels were set conservatively in the beginning starting at the default settings. After approximately 1 month of wear, the family reported some instances they felt were not appropriately masked. At that time, they requested the masking levels be increased slightly. Speech recognition testing while wearing the devices revealed that LR could still follow simple commands presented via monitored live voice at a soft input level of 35 dB hearing loss (HL).

4. **Will the current hearing aid settings remain appropriate forever?**

The levels of the tinnitus masking have been increased one time after a month of wear. After an additional 6 months of wear, no more settings have been changed. Because these particular hearing aids have several sound options, the type of sound can be changed should LR become acclimated to a particular sound.

5. **Should any additional therapies be considered for LR?**

After noting the ability to follow some commands and her ability to point to some body parts, it was recommended that LR see a speech pathologist that specializes in augmentative communication devices. LR completed an evaluation for a device, and it was determined she could utilize this technology to help her communication. She also received an occupational therapy evaluation.

21.5 Outcomes

- LR was fit with an Oticon Ria2Ti 2 months after her audiological evaluation. Hearing aid microphones are turned off,

and only the tinnitus masking feature is utilized. Initial settings for masking levels were set conservatively, and numerous follow-up appointments have been used to determine an appropriate loudness for the masking. To determine appropriate loudness levels for the masking, LR was asked to point to body parts and do other simple commands in a quiet room by her mother using a regular conversational level voice. This task was also completed in the sound booth at 50 and 35 dB HL to determine if LR could complete the task with greater than 80% accuracy before leaving the masking levels set.

- At the initial fitting, LR did amazingly well and did not pull off the hearing aids. LR's father sneezed during the same appointment, and per family report that this would have usually caused a seizure. LR did not have a seizure that day while newly wearing the aids.

- After the fitting appointment, the family went to lunch at a restaurant with an open kitchen. This specific restaurant previously caused lots of seizure activity with the loudness of the kitchen. LR did not have a seizure during the visit to the restaurant wearing her aids.

- LR was evaluated for an augmentative communication device shortly after her seizures were more controlled.

- Since the fitting, parents have noticed a great reduction in seizure activity on a daily basis and are happy with the results.

References

[1] Manford MR, Fish DR, Shorvon SD. Startle provoked epileptic seizures: features in 19 patients. J Neurol Neurosurg Psychiatry. 1996; 61(2):151–156

[2] Klinkenberg S, Ubbink S, Vles J, et al. Noninvasive treatment alternative for intractable startle epilepsy. Epilepsy Behav Case Rep. 2014; 2:49–53

22 Hyperbilirubinemia

Karen Muñoz and Elizabeth Preston

22.1 Clinical History and Description

Mason was born at 32 weeks' gestational age and spent 6 weeks in the neonatal intensive care unit (NICU) because of hyperbilirubinemia,[1,2] an identified risk factor for hearing loss,[3] and anemia. He required a blood transfusion and was receiving antibiotics. When he was 5 weeks of age, he received a two-stage newborn hearing screening. He passed a screening using transient-evoked otoacoustic emissions (TEOAEs), but he had no response on an Automated Auditory Brainstem Response (A-ABR) screening, for either ear. A diagnostic ABR was performed the same day. The report indicated thresholds obtained for a click stimulus were 70 dB nHL, and for tone burst stimuli, estimated thresholds were 55 dB eHL at 500 Hz and 65 dB eHL at 4,000 Hz, for both ears. The waves I–V interpeak latencies were within norms for his age (5.12 ms right; 5.06 ms left), and the cochlear microphonic was present with wave V remaining intact with the change in polarity. Based on these results, Mason was diagnosed with a bilateral moderate to moderately severe loss of hearing, with the report indicating that "the presence of the TEOAEs and elevated ABR thresholds suggested inner hair cell loss." It was recommended he be reevaluated in 2 to 4 weeks.

22.2 Audiologic Testing

Mason was 2 months of age at the time of his first visit to the pediatric audiology clinic, when he came for a diagnostic reevaluation.[4] His tympanometry results were consistent with normal tympanic membrane mobility, for each ear, when assessed using a 1,000-Hz probe tone. His ipsilateral acoustic reflexes were absent bilaterally with the exception of a response at 105 dB at 2,000 Hz in the left ear. Distortion product otoacoustic emissions (DPOAEs), assessed with a 12-frequency protocol (65/55), were present at all 12 frequencies evaluated in the right ear, and at 11 of the 12 frequencies evaluated in the left ear. The click ABR (▶ Fig. 22.1) was initially done at 80 dB nHL using a 33.3 click rate. Results showed a large cochlear microphonic; however, wave I was difficult to interpret when looking at rarefaction and condensation together because the waveform morphology was poor. Testing was then done using an alternating click at a slow click rate (13.3), and resulted in the ability to identify waves I, III, and V. The absolute wave and interwave latencies were within normal limits. Toneburst results revealed estimated thresholds at 20 dB eHL at 500 Hz in both ears, 40 dB eHL at 4,000 Hz in the right ear, and 60 dB eHL at 4,000 Hz in the left ear. Based on his test results (i.e., present OAEs; some improvement in hearing thresholds; slightly larger cochlear microphonic than typical), the recommendation was to continue monitoring his hearing before making any decisions related to use of hearing aids. Early intervention (EI) was discussed with the parents, and a referral was made to the local EI program.

22.3 Questions for the Reader

1. Why would slowing down the click rate improve responses?
2. When a hearing loss is identified, what recommendations/referrals are appropriate?

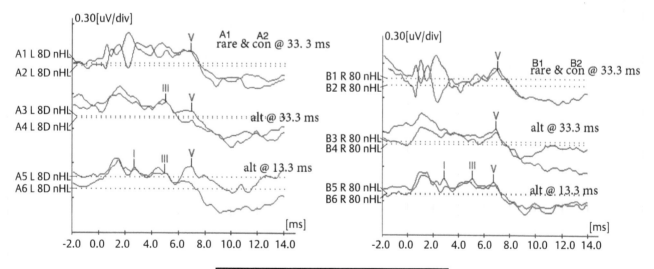

Latencies (ms)					
Label Index	I	II	III	IV	V
A1					6.91
A3			5.03		6.97
A5	2.66		4.07		6.97
B1					7.03
B3					6.01
B5	2.85		5.03		6.74

Fig. 22.1 Click ABR tracings at 8 weeks of age.

3. Why do you think hearing aids were not recommended at this time?
4. What audiological testing is appropriate at this point?

22.4 Discussion of Questions

1. **Why would slowing down the click rate improve responses?**

Many clinics use a click rate between 27.7 and 33.3 per second or even faster in order to be more efficient in the collection process[5]; however, for babies born prematurely, this fast rate can tax the system and result in poor waveform morphology and amplitude. This problem occurs because their auditory pathway is less mature and has less myelination than babies born full-term. The latencies and amplitudes with the click ABR do not become adultlike until around the age of 3 years.[6] Slowing the click rate can help improve morphology, amplitude, and latency of the waveforms, which makes it easier to interpret accurately.

2. **When a hearing loss is identified, what recommendations/referrals are appropriate?**

Federal law states that a child diagnosed with a hearing loss must be referred for EI within 7 days of the diagnosis.[7] This law is part of the U.S. Department of Education's Individuals with Disabilities Education Act (IDEA) Part C, which "requires states to provide children with disabilities with free and appropriate education in the least restrictive environment."[8] Once the referral is received, the agency providing EI must complete a full assessment and hold an Individualized Family Service Plan (IFSP) within 45 days.

Medical referrals are critical for determining the cause of hearing loss, to determine if there are other comorbid conditions, and to obtain medical clearance for amplification, if applicable.[3,9] Referrals to the primary care physician and an otolaryngologist are essential for a full medical evaluation (thorough case history, evaluation of head and neck, scans of ears to look for structural abnormalities, and possibly other blood work). Referrals to an ophthalmologist for an assessment of vision and to a geneticist are recommended. If needed, further medical referrals may be made, usually by the child's medical home, to a developmental pediatrician, cardiologist, nephrologist, and neurologist.

Follow-up audiological testing is also necessary to monitor hearing stability and, if needed, to obtain additional diagnostic detail. When ABR testing is conducted with infants, it is done during natural sleep. The baby may wake up, necessitating additional testing to obtain further frequency-specific results or to complete bone conduction testing. If tympanometry, reflexes, OAEs, click, and toneburst ABR were completed,[4] then repeating the testing in 1 to 2 months is appropriate.

When a hearing loss is identified, parents need access to accurate information on many topics (e.g., communication options, hearing technology). They will need support, not only for learning new information and skills, but also emotional support.[10] An important avenue of support is access to other parents of children who are deaf or hard of hearing.[11] Connecting parents to parent support organizations (e.g., Hands and Voices [http://www.handsandvoices.org/]; AG Bell Association for the Deaf and Hard of Hearing [AGBell.org]) or other parent groups in the local area helps parents know that they are not alone and can provide hope and encouragement.

3. **Why do you think hearing aids were not recommended at this time?**

Hearing aids were not recommended because of the improvement in hearing that was observed when the outpatient diagnostic test was completed, in conjunction with the presence of OAEs and the larger than typical cochlear microphonic. Collectively, this information suggested the possibility that hearing may continue to improve and that further monitoring was needed before decisions related to hearing technology could be considered.

4. **What audiological testing is appropriate at this point?**

One month later, Mason received a full diagnostic evaluation that included tympanometry, acoustic reflexes, OAEs, and an ABR to continue to monitor his hearing.[12] It is important to monitor Mason in a timely manner to determine needed interventions. If his hearing improves to within normal limits, additional audiological monitoring is important to determine the stability of his hearing and to rule out any fluctuations in hearing. Once a fluctuating hearing loss can be ruled out, another follow-up by 24 months would be appropriate because of Mason's risk factors at birth.[4]

22.5 Audiologic Monitoring

Mason returned for a reevaluation at 3 months of age. Toneburst testing was done using a slow rate (13.3), and results revealed thresholds within the range of normal at 500, 2,000, and 4000 Hz in the right ear, and at 500 and 4,000 Hz in the left ear (2,000 Hz was not assessed). Tympanometry, assessed using a 1,000-Hz probe tone, was consistent with normal middle ear function for each ear. Based on the continued improvement in hearing thresholds, continued monitoring was recommended. It was recommended he return in 2 months, so a sleep-deprived ABR could be attempted to confirm the stability of his hearing.

Mason was scheduled for a sleep-deprived ABR at 5 months of age; however, he would not sleep, and the test could not be completed. Other test results revealed continued presence of OAEs, assessed using a 12-frequency DPOAE protocol, in each ear. Tympanometry, assessed using a 1,000-Hz probe tone, was consistent with normal middle ear function for each ear. His ipsilateral acoustic reflexes were now present but elevated in each ear. At 6 months of age, another sleep-deprived ABR was attempted; however, Mason would not sleep. He also would not condition to visual reinforcement audiometry (VRA). Therefore, behavioral testing was recommended in 1 month, and if at that time Mason's hearing could not be reliably assessed, a sedated ABR would be considered.

At 9 months of age, Mason returned for a reevaluation. His mother expressed no concerns regarding his hearing and felt he was responding well to his parents' voices as well as to environmental sounds. Behavioral testing (VRA) was completed in the sound field (▶ Fig. 22.2). Results were within normal limits in the better ear at 250, 2,000, and 4,000 Hz, and a speech detection

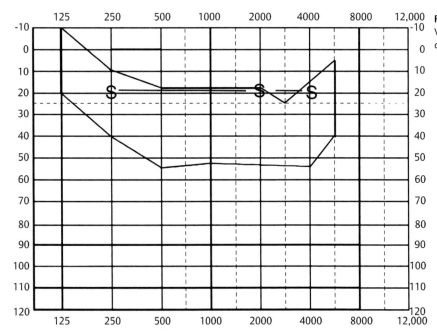

Fig. 22.2 Behavioral thresholds obtained using VRA at 9 months of age. S, soundfield air conduction.

threshold was observed at 15 dB HL. Tympanometry, using a 226-Hz probe tone, revealed a slightly restricted tympanic mobility (Type A$_s$) in the right ear and normal mobility (Type A) in the left ear. Ipsilateral acoustic reflexes were present within normal limits in both ears for 500, 1,000, 2,000 Hz, and when using a broadband noise, with the exception of no response for 500 Hz at 100 dB in the right ear. DPOAEs were present in the high frequencies and absent in the midfrequencies in the right ear and were present in the left ear. It was recommended he return in 3 months to continue to monitor his hearing. If at that time his hearing is still normal, then a 6-month follow-up would be recommended. The reason for the continued follow-up is because of the presence of risk factors, which can cause a progressive hearing loss. Those risk factors are (1) premature birth, (2) greater than 5 days in NICU, and (3) blood transfusion. Additionally, given the abnormal results obtained with initial ABR assessments, continued monitoring will allow the clinician to probe for delays in audition, speech, and language related to the early delays in auditory maturation.

References

[1] Abdollahi FZ, Ahmadi T, Manchaiah V, Lotfi Y. Auditory brainstem response improvements in hyperbillirubinemic infants. J Audiol Otol. 2016; 20(1):13–16

[2] Khalid S, Qadir M, Salat MS. Spontaneous improvement in sensorineural hearing loss developed as a complication of neonatal hyperbilirubinemia. J Pak Med Assoc. 2015; 65(9):1018–1021

[3] American Academy of Pediatrics, Joint Committee on Infant Hearing. Year 2007 position statement: Principles and guidelines for early hearing detection and intervention programs. Pediatrics. 2007; 120(4):898–921

[4] American Speech-Language-Hearing Association. Permanent childhood hearing loss: assessment.. Available at: www.asha.org/Practice-Portal/Clinical-Topics/Permanent-Childhood-Hearing-Loss. Accessed July 12, 2016

[5] Picton T. Auditory brainstem responses: peaks along the way. In: Human Auditory Evoked Potentials. San Diego, CA: Plural Publishing; 2010:213–245

[6] Atcherson SR, Stoody TM. The auditory brainstem response. In: Auditory Electrophysiology: A Clinical Guide. New York, NY: Thieme Medical Publishers, Inc; 2012:68–83

[7] Office of Special Education and Rehabilitative Services, Department of Education. Early intervention program for infants and toddlers with disabilities. Federal Register: vol. 76; 188. Available at: https://www.federalregister.gov/documents/2011/09/28/2011–22783/early-intervention-program-for-infants-and-toddlers-with-disabilities. Effective September 2011. Accessed July 2016

[8] White KR. Early intervention for children with permanent hearing loss: finishing the ehdi revolution. Volta Rev. 2006; 106(3):237–258

[9] American Academy of Pediatrics. Early Hearing Detection and Intervention (EHDI) guidelines for pediatric medical home providers. Available at: https://www.aap.org/en-us/advocacy-and-policy/aap-health-initiatives/PEHDIC/Documents/Algorithm1_2010.pdf. Published February 2010. Accessed July 22, 2016

[10] American Speech-Language-Hearing Association. Guidelines for audiologists providing informational and adjustment counseling to families of infants and young children with hearing loss birth to 5 years of age. Available at: www.asha.org/policy. Published 2008. Accessed July 12, 2016

[11] Henderson RJ, Johnson AM, Moodie ST. Revised conceptual framework of parent-to-parent support for parents of children who are deaf or hard of hearing: A modified Delphi study. Am J Audiol. 2016; 25(2):110–126

[12] Gravel JS. Audiologic assessment for the fitting of hearing instruments: big challenges from tiny ears. In: Seewald RC, ed. A Sound Foundation through Early Amplification: Proceedings of an International Conference. Stäfa, Switzerland; 2000:33–46

23 CHARGE Syndrome

Karen Muñoz and Cache Pitt

23.1 Clinical History and Description

The patient, Grace, received audiology services at a pediatric audiology clinic in the United States, after moving from another country. She was diagnosed with CHARGE syndrome (coloboma of the eye, heart defects, atresia of the choanae, retardation of growth and development, and ear abnormalities) shortly after her birth. Decisions about hearing technology to provide her with optimal auditory brain access were addressed by a multidisciplinary team.

Grace was born full-term. There was no family history of hearing loss, and her mother experienced no complications during pregnancy.[1] During the delivery, however, the umbilical cord was around her neck, and she subsequently spent 9 days in the neonatal intensive care unit. She failed her newborn hearing screening, and a follow-up auditory brainstem response test at 3 weeks of age revealed a severe-to-profound hearing loss in her right ear and a profound hearing loss in her left ear. Grace received binaural hearing aids at 8 weeks of age. Her parents chose to communicate with Grace using listening and spoken language, and Grace was enrolled in a specialized auditory/oral early intervention program.[2]

23.2 Audiologic Testing and Radiologic Imaging

Grace was 19 months of age when her family began receiving services for her hearing in the United States. At this time, she demonstrated some awareness to sound while wearing her hearing aids. Unaided visual reinforcement audiometry results indicated a severe to profound hearing loss in the right ear, and a profound hearing loss in the left ear, and her aided thresholds ranged from 45 to 60 dB HL (▶ Fig. 23.1). Her parents decided to explore cochlear implantation. At the medical evaluation, scans of the cochleae indicated they were malformed (1½ turns). In addition, Grace had narrow internal auditory canals, poorly developed semicircular canals, and small vestibules. Additionally, no auditory nerve could be visualized on the left side, and the presence of an auditory nerve on her right side was questionable (▶ Fig. 23.2).

Ongoing audiologic monitoring demonstrated that Grace was consistent in her responses to sound. Grace also continued to demonstrate awareness to sound at home when wearing her aids, and she was responding to intervention. By 24 months of age, she began making vocal attempts, and language scores based on the HELP (Hawaii Early Learning Profile) placed her in the 12- to 18-month age range. Although she was making progress, it was determined that her rate of progress was inadequate for developing typical language, and a cochlear implant was considered. Potential benefit from cochlear implantation was in question because the results from the radiologic scans were contradictory to the audiologic test results and observed aided benefit. As a result, Grace's parents decided to obtain an electrical auditory brainstem response (eABR) test in hopes of better understanding how her cochlear nerves may respond to electrical stimulation.[3] In both ears, a wave V response was initially identified but it attenuated to the point of almost complete absence as testing continued on subsequent runs, with the right ear having a slightly stronger response than the left. The eABR test results were, therefore, similar to radiologic findings and indicated that cochlear nerves were present bilaterally, but hypoplastic, or underde-

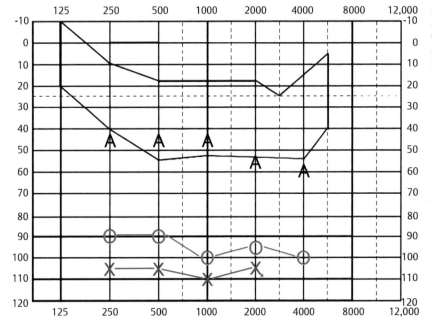

Fig. 23.1 Visual reinforcement audiometry air conduction thresholds, and binaural aided thresholds, at 19 months of age. O, right ear air conduction; X, left ear air conduction; A, binaural hearing aids behind the ear; Arrows, no response.

veloped, suggesting that the auditory nerve development may be insufficient to support cochlear implantation. Based on the findings of the eABR results, it was assumed that continuous electrical stimulation from the cochlear implant would result in rapid adaptation to signals, much like was discovered during the eABR testing, suggesting that if implanted, programming needs may change frequently requiring frequent mapping appointments. Based on the eABR results, Grace's parents were told that the right ear was a marginal candidate for cochlear implantation, and the left ear was not a candidate. They decided not to pursue a cochlear implant for Grace and to continue with hearing aid use and listening and

spoken language intervention. Her language development was progressing; however, it was delayed compared to typically hearing children (Preschool Language Scale Age Equivalent score of 21 months, at 32 months of age).

At 3 years of age, Grace experienced a sudden and complete loss of hearing (▶ Fig. 23.3). Following an immediate medical referral, Grace began treatment with steroids; however, even though it did result in some improvement of hearing, it was not to her previous degree of loss. Grace no longer received benefit from her hearing aids. Grace repeatedly told her parents that the hearing aids were broken, suggesting that the sudden loss of hearing was traumatic. The family was faced with the decision to either try cochlear implantation despite the possibility that benefit may be limited because of her hypolastic cochlear nerves or learn American Sign Language and use a manual mode of communication with Grace.

23.3 Questions for the Reader

1. Would you recommend a cochlear implant for Grace?
2. What medical complications are a concern for considering a cochlear implant for Grace?
3. What follow-up decisions would you anticipate needing to have in place if Grace were to receive a cochlear implant?

23.4 Discussion of Questions

1. **Would you recommend a cochlear implant for Grace?**
   Yes, a cochlear implant was recommended for her right ear for several reasons. Grace's sudden decrease in hearing resulted in a complete loss of speech audibility and ability to communicate using spoken language. By the age of 3, her parents had already committed to an oral mode of communication. Grace was also influential in the decision process because she continually demonstrated a desire to hear by requesting hearing aids prior to the sudden loss and her

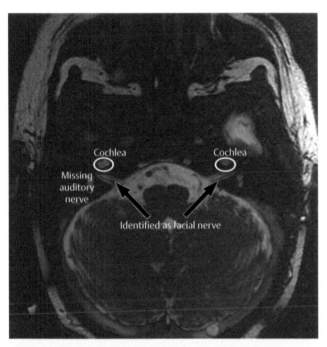

Fig. 23.2 Radiologic imaging of the auditory and facial nerves.

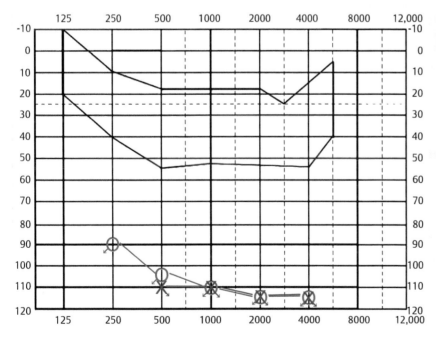

Fig. 23.3 Hearing evaluation results for air conduction testing at 3 years of age. O, right ear air conduction; X, left ear air conduction; Arrows, no response.

persistent report that her hearing aids were broken after the sudden hearing loss. As very well-informed parents, they understood the risks that had been presented to them, including the concern of facial nerve trauma during surgery, potential persistent programming changes due to neural fatigue, and potential limited benefit from a cochlear implant given the status of her poorly developed auditory nerves. Because of the commitment and efforts already devoted to spoken language, the family felt that cochlear implantation was worth the risks. Several factors influenced the recommendation and included her sudden decrease in hearing, her prior ability to respond to speech and sound, her development of spoken language, her own desire to hear, and the family's commitment to maximize her spoken language development that resulted in a recommendation to pursue cochlear implantation. Even if the family decided to move Grace to a sign language program in the future, the ability to use hearing, even at reduced levels, would improve awareness of sound and potentially improve communication.

2. **What medical complications are a concern for considering a cochlear implant for Grace?**

The peer-reviewed literature indicates varying outcomes for children with auditory nerve deficiency and cochlear implantation, ranging from an absence of sound awareness to an ability to discriminate speech, although with less benefit when compared to implanted peers with typical auditory nerves.[4,5,6] Specifically for Grace, eABR testing identified wave V's for each ear that diminished significantly with repeated stimulation, presenting significant concern that the electrical stimulation from the cochlear implant may result in similar behavior of continuous adaptation to the electrical signal. The reports of Grace's eABR testing suggest that if she were to receive a cochlear implant, then she may need to have more frequent follow-up programming to accommodate the rapid changes of the auditory nerve in response to the electric signal from the cochlear implant. Of potential more concern than more frequent mapping, the rapid changes to an electrical stimulus may provide inconsistent access to sound, decreasing the benefit for spoken language development. Facial nerve trauma is a risk of any cochlear implant surgery because of its proximity to the surgical site. While facial nerve monitoring is routine in any cochlear implant surgery, it is imperative that extra precautions take place in cases of CHARGE syndrome because of the unpredictable location of the facial nerve. With careful facial nerve monitoring during the surgery, the otologist is typically able to avoid facial nerve injury. The medical risks that the implant team and the parents must consider are potential limited benefit from a cochlear implant due to the lack of development of the auditory nerve as well as an increased risk of potential harm to the facial nerve.

3. **What follow-up decisions would you anticipate needing to have in place if Grace were to receive a cochlear implant?**

In order to be considered a candidate for a cochlear implant, expectations, although unclear, must be appropriate. Listening and language intervention and treatment need to be accessible, and both the programming center and the parents need to be prepared for routine as well as unanticipated programming. School and/or therapists need to be prepared for a variety of potential outcomes with the expectation to maximize intervention. Parents need to be prepared to accept any outcome, ranging from no benefit from a cochlear implant to some auditory brain access, but parents of children with exceptional needs (e.g., CHARGE syndrome) need to be better prepared than most for a need to be patient and persistent. Counseling should include the potential need to endure through a variety of unknowns including medical complications, a lack of response to sound, and consistent therapy.

23.5 Recommended Treatment

Surgical implantation of a Nucleus Freedom cochlear implant resulted in a complete insertion without any negative medical consequences to the facial nerve. Prior to cochlear implantation, Grace was an excellent participant in conditioned play audiometry. Initial mapping was done over two appointments. Approximately 4 weeks after surgery at the time of the activation, Grace did not respond to any electrical stimulus during T level measurement, despite changing parameters. She also did not respond to stimulation in live mode, despite changing parameters. Neural response telemetry (NRT) is an evoked potential from the cochlear nerve (i.e., the electrically evoked compound action potential). There was no NRT response obtained on the first day of activation. With no responses of any kind, a flat map using ACE 900 Hz, 25 µs pulse width was used to try to stimulate her auditory system. At the second day of activation, there continued to be no response to stimuli for measuring T levels, but NRT thresholds were obtained. NRT thresholds were used to estimate her T levels and to create an objectively fit map, but Grace persisted in her inability to perceive any sound. After her day 2 activation appointment, Grace's family then went on vacation for 1 month. They left assuming that Grace would not receive benefit from her cochlear implant, but they were committed to having her wear the implant.

During the family vacation, after continuing to wear her processor for 2 weeks, Grace suddenly demonstrated awareness to sound by answering the telephone when it rang. She continued to demonstrate some awareness to sound, and 4 weeks after her activation she suddenly started repeating the Ling Six sounds. Upon returning home from vacation, Grace participated in her programming to measure T levels, and one threshold was obtained. Two weeks later, Grace was able to complete T level measurement for every other electrode.

For the next several months, Grace's electrical thresholds changed repeatedly, requiring significant changes in programming parameters. Nine months after Grace received her cochlear implant, her programming stabilized, and despite minor anticipated changes in programming, Grace's program parameters have not strayed from use of the ACE signal coding strategy with a 500 pulses per second stimulation rate and a 50 µs pulsewidth. Aided warbled tone testing was repeatedly in the 15 to 20 dB HL range from 250 to 6,000 Hz. Grace continued to wear a hearing aid in her left ear, although she received no observable benefit. Her parents considered implanting the left ear, but chose not to pursue it

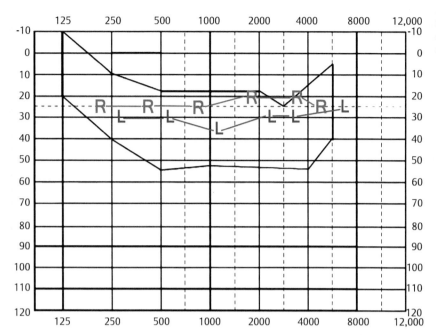

Fig. 23.4 Aided hearing thresholds for each cochlear implant. L, left ear hearing aid; R, right ear hearing aid.

because of the radiologic scans and eABR test findings suggested that she would be unlikely to benefit from an implant in her left ear.

23.6 Outcome

When Grace was 5 years of age, her parents had her cortical auditory responses assessed to help them consider if implanting the left ear would benefit Grace. They were told that the right ear had replicable P1 response, suggesting "auditory cortical pathways are present and developing typically for the patient's age." Her left ear had no P1 responses, suggesting a lack of typical development of the auditory cortical pathways. When Grace was 7 years of age, and after several years of considering a cochlear implant, her parents decided to have her left ear implanted. Her parents observed that Grace always wanted to wear her hearing aid on the left ear, even though she had no observable benefit. She received a CI 24RE Straight. Her mapping had variable pulse widths using ACE 500 Hz. She gradually began to have speech detection, but not discrimination. Three years after her surgery, she reported hearing cars going by in her left ear. She can now discriminate the Ling Six sounds with her left implant.

At age 10, Grace had routine audiologic and speech/language assessments. Her aided thresholds were 20 and 35 dB HL for the right and left ears, respectively (▶ Fig. 23.4). Her aided recognition scores for the right ear on the CNC word test are 56% for words and 76% for phonemes, and 84% for pediatric AZ Bio sentences. She scored 42% correct on the

NU-CHIPS with her left ear. Results of the Goldman Fristoe Test of Articulation and the CELF-5 language assessment indicate that she is just below 1 standard deviation lower than typically developing peers (Goldman Fristoe, 79 and CELF-5, 73–91). Grace is mainstreamed in a public charter school with no support, and her parents and teachers are pleased with her academic progress. She receives regular speech and language therapy pullout services at school. Grace is taking and enjoying piano lessons and is "loving life" as described by her parents.

References

[1] American Academy of Pediatrics, Joint Committee on Infant Hearing. Year 2007 position statement: Principles and guidelines for early hearing detection and intervention programs. Pediatrics. 2007; 120(4):898–921

[2] Muse C, Harrison J, Yoshinaga-Itano C, et al. Joint Committee on Infant Hearing of the American Academy of Pediatrics. Supplement to the JCIH 2007 position statement: principles and guidelines for early intervention after confirmation that a child is deaf or hard of hearing. Pediatrics. 2013; 131(4):e1324–e1349

[3] Birman CS, Brew JA, Gibson WPR, Elliott EJ. CHARGE syndrome and Cochlear implantation: difficulties and outcomes in the paediatric population. Int J Pediatr Otorhinolaryngol. 2015; 79(4):487–492

[4] Shelton C, Luxford WM, Tonokawa LL, Lo WW, House WF. The narrow internal auditory canal in children: a contraindication to cochlear implants. Otolaryngol Head Neck Surg. 1989; 100(3):227–231

[5] Bamiou DE, Worth S, Phelps P, Sirimanna T, Rajput K. Eighth nerve aplasia and hypoplasia in cochlear implant candidates: the clinical perspective. Otol Neurotol. 2001; 22(4):492–496

[6] Warren FM, III, Wiggins RH, III, Pitt C, Harnsberger HR, Shelton C. Apparent cochlear nerve aplasia: to implant or not to implant? Otol Neurotol. 2010; 31(7):1088–1094

24 Enlarged Vestibular Aqueduct with Fluctuating Hearing Loss

Kimberly Auerbach

24.1 Clinical History and Description

Sarah's journey began when she was 8 years old, when she failed a school hearing screening in January 2013. Sarah reportedly passed all of her previous hearing screenings. Her first formal audiological evaluation in January 2013 demonstrated a bilateral moderate to severe sensorineural hearing loss, worse in the right ear, and decreased word recognition ability (▶ Fig. 24.1). Sarah reported she was not hearing as well as usual and her mother also indicated that there was an increased need for repetition. However, there were no speech-language or academic concerns at the time of the initial diagnosis most likely due to the sudden nature of the hearing loss. Sarah received a computed tomography (CT) scan at the end of January 2013, which revealed enlarged vestibular aqueduct with the right worse than the left. Sarah received her first set of hearing aids in March 2013.

24.2 Audiologic Testing

Audiological evaluations throughout 2013 demonstrated bilateral fluctuations in hearing (▶ Fig. 24.2, ▶ Fig. 24.3). In May the following year, Sarah's hearing dropped to a profound sensorineural hearing loss bilaterally. Subsequent treatment with steroids did not show any recovery in hearing. She was seen for a cochlear implant (CI) evaluation in June 2014 (▶ Fig. 24.4) and was subsequently implanted with a right CI in July 2014. Sarah adjusted quickly to her CI and started receiving good benefit as she had better access to sounds and improved word recognition

with use of the CI only a few months after her initial stimulation (▶ Fig. 24.5). Sarah continued to use her left hearing aid alongside her right CI (▶ Fig. 24.5). Audiological monitoring of her left ear hearing was performed through the end of 2014 and 2015. Improvement in her left ear hearing was noted in fall of 2014, and by September 2015, it had recovered to normal hearing levels through 2,000 Hz, dropping to moderately severe hearing levels (▶ Fig. 24.6). Throughout Sarah's journey, there have been many fluctuations in her pure tone audiometry (PTA) for each ear (▶ Table 24.1). ▶ Table 24.1 demonstrates the fluctuations in hearing as well as its implications on word recognition ability. Sarah's word recognition fluctuated between 52 and 100%; at times, output limitations of the audiometer may have had a negative effect on the word recognition scoring.

24.3 Questions for the Reader

1. Was a CI for the right ear necessary?
2. Why did Sarah adjust so quickly to the CI? What may have happened if surgery was delayed?
3. Would a CI be a good choice for the left ear?

24.4 Discussion of Questions

1. **Was a CI for the right ear necessary?**
   Sarah was not receiving adequate benefit from her hearing aids at the time of the CI evaluation. She was in school and needed to maintain her academics and ability to communicate in everyday life. There is no way to predict if

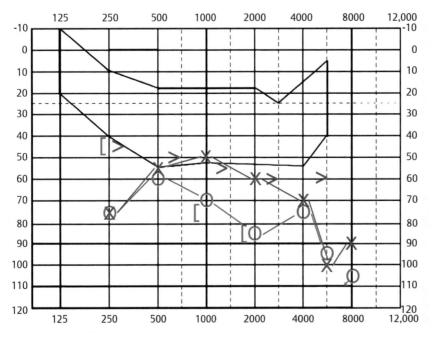

Fig. 24.1 Audiogram from January 2013. O, right ear air conduction; X, left ear air conduction; >, left ear bone conduction; [, right ear bone conduction masked.

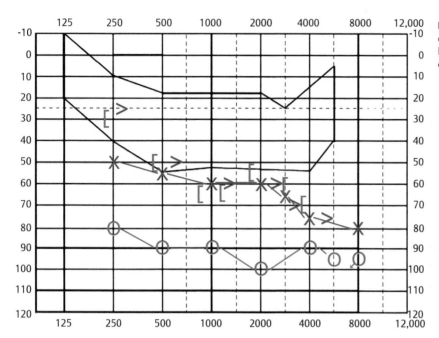

Fig. 24.2 Audiogram from June 2013. O, right ear air conduction; X, left ear air conduction; >, left ear bone conduction; [, right ear bone conduction masked.

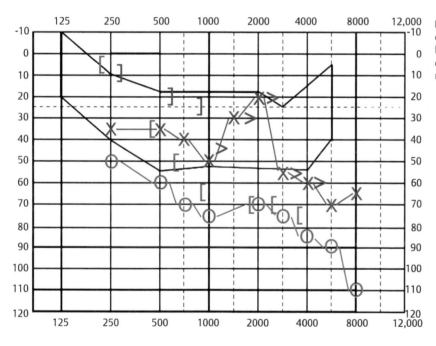

Fig. 24.3 Audiogram from August 2013. O, right ear air conduction; X, left ear air conduction; >, left ear bone conduction; [, right ear bone conduction masked;], left ear bone conduction masked.

the right ear hearing would have ever recovered. Waiting to see if the hearing recovered would have delayed her brain access to auditory information at the time.

2. **Why did Sarah adjust so quickly to the CI? What may have happened if surgery was delayed?**
Sarah had normally developing speech and was doing well academically, so it is very likely she had normal hearing in her early years, and therefore she relied on audition for language access and her brain had been developed with auditory information. She had been quickly introduced to hearing aids, and therefore, her auditory system had been flooded with sound, keeping the brain pathways active. Her auditory system quickly adjusted from acoustic sound with the hearing aid to electrical sound with the CI because her

brain had been developed with auditory information, and the drop in hearing happened fairly quickly. If surgery was delayed and her hearing remained in the profound range, her brain may not have received enough auditory input from hearing aids. This lack of auditory information may have resulted in auditory neural deprivation and may have had negative effects on Sarah's ability to interpret auditory information from the CI.

3. **Would a CI be a good choice for the left ear?**
At this time, the left ear is not a candidate for a CI. The left ear hearing will continue to be monitored. However, if the hearing sensitivity of the left ear hearing decreases and/or continues to fluctuate, a CI may be considered if the hearing aid is not providing enough consistent benefit.

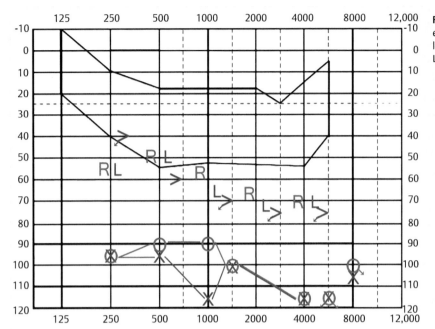

Fig. 24.4 Audiogram from June 2014. O, right ear air conduction; X, left ear air conduction; >, left ear bone conduction; R, right ear hearing aid; L, left ear hearing aid.

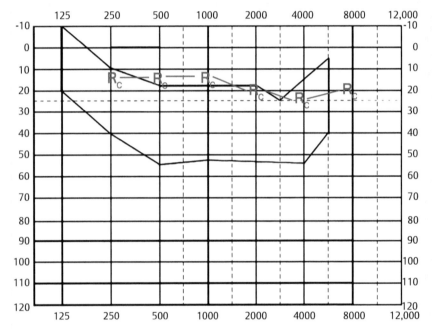

Fig. 24.5 Testing with right cochlear implant from April 2015. RC, right cochlear implant.

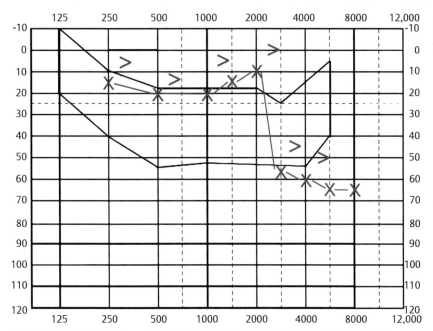

Fig. 24.6 Audiogram from September 2015. X, left ear air conduction; >, left ear bone conduction.

Table 24.1 Unaided PTA and word recognition scores

Date of test	PTA (dB)	Word recognition score	PTA (dB)	Word recognition score
	Right	Right	Left	Left
January 15, 2013	72	60% at 75 dB	55	80% at 70 dB
June 28, 2013	93	52% at 95 dB	85	88% at 80 dB
August 26, 2013	68	90% at 90 dB	35	100% at 75 dB
June 16, 2014	93	88% at 100 dB	103	88% at 100 dB
September 28, 2015	DNT	DNT	16	100% at 55 dB

Abbreviations: DNT, did not test; PTA, pure tone audiometry.

24.5 Outcome

Sarah is currently utilizing her CI on the right ear and her hearing aid on the left ear. Audiological monitoring of the left ear hearing and hearing aid, and CI mapping of the right ear continue. Sarah uses a remote microphone system at school and is doing well academically.

25 Complex Audiologic Diagnostic Case

Joan Hewitt

25.1 Clinical History and Description

Sam was a 4.10-year-old boy who was referred by his parents for a second opinion on behavioral audiological testing. According to parent report, he appeared to have normal hearing and normal speech and language development until 16 months of age when he received nine vaccinations at once. Over the next 2 months, he seemed to develop "total hearing loss."

The family lives in a rural area where pediatric resources are limited. At age 2 years, Sam was referred to a regional center for audiological testing. The audiological testing reports type A tympanograms and no conditioned response. The audiologist reported that he had poor eye contact and no response to sound. A referral to autism specialist was recommended for evaluation.

The family followed through with the audiologist's recommendation, and Sam was subsequently diagnosed with an autism spectrum disorder (ASD). At the age of 2.5 years, he began receiving 15 + hours of applied behavioral analysis (ABA) therapy and preschool intervention per week. At age 4.6 years, his ABA therapist changed. The new therapist felt Sam's lack of response to sound and lack of language development were different than that of other children with autism and recommended audiological testing.

25.2 Audiologic Testing

Audiological testing in the sound field indicated a flat 40 dB HL loss bilaterally. Although the audiogram does not indicate the testing method used, the parents reported that, when Sam turned his head in the direction of the sound, a box lit up (▶ Fig. 25.1). The audiological report states, "Testing suggests a mild to moderate sensorineural hearing loss in both ears." Auditory brainstem response (ABR) testing was recommended, but because of concerns about sedation, the parents sought a second opinion on behavioral results.

At age 4.10 years, Sam was seen for a second opinion. Although he was observed to vocalize a vowel-like hum, he had no oral receptive or expressive language according to both parent and teacher of the deaf observation. He used gestures and three formal signs that had recently been introduced to him. He engaged easily with the audiologists, made appropriate eye contact, and was not tactilely defensive to any of the testing. Behavioral audiological testing with insert earphones using conditioned play audiometry revealed a profound to moderate reverse slope hearing loss in the right ear, and a profound to severe reverse slope hearing loss in the left ear. Unmasked bone conduction testing indicated that the loss was sensorineural (▶ Fig. 25.2). Sam was referred for otoacoustic emissions (OAE) and ABR testing at a facility that was willing to attempt an unsedated ABR.

OAE testing revealed present robust emissions in the right ear and absent emissions in the left ear. An unsedated ABR revealed no responses to click or tone-burst stimuli and no cochlear microphonic in either ear. However, although the waveforms in the right ear indicated no response, they were unusual. The audiologist then asked several experts from other facilities to review the results. The consensus of those experts was that "the continued presence of otoacoustic emissions in the right ear indicates the presence of outer hair cell function

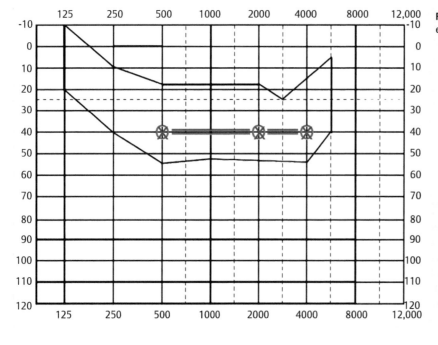

Fig. 25.1 Initial evaluation, age 6 years. O, right ear air conduction; X, left ear air conduction

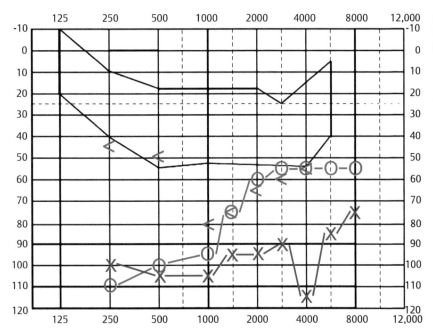

Fig. 25.2 Test results obtained at age 10 years. O, right ear air conduction; X, left ear air conduction; <, right ear bone conduction.

within the cochlea. Despite no evident cochlear microphonic, some waveforms appear to reveal possible early response which suggests auditory neuropathy spectrum disorder in this right ear. Left ear ABR results coupled with absence of otoacoustic emissions suggest unspecified sensorineural hearing loss."

25.3 Diagnosis

Right ear responses suggest auditory neuropathy spectrum disorder (ANSD). Left ear responses are consistent with profound to severe reverse slope sensorineural hearing loss.

25.4 Questions for the Reader

1. Do you agree with the recommendations of the first audiologist (at age 2 years)? Why or why not? If not, what would your recommendations have been?
2. Review the testing and findings of the second audiologist (at age 4.6 years). Identify at least three concerns with the testing and findings.
3. What are the benefits of using insert earphones with this type of patient?
4. How would you teach conditioned play audiometry to a child who has no language?
5. Are the second opinion behavioral results consistent with the electrophysiological results (at age 4.10 years)? Why or why not?
6. Why is the diagnosis in the right ear different than the diagnosis in the left ear?

25.5 Discussion of Questions

1. **Do you agree with the recommendations of the first audiologist (at age 2 years)? Why or why not? If not, what would your recommendations have been?**

We do not agree with the recommendations of the first audiologist. These parents presented with specific concerns and examples that their 2-year-old had previously responded to sound but was no longer doing so at the time of the appointment. Moreover, the audiologist was unable to elicit any responses to sound. The parents' observations coupled with the audiologist's findings necessitated an immediate referral for ABR and OAE testing. In addition, children with hearing impairment can display behaviors such as lack of attention, lack of eye contact, speech and language impairments, and clumsiness, which are similar to those of children on the autism spectrum.[1] Because hearing impairment can have such a profound effect on early development and can mimic ASD, it is extremely important to fully define a child's hearing status prior to assessing for ASD (or other developmental disabilities).[2]

2. **Review the testing and findings of the second audiologist (at age 4.6 years). Identify at least three concerns with the testing and findings.**
   - Type of behavioral testing used: Based upon the parent's description, Sam was assessed using visual reinforcement audiometry. Visual reinforcement audiometry is recommended for use with children from 6 months to 3 years of age. Conditioned play audiometry becomes developmentally appropriate between 2 and 3 years of age. Sam was 4.6 years at the time of testing. Visual reinforcement audiometry would not have been developmentally appropriate. We would anticipate that Sam would become bored with the reinforcers very quickly and would not respond at threshold levels. Thus, the reliability of the testing would be questionable.
   - Method of presentation of stimuli: According to the audiogram, all stimuli were presented in the sound field. Sound field testing does not provide ear-specific information. Thus, recording these results as right and left ear results is inaccurate.

- Thresholds obtained: We find it unusual and concerning that every threshold is at 40 dB HL. Moreover, the impedance measurements indicate absent acoustic reflexes. All thresholds at 40 dB HL would appear to be inconsistent with absent acoustic reflexes.
- Degree of hearing loss: Although the report stated that testing suggested a mild to moderate hearing loss in both ears, ear-specific information cannot be obtained from sound field testing. Thus, at best, the testing suggests the response of the better ear at each frequency tested.
- Type of hearing loss: Although the report states that hearing loss appears to be sensorineural, type A tympanograms with sound field testing are not sufficient to determine the type of hearing loss. Ear-specific air conduction and bone conduction testing are needed to determine to type of hearing loss.

3. **What are the benefits of using insert earphones with this type of patient?**

Insert earphones can be very helpful when testing young children. With them, we are able to obtain ear-specific information and, at the same time, minimize the equipment on the child's head. For children with ASD or other sensory disorders, which can create tactile defensiveness, minimizing the amount of equipment that touches the child can be essential to successfully obtaining complete results.

4. **How would you teach conditioned play audiometry to a child who has no language?**

Children do not need to have receptive or expressive language in order to learn conditioned play audiometry. Remember that we are just teaching a conditioned *behavioral* response. For children like Sam, it is essential to have a skilled test assistant to guide the child through the conditioning process. It is also essential that stimuli used for conditioning be loud enough for the child to hear. If a child cannot hear sound field or earphone stimuli, vibrotactile stimulation using a bone vibrator can be used to train the task. We have found that live voice is often the best stimulus to use for developing the conditioned response. Once the response to speech is conditioned and consistent, we have found that children can often easily transition the conditioned response to pure-tone threshold testing. Finally, it is important to be aware that children often produce their own conditioned response that may not be the one we are attempting to teach. In Sam's case, he initially held the toy to his ear, but rather than putting it down when he heard a sound, he would raise his eyebrows, say "Uh!" and turn to the test assistant. While this was not the targeted response, Sam consistently exhibited this behavior in response to the stimulus presentation, so the response was deemed to be a reliable conditioned response.

5. **Are the second opinion behavioral results consistent with the electrophysiological results (at age 4.10 years)? Why or why not?**

Yes. We can easily see that the left ear behavioral and electrophysiological results are consistent with a severe to profound sensorineural hearing loss. At first glance, the right ear behavioral results might seem inconsistent with the electrophysiological results, but we must remember that, with ANSD, electrophysiological results are not predictive of behavioral thresholds. It is also important to remember that bone conduction results at 250 and 500 Hz can be vibrotactile, so the presence of bone conduction responses at those frequencies is still consistent with a severe to profound sensorineural hearing loss or ANSD.

6. **Why is the diagnosis in the right ear different than the diagnosis in the left ear?**

AE were consistently present and robust in the right ear, but they were absent in the left ear. Although the right ear ABR results did not provide a clear reversal of the cochlear microphonic, the experts who reviewed the case felt that the consistent presence of OAEs strongly indicated normal outer hair cell function. In the left ear, the absence of OAEs combined with the ABR and behavioral results was not consistent with ANSD.

25.6 Outcome

Sam was fitted with loaner behind-the-ear hearing aids using Desired Sensation Level (DSL) v.5.0 pediatric targets. The settings were verified with simulated real ear measurements because Sam would not tolerate the probe tube in his canal. Sam readily accepted the hearing aids, consistently wore them every day, and even asked to have them put on in the morning. His parents reported increased awareness of sound, but responses were very inconsistent. They also reported an increase in negative behaviors and angry outbursts. Aided testing revealed inconsistent results. Right-ear-aided results were interesting, as no responses were obtained above 1,000 Hz and no response to speech was noted. In addition, frustration was observed to increase dramatically with the right hearing aid alone.

Although a CT (computed tomography) scan revealed normal cochlear anatomy, initially Sam was not deemed an appropriate candidate for cochlear implantation because of his age and additional disabilities. However, after consultation with a number of medical and audiological professionals, simultaneous bilateral cochlear implantation was recommended. The general recommendation was to initially activate the left (sensorineural) cochlear implant, observe behavior and auditory development for a period of time, and then activate the right (ANSD) implant. Sam was simultaneously bilaterally implanted at the age of 5.10 years.

At activation, neural responses with good morphology were obtained with the left implant using Neural Response Telemetry (NRT); no neural responses were obtained with the right implant. The left implant was activated. Sam tolerated the activation of the left implant well, but showed no awareness of sound. The activation of the left went so quickly and easily that activation of the right was attempted. Within minutes of activating the right implant, Sam began pointing to his ear and vocalizing to indicate that he had heard a sound. By the second day of activation, Sam could replicate pattern perception with the right CI. Since that time, performance with the right CI has consistently surpassed performance with the left CI. Programming of the left CI has required a wider pulse width than the right, but otherwise, the MAPs are unremarkable. In addition, while sound field speech awareness thresholds (SAT) are consistently obtained at 20 to 25 dB HL with the right and left implants independently, a speech reception threshold (SRT) using a closed set of objects has only been obtained with the right CI, indicating clearer speech perception with the right CI.

Nevertheless, from the first day, Sam has worn his cochlear implants all his waking hours. He loves to listen and understands some words and phrases with audition alone. He uses a combination of words and signs to express himself and, according to his parents and teachers, "is so much happier" now that he can hear.

25.7 Additional Questions for the Reader

1. Why might observation and testing of Sam's aided responses be inconsistent?
2. Why might use of the hearing aids, especially the right hearing aid, lead to an increase in negative behaviors?
3. Why do you think implantation of both ears was recommended with activation of the left cochlear implant first and then a later activation of the right ear?
4. How did Sam's results with his cochlear implants coincide and differ from the expected results?
5. Would you have recommended implanting a 5-year-old with ASD? Why or why not?
6. Do you think Sam really had ASD, a hearing loss, or both? Why?

25.8 Discussion of Additional Questions

1. **Why might observation and testing of Sam's aided responses be inconsistent?**

   Sam has a very significant hearing loss. Even with appropriately fitted amplification, he may not hear soft or distant sounds, speech in noise, or sounds in frequency ranges where his hearing is poorest. In addition, according to the history the parents provided, Sam has not heard for at least 3 years. During that time, his brain has developed without recognizable, meaningful auditory input. Some sounds, especially speech, may be audible, but meaningless to Sam. If sounds are meaningless to him, he is unlikely to respond to them consistently.

2. **Why might use of the hearing aids, especially the right hearing aid, lead to an increase in negative behaviors?**

   While hearing aids may provide significant amplification of sounds, they may not overcome the distortion present in a severe to profound hearing loss. Moreover, with ANSD in his right ear, we know nothing about the quality of the sound Sam hears in that ear. It is interesting that, although his unaided thresholds in the right ear are better in the high frequencies, he had no aided responses above 1,000 Hz. He also had no response to speech with the right hearing aid. We believe children's behaviors often provide significant information that they may be unable to express. For Sam, the consistent increases in negative behaviors when he wore his right hearing aid alone strongly indicated that amplified sound in the right ear was unintelligible and disturbing. In addition, right ear amplification may have interfered with the information he was receiving from the left hearing aid.

3. **Why do you think implantation of both ears was recommended with activation of the left cochlear implant first and then a later activation of the right ear?**

   Even though Sam's age was past the optimal age of implantation, the team believed that he could benefit from implantation, especially because he readily accepted and even requested hearing aid amplification. When discussing which ear to implant, the consensus was that the left ear with sensorineural hearing loss should have a predictively positive outcome. On the other hand, the response and benefit in the right ear with ANSD was more difficult to predict because an MRI (magnetic resonance imaging) had not been completed to assess the integrity of the auditory nerve. However, all the experts were concerned that, if the right auditory nerve was functional and the right ear remained unimplanted, the auditory input could interfere with information from a well-functioning left ear cochlear implant. Thus, it was decided that the right ear be implanted along with the left ear to minimize the ability of the right ear to provide input that interfered. The same arguments were used to support activation of the left implant first because that ear had a sensorineural hearing loss so outcomes could be more easily predicted. The right ear would then be activated at a later date because the outcomes with it were more difficult to predict.

4. **How did Sam's results with his cochlear implants coincide and differ from the expected results?**

   First, Sam had no negative reactions to any of the assessments or activation of the left cochlear implant, which was an unexpected surprise for a child with ASD and little to no language. In addition, the presence of replicable neural responses made programing fairly easy with a patient who could not provide feedback about what he was hearing because the NRT provided an estimate of appropriate stimulation levels. However, it was interesting, but not unusual, that Sam did not respond to any sound with the activation of the left implant. Nevertheless, Sam's acceptance made activating the right implant during the initial stimulation a possibility, which was not originally considered. A lack of neural responses with the right implant made initial stimulation more challenging. However, Sam's immediate responses to sound and his quick recognition of pattern perception indicated that the right implant was providing meaningful input. Delaying activation of the right implant as recommended would have delayed Sam's brain access to meaningful sound/ auditory information. Finally, while Sam's auditory and speech/language development is not comparable to early implanted children, it has surpassed expectations.

5. **Would you have recommended implanting a 5-year-old with ASD? Why or why not?**

   With appropriate expectations and support, we believe cochlear implantation of children with multiple disabilities should be a consideration. While traditional outcomes may not be realized, improved eye contact, awareness of the environment, responsiveness, speech development, language development (including sign language), and quality of life are some of the benefits that have been documented in implanted children with complex needs.[3]

6. **Do you think Sam really had ASD, a hearing loss, or both? Why?**

This case (and others we have seen like it) in which a child has been diagnosed first with ASD or other developmental disorders and then later with a significant hearing loss is extremely distressing to us. Because, when we met him, Sam had no language and had spent the critical period of auditory brain development in programs with strict ABA intervention and only peers on the autism spectrum, it is impossible for us to know if the initial behaviors that led to his diagnosis of ASD were from auditory deprivation or a combination of auditory deprivation and autism. Moreover, if he had received minimal sound input from the left sensorineural ear and a degraded or unrecognizable signal from the right ANSD ear, then it would not be surprising that Sam's behavior and responses might look unusual. Our observations of Sam's consistent willingness and eagerness to engage with others despite his extreme lack of language have caused us to seriously question the diagnosis of ASD. In addition, experts who have assessed Sam do not know if his remaining "quirky" behaviors stem from ASD or from years of inappropriate intervention with no language development. While we may never have a definitive answer to this question, in our opinion Sam acts more like a child with a significant hearing loss who experienced extreme language deprivation and was immersed in rigid ABA intervention with minimal interaction with typically developing peers.

References

[1] Birath AL, Robbins AM, Beau VV. Autism and Hearing Loss: What you need to know to help your families. Loud & Clear. 2014(1):1–5

[2] Worley JA, Matson JL, Kozlowski AM. The effects of hearing impairment on symptoms of autism in toddlers. Dev Neurorehabil. 2011; 14(3):171–176

[3] Edwards LC. Children with cochlear implants and complex needs: a review of outcome research and psychological practice. J Deaf Stud Deaf Educ. 2007; 12(3):258–268

26 Auditory Processing Evaluation: 8-Year-Old Female

Shelby L. Landes and Erin C. Schafer

26.1 Clinical History and Description

Katie, an 8-year-old second-grade female student, was seen for a complete auditory processing evaluation. Her medical history includes frequent ear infections at an early age that subsided spontaneously prior to the placement of pressure equalization tubes. Katie has been diagnosed with a receptive and expressive language disorder and currently receives speech therapy, cognitive therapy, and resource instruction for reading and writing. Her mother has a history of speech and learning disorders, and her sister has been diagnosed with dyslexia. Katie's mother reports that Katie often lacks self-confidence because she does not meet the high expectations she sets for herself. Katie is outgoing and hardworking, but she has problems expressing herself and can become frustrated because of these problems. Katie has also difficulty following complex directions, especially in the presence of background noise.

26.2 Diagnostic Auditory Processing Evaluation Results

26.2.1 Audiologic Testing

Otoscopy revealed clear ear canals with good visualization of a healthy tympanic membrane bilaterally, with some redness visualized on the walls of both ear canals. Immittance results yielded a type A tympanogram in both ears, which is consistent with normal middle ear function. Responses to pure tone stimuli were within normal limits bilaterally, and speech reception thresholds (SRTs) were obtained at 10 dB HL in both ears. Word recognition scores at 40 dB SL using Phonetically Balanced Kindergarten (PBK-50) word lists in quiet were 100% bilaterally.

26.2.2 Speech Perception in Noise

The Bamford-Kowal-Bench Speech-in-Noise test (BKB-SIN) was used to estimate Katie's speech recognition at the 50% correct level. In other words, this test determines the signal-to-noise ratio (SNR) that is required by the listener to understand 50% of key words in the presence of background noise. Sentences were presented at 0-degree azimuth (directly in front of the listener), and noise was presented from two locations: 0 and 180 degrees. Katie's thresholds in noise were +2 dB SNR with noise at 0-degree azimuth and –2 dB SNR with noise at 180-degree azimuth. These results are within normal limits for the 0-degree noise condition. The 180-degreee noise condition results suggest that her performance will improve when background noise is spatially separated from the sentences, which is a skill achieved by most listeners.

26.2.3 Binaural Integration

Katie's binaural integration skills were tested to determine her ability to process different stimuli when they were presented to each ear at the same time. Deficits in binaural integration often demonstrate a large right ear advantage, and can result in increased difficulty understanding speech in the presence of background noise or when there are multiple talkers.

The Dichotic Digits Test (DDT) is a method of assessing binaural integration by presenting four digits dichotically (two different digits per ear) and asking the child to repeat each number heard using free recall. Katie's scores for 50 stimuli sets in the right and left ears were 82% (norm = 79.9 ± 8.2%) and 66% (norm = 70.6 ± 8.2%), respectively, suggesting performance within normal limits in both ears. There was an ear difference score of 16 (norm = 9.4 ± 3.1), suggesting a right ear advantage just over two standard deviations above the mean.

The Competing Words–Directed Ear (CW-DE) subtest of the SCAN-3 was also used to assess binaural integration. This test involves presenting words dichotically and asking the child to repeat both words. The DE component asks the child to repeat the words in a specific order based on which ear heard each word. This test is a means of identifying the large right ear advantage common to the auditory processing disorder (APD) diagnosis. Katie's total scaled score of 1 places her in the 0.1 percentile, which is in the disordered range. A typical right ear advantage was seen in the Directed Right Ear task, and a typical left ear advantage was seen in the Directed Left Ear task.

26.2.4 Binaural Separation

The Competing Sentences (CS) subtest of the SCAN-3 was used to evaluate Katie's binaural separation abilities. Binaural separation is the ability to ignore a stimulus in one ear and focus on a different stimulus in the other ear when both stimuli are presented simultaneously. Abnormal results in this domain typically are associated with increased difficulty understanding speech in background noise or when there are multiple talkers.

Katie's scaled score on the CS subtest was 7. This score falls in the lower range of normal limits in the 16th percentile. A typical right ear advantage was observed for this measure. These results are consistent with normal binaural separation abilities.

26.2.5 Temporal Processing

The Random Gap Detection Test (RGDT) was used to determine Katie's temporal processing abilities by asking her to identify whether two stimuli were perceived as one sound or two. Abnormality in the ability to detect small fluctuations in the timing of speech cues is consistent with temporal processing deficits and can increase difficulty with speech perception.

The composite gap detection threshold is calculated by averaging the lowest identifiable gap for pure tones 500 to 4,000 Hz. A reliable gap detection threshold could not be identified due to inconsistent responses during the test. Katie's temporal processing abilities could not be determined with the test results; this is a difficult task for some children.

26.2.6 Temporal Patterning

The Pitch Pattern Sequence (PPS) test was used to examine Katie's temporal-patterning abilities, which are the recognition of presentation patterns of nonlinguistic auditory stimuli (▶ Table 26.1). The PPS requires children to discriminate between high and low pitches in sets of three tones (e.g., high-high-low, high-low-high, low-low-high) that are presented monaurally. A percentage of the pitch patterns correctly identified is calculated. Katie's temporal patterning abilities could not be determined because she did not provide reliable responses. She would respond appropriately to the first few patterns, but then repeatedly responded with the same answer, despite reinstruction. This test was conducted near the end of the evaluation; therefore, it is possible that fatigue contributed to the inconsistent responses.

26.2.7 Spatial Stream Segregation

Auditory stream segregation is the listener's ability to separate simultaneous incoming auditory signals and attach meaningful representations to those signals. The Listening in Spatialized Noise—Sentences Test (LiSN-S) evaluates these skills by varying the spatial and pitch characteristics of incoming stimuli and by calculating speech recognition thresholds in noise as well as advantage scores for each of the test conditions. Sentences are presented in the presence of distracter stories, with the intensity level of the phrase adjusted to find the patient's SRT in noise at the 50% correct level. The distracter stories are varied in regard to their position in space

Table 26.1 Summary of Katie's performance on speech perception in noise, binaural listening, and temporal processing/patterning tasks

Speech perception in noise			
BKB-SIN	+2 dB SNR (0-degree azimuth)	−2 dB SNR (180-degree azimuth)	WNL
Binaural integration			
DDT	82%—RE 66%—LE	16% difference	WNL Strong right ear advantage
CW-DE	1 (0.1 percentile)	No significant cumulative preference	Outside normal limits No ear advantage
Binaural separation			
CS	7 (16th percentile)	No significant cumulative preference	WNL No ear advantage
Temporal processing/patterning			
RGDT	Unable to be determined	n/a	
PPS	Unable to be determined	n/a	

[Abbreviations: BKB-SIN, Bamford-Kowal-Bench Speech-in-Noise; CW-DE, Competing Words–Directed Ear; DDT, Dichotic Digits Test; PPS, Pitch Pattern Sequence; RGDT, Random Gap Detection Test; WNL, within normal limits.]

(±0-degree azimuth vs. ±90-degree azimuth) and the vocal quality of the speakers (same voice vs. different voices). The low-cue SRT represents listening skills when no spatial or vocal cues are available, while the total advantage and high-cue SRT represents listening skills when both vocal and spatial cues are available. Talker advantage indicates the listener's ability to use differences in vocal quality to distinguish the signal of interest, and spatial advantage reflects a listener's ability to use differences in the physical location of incoming stimuli to perceive the signal of interest amidst competing signals.

This combination of scores is considered unusual according to the LiSN-S test manual (▶ Table 26.2).

26.2.8 Informal Evaluation

The Children's Auditory Performance Scale (CHAPS) is a teacher questionnaire designed to examine the listening difficulties of a child compared with age-matched, typically functioning peers. Six listening conditions are evaluated, including noise, quiet, ideal, multiple inputs (i.e., auditory, visual, tactile), auditory memory (i.e., recalling spoken information), and auditory attention span. Katie's teacher completed the survey. Her responses indicate that Katie is in the at-risk range for the noise, multiple inputs, auditory memory, and overall listening conditions, and borderline at-risk in quiet listening conditions. These responses suggest that Katie has substantially greater difficulties listening in the classroom than her peers.

The Children's Communication Checklist-2 (CCC-2) is a comprehensive parent/caregiver survey of a child's communication skills across language and pragmatic domains. Based on responses from Katie's mother, the General Communication Composite score was 74, indicating an overall communicative competence in the 4th percentile. Typical scores of other children are around 100 (standard deviation = 15), which places Katie's scores 2 standard deviations below the mean. The Social Interaction Difference Index (SIDI) was 27, suggesting the communicative profile of a specific language disorder. This is consistent with Katie's confirmed diagnosis of an expressive and receptive language disorder.

Fisher's Auditory Problems Checklist collects information from the parent/caregiver about the perceived auditory problems experienced by the child and is often used as an informal screening tool for APD. Responses from Katie's mother were converted into a score of 36%. This suggests that she has a range of auditory difficulties well below the mean for peers of the same age, with the average score for 8-year-olds being 85.6%.

Table 26.2 Katie's average test scores and normal test scores on the Listening in Spatialized Noise—Sentences Test (LiSN-S)

Measure	Average score for age	Katie's score (dB)	Normal limits	Standard deviation
Low-cue SRT	−0.2	0.4	Within	−0.6
High-cue SRT	−10.4	−7.4	Within	−1.4
Talker advantage	5.1	0.1	Outside	−2.3
Spatial advantage	9.1	4.7	Outside	−2.7
Total advantage	10.2	7.8	Within	−1.2

Abbreviation: SRT, speech reception threshold.

26.3 Questions for the Reader

1. What were the strengths and deficit areas identified in the auditory processing evaluation?
2. Would you diagnose Katie with an auditory processing disorder? Why or why not?
3. How did Katie's language disorder impact her performance on auditory processing tasks?
4. Would you recommend any additional testing for Katie?

26.4 Discussion of Questions

1. **What were the strengths and deficit areas identified in the auditory processing evaluation?**

   The comprehensive test results are indicative of normal auditory processing abilities for speech perception in noise and binaural separation. Deficits were seen in Katie's auditory processing abilities for binaural integration and spatial stream segregation. Temporal processing and patterning abilities could not be determined from the results, likely due to a lack of sustained attention rather than a reflection of impaired temporal resolution.[1] According to informal evaluations completed by Katie's mother and teacher, she has substantial listening difficulties both at home and in the classroom.

2. **Would you diagnose Katie with an auditory processing disorder? Why or why not?**

   No. The deficits seen in this evaluation cannot be confirmed as an auditory processing disorder independent of Katie's known language disorder. The American Speech-Language-Hearing Association holds that "(C)APD is best viewed as a deficit in the neural processing of auditory stimuli that may coexist with, but *is not the result of,* dysfunction in other modalities," including language impairments.[2] Despite Katie's known language disorder, an auditory processing evaluation was completed to compare her auditory performance to that of age-matched, typically developing peers to generate recommendations about how to improve her ability to attend to auditory stimuli. In the presence of a language disorder, we concluded that her auditory performance is markedly different than that of age-matched, typically developing peers in the domains of binaural integration and spatial stream segregation.

3. **How did Katie's language disorder impact her performance on auditory processing tasks?**

   The difference in Katie's performance on binaural integration tasks between the two tests could be due to the fact that the CW-DE subtest is much more linguistically loaded than the DDT.[3] Therefore, in our opinion, the remarkably different performance on the two tests is a result of Katie's language impairment. An atypical right ear advantage was observed for the DDT but none of the other dichotic listening tasks. Considering this ear advantage was only slightly outside of two standard deviations from the mean and not replicated in other measures, it is likely not associated with the strong right ear advantage common to the diagnosis of APD. Additionally, an unusual pattern of scores on the LiSN-S was observed. It is possible that Katie's language disorder influenced the results in a pattern that is not characteristic of the listening profiles typically seen on the LiSN-S for children with APDs independent of other impairments, including language disorders.

4. **Would you recommend any additional testing for Katie?**

   Given that Katie has already been evaluated for speech and language and is receiving both speech and cognitive therapies and resource instruction at school, it is likely that no outside referrals are necessary. A follow-up appointment could be recommended to obtain more complete data about Katie's temporal processing and patterning abilities. There were several other auditory processing test measures that were not utilized in our test protocol; however, we attempted to address each domain of auditory processing with one to two measures.[4,5] In an ideal world, our protocol would also include electrophysiological measures from the level of the brainstem to the cortex in response to speech stimuli, which could corroborate behavioral results with objective data about the functional integrity of the auditory system relative to age-matched, typically functioning peers.[4]

26.5 Recommended Treatment

The deficits seen in this evaluation cannot be confirmed as an APD independent of Katie's known language disorder. Therefore, the following recommendations were provided to attempt to improve Katie's ability to attend to auditory stimuli:

1. Continue with recommended language and cognitive therapies.
2. Consider the use of remote microphone technology (e.g., ear-level frequency modulation system) in the classroom.

Note: Although a formal diagnosis of APD was not made and Katie's speech-in-noise understanding was within normal limits, she did perform better when the background noise was spatially separated from the sentences. There is evidence to support the use of remote-microphone technology for children with auditory difficulties as the result of various disorders, such as attention-deficit hyperactivity disorder (ADHD), autism spectrum disorder (ASD), and language impairments.[6] The family was highly motivated to seek out any type of intervention that may help Katie in the classroom; therefore, in this case, we recommended the use of remote microphone technology, which may be provided at school as part of her special educational services after an assistive technology evaluation documents her educational need.

3. Use of strategic seating in the classroom (close to the teacher, away from distracting outside noises such as hallways, projectors, fans, etc.).
4. Allow extra time for processing information.
5. Reduce visual distractions.
6. Check for understanding during verbal classroom instruction.
7. Repeat or rephrase information when necessary.
8. Use hearing protection whenever in the presence of loud sounds.

References

[1] Loo JH, Bamiou DE, Rosen S. The impacts of language background and language-related disorders in auditory processing assessment. J Speech Lang Hear Res. 2013; 56(1):1–12

[2] (Central) Auditory Processing Disorders [Technical report]. American Speech-Language-Hearing Association. Available at: http://www.asha.org/policy/TR2005–00043/. Published 2005. Accessed July 27, 2016

[3] Lawson GD, Peterson ME. Assessment of auditory processing disorders. In: Hall JW, Ramachandran V, eds. Speech Audiometry. San Diego, CA: Plural Publishing; 2011: 77–104

[4] Jerger J, Musiek F. Report of the consensus conference on the diagnosis of auditory processing disorders in school-aged children. J Am Acad Audiol. 2000; 11(9):467–474

[5] Cameron S, Dillon H. Essays in audiology: auditory processing disorder – from screening to diagnosis and management – a-step-by-step guide. Audiology Now. 2005; 21:47–55

[6] Schafer EC, Traber J, Layden P, et al. Use of wireless technology for children with auditory processing disorders, attention-deficit hyperactivity disorder, and language disorders. Semin Hear. 2014; 35(3):193–205

Additional Readings

[1] Sharma M, Purdy SC, Kelly AS. Comorbidity of auditory processing, language, and reading disorders. J Speech Lang Hear Res. 2009; 52(3):706–722

[2] Miller CA, Wagstaff DA. Behavioral profiles associated with auditory processing disorder and specific language impairment. J Commun Disord. 2011; 44 (6):745–763

27 Unilateral Auditory Neuropathy Spectrum Disorder/ Cochlear Nerve Aplasia

Jane Burton and Meredith Holcomb

27.1 Clinical History

Luke presented to our clinic for repeat newborn hearing screen. He was born full-term after uncomplicated pregnancy, and he passed the left ear and referred on the right ear with an auditory brainstem response (ABR) newborn hearing screen prior to discharge from the hospital. His mother reported he startles to sounds, and there is no family history of childhood hearing loss.

27.2 Audiologic Testing

He was tested in our clinic at 1 month of age. Distortion product otoacoustic emission (DPOAE) testing was initially used for rescreen because he would not sleep for ABR testing. DPOAEs were present and robust for both ears (▶ Fig. 27.1; ▶ Fig. 27.2). Tympanometry results suggested normal middle ear function (type A tympanograms), bilaterally. He returned 1 week later for a diagnostic ABR test using tone bursts and click stimuli. Tone burst ABR results were consistent with normal hearing in the left ear and no responses in the right ear (500, 1,000, and 4,000 Hz). Click ABR results revealed a cochlear microphonic for the right ear (▶ Fig. 27.3).

27.3 Questions for the Reader

1. Why was Luke rescreened with both OAE and ABR testing? He passed the bilateral OAE rescreen, so was ABR testing warranted?
2. What possible diagnosis could be made based on the presented audiology testing alone?

3. What recommendations are necessary for the child at this point?
4. Why should Luke undergo radiographic imaging as part of the ENT evaluation?
5. What amplification options are available for the right ear in the future?

27.4 Discussion of Questions

1. **Why was Luke rescreened with both OAE and ABR testing? He passed the bilateral OAE rescreen, so was ABR testing warranted?**

OAE testing was completed initially because Luke would not sleep for ABR testing. OAE results suggested normal cochlear function, bilaterally. However, because he referred in the right ear on an ABR newborn hearing screen, it was necessary to retest him with ABR to assure correct diagnosis and recommendations for the right ear.[1] While OAEs assess the function of the outer hair cells in the cochlea, they do not provide information regarding function of higher levels of the auditory system, including the integrity of the auditory nerve and the brainstem's response to sound. If ABR testing was not completed, Luke likely would be recorded as a "pass" for both ears on the rescreen.

2. **What possible diagnosis could be made based on the presented audiology testing alone?**

Diagnosis of unilateral auditory neuropathy spectrum disorder (ANSD) was made following ABR testing. ANSD is characterized by the presence of or history of OAE responses and

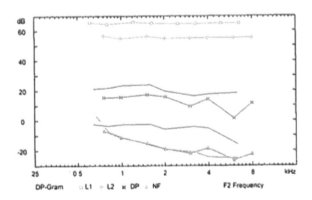

Fig. 27.1 DPOAE test results for left ear.

Left:		-: 750-8000 Hz Diagnostic Test - High Noise:				OAE	
L1(dB)	L2(dB)	F1(Hz)	F2(Hz)	GM(Hz)	DP(dB)	NF(dB)	DP-NF(dB)
64.9	55.2	6516	7969	7206	11.5	-22.5	34.0
64.9	55.0	4922	6000	5434	1.4	-26.6	28.0
64.5	55.0	3281	3984	3616	14.2	-18.7	32.9
64.6	55.0	2484	3000	2730	9.5	-22.2	31.7
64.9	54.8	1641	2016	1818	15.9	-19.1	35.0
65.8	56.2	1219	1500	1352	17.1	-15.3	32.4
64.2	54.8	797	984	886	15.5	-11.6	27.1
65.4	56.4	609	750	676	15.3	-6.9	22.2

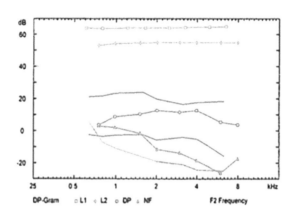

Fig. 27.2 DPOAE test results for left ear .

Right:		-: 750-8000 Hz Diagnostic Test:			OAE		
L1(dB)	L2(dB)	F1(Hz)	F2(Hz)	GM(Hz)	DP(dB)	NF(dB)	DP-NF(dB)
64.8	54.9	6516	7969	7206	3.7	-17.6	21.3
64.7	54.9	4922	6000	5434	5.2	-26.5	31.7
64.2	54.8	3281	3984	3616	12.4	-18.7	31.1
64.0	54.8	2484	3000	2730	11.5	-14.0	25.5
64.1	54.7	1641	2016	1818	12.6	-11.8	24.4
64.0	54.6	1219	1500	1352	10.2	-1.7	11.9
63.7	54.2	797	984	886	8.7	1.8	6.9
64.1	53.1	609	750	676	3.6	2.6	1.0

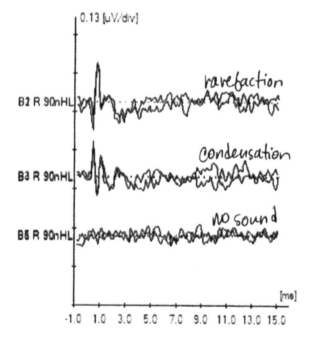

Fig. 27.3 Click stimulus ABR results for right ear with cochlear microphonic.

absent or grossly abnormal ABR results, often with the presence of a cochlear microphonic.[2] Site of lesion may be located at the level of the inner hair cells (IHCs), the synapse between the IHCs and the auditory nerve, or at the auditory nerve.[3] According to one study, prevalence of ANSD is thought to range from 7 to 10% in children with permanent hearing loss.[4] Of this population, only 6% of cases are unilateral.[2] Audiometric configurations can vary from normal hearing sensitivity to profound hearing loss. For this reason, ANSD is considered a spectrum disorder, with some patients exhibiting no overt delays or auditory complaints until adulthood to a complete lack of sound awareness.[2]

3. **What recommendations are necessary for the child at this point?**

Luke should be referred for a medical evaluation to an otologist or a pediatric otolaryngologist with extensive experience in pediatric hearing loss. Medical work-up should include, but is not limited to, radiographic imaging, speech evaluation, and genetics consultation. Once the child is developmentally capable of performing behavioral audiological testing, ear-specific hearing thresholds should be obtained. In the case of ANSD, frequent audiological testing is recommended until stable thresholds are obtained. Follow-up audiological evaluations should occur every 3 months after obtaining stable thresholds due to increased risk of fluctuating hearing loss. Amplification is not recommended at this time due to limited knowledge of hearing sensitivity of the right ear. Children with ANSD should not be fitted with amplification until consistent behavioral hearing thresholds are obtained.

4. **Why should Luke undergo radiographic imaging as part of the ENT evaluation?**

Magnetic resonance imaging (MRI) is strongly recommended in the case of ANSD to appropriately evaluate both inner ear anatomy and, most importantly, the status of the cochlear nerve. Previous studies found cochlear aplasia or cochlear nerve deficiency in 18 to 38% of children presenting with ANSD, and all noted it was more common in cases of unilateral ANSD.[2,5] Aural rehabilitation options will be altered based on MRI results.

5. **What amplification options are available for the right ear in the future?**

Results from the MRI and behavioral testing will dictate recommended amplification options for this child. A traditional hearing aid will likely be considered if hearing thresholds are in the mild to moderately severe hearing loss range. Frequent monitoring and adjustments are recommended, as behavioral thresholds do not reflect functional hearing in patients with ANSD. Of note, amplification is found to be beneficial in only a small percentage of patients, due to the nature of ANSD pathology.[3] Unilateral cochlear implantation is a possible consideration if the cochlear nerve is present and if hearing thresholds are severe to profound. However, cochlear nerve aplasia is a contraindication for a traditional hearing aid or a cochlear implant. An osseointegrated device or contralateral routing of the off-side signal (CROS) hearing system are potential options if hearing thresholds are

severe and/or if the cochlear nerve is absent. A remote microphone system should also be recommended in conjunction with any of the aforementioned options because ANSD patients, generally, have very poor ability to understand speech in background noise.[3] Parents may also wish to forgo any type of amplification because the normal-hearing left ear may be adequate for successful communication.

27.5 Diagnosis and Recommended Treatment

Luke was diagnosed with right ear unilateral ANSD. Initial recommendations included medical evaluation with a pediatric otolaryngologist with extensive experience in pediatric hearing loss. Radiographic imaging was recommended to assess inner ear anatomy of the right ear. An MRI was completed and revealed an absence of the right cochlear nerve (cochlear nerve aplasia) and normal left inner ear anatomy. The child began behavioral testing at 7 months of age to confirm ABR and MRI results. By age 12 months, behavioral testing confirmed the right ear was unresponsive to sound; therefore, no amplification options were recommended at that time.

27.6 Outcome

Luke is now 7 years old and is struggling academically. He was recently fit with a CROS hearing system and is performing/attending better in school. A remote microphone system has not been trialed in the classroom, but should certainly be considered to improve acoustic accessibility of instruction.

References

[1] American Academy of Pediatrics. Joint Committee on Infant Hearing 2007. Year 2007 Position Statement: Principles and Guidelines for Early Hearing Detection and Intervention Programs. Pediatrics. 2007; 120(4):896–921

[2] Berlin CI, Hood LJ, Morlet T, et al. Multi-site diagnosis and management of 260 patients with auditory neuropathy/dys-synchrony (auditory neuropathy spectrum disorder). Int J Audiol. 2010; 49(1):30–43

[3] Hood LJ. Auditory neuropathy/dys-synchrony disorder: Diagnosis and management. Otolaryngol Clin North Am. 2015; 48(6):1027–1040

[4] Roche JP, Huang BY, Castillo M, Bassim MK, Adunka OF, Buchman CA. Imaging characteristics of children with auditory neuropathy spectrum disorder. Otol Neurotol. 2010; 31(5):780–788

[5] Buchman CA, Roush PA, Teagle HF, Brown CJ, Zdanski CJ, Grose JH. Auditory neuropathy characteristics in children with cochlear nerve deficiency. Ear Hear. 2006; 27(4):399–408

Suggested Reading

[1] Guidelines for Identification and Management of Infants and Young Children with Auditory Neuropathy Spectrum Disorder. Available at: https://www.childrenscolorado.org/contentassets/728eca7b14724f318fbb60a5047ffc93/ansd-monograph-bill-daniels-center-for-childrens-hearing.pdf

[2] Roush P, Frymark T, Venediktov R, Wang B. Audiologic management of auditory neuropathy spectrum disorder in children: a systematic review of the literature. Am J Audiol. 2011; 20(2):159–170

28 Bilateral Microtia/Atresia with Mixed Hearing Loss

Michele DiStefano

28.1 Clinical History and Description

Jay is 1 year 3 months old with bilateral microtia/atresia. She was born with lower facial nerve palsy, a neck nodule, simian crease, and bilateral microtia/atresia, and her right eye did not close fully due to possible muscle aplasia. Reportedly, there is a positive gestational history of maternal use of isotretinoin during the first 5 weeks of gestation. Her mother reported that both the magnetic resonance imaging (MRI) and genetic testing were normal. She further reported that Jay possibly had a stroke in utero. Jay is enrolled in the early intervention program, receiving speech therapy, physical therapy (PT), and occupational therapy (OT). She is not progressing in speech and language, using only limited words and mostly gestures.

28.2 Audiologic Testing

Jay has been followed audiologically since she was 3 months old. Her most recent hearing test revealed profound hearing loss bilaterally with bone conduction thresholds at moderately severe hearing loss levels. Bone conduction thresholds could not be masked. Sensorineural acuity level (SAL) could not be performed due to Jay's inability to perform task (▶ Table 28.1).

28.3 Questions for the Reader

1. What further testing, if any, would you perform?
2. What amplification, if any, would you fit on this child?
3. What educational program would you recommend for this child?
4. What medical workup, if any, would you recommend for this child?

28.4 Discussion of Questions

1. **What further testing, if any, would you perform?**
   Further testing with the Cochlear Baha 5 SP is to be performed in order to further assess any possible benefit from a stronger hearing aid. Additionally, further unaided testing to obtain a full audiogram has been performed.

2. **What amplification, if any, would you fit on this child?**
   The child is currently using bilateral Cochlear Baha BP110 with softband pending aided test results with the Cochlear Baha 5 SP. However, it is felt that the child should undergo cochlear implant evaluation to further assess candidacy for cochlear implant.

3. **What educational program would you recommend for this child?**
   The child is currently receiving speech–language therapy, OT, PT and special instruction in a home-based setting through early intervention. Educational options have been discussed with her mother, including the child being taught American Sign Language (ASL). However, her mother would like her to be verbal and has not agreed to ASL at this time. The family is having an educational consultation.

4. **What medical workup, if any, would you recommend for this child?**
   The child received a computed tomography (CT) scan revealing bilateral cochlear dysplasia. Further testing could include an MRI to further assess the cochlear and facial nerves. Additionally, further genetic testing could be performed.

28.5 Additional Testing

A tonal auditory brainstem response was performed on Jay, revealing abnormal bone conduction results, which could not be masked indicating some degree of a mixed hearing loss. Jay was then initially bilaterally fit with Cochlear Baha 4 hearing aids with softband at 8 months of age. Aided testing with the Baha 4 s revealed limited benefit. At 1 year old, Jay was fit with bilateral BP110 aids with softband. Aided Ling 6 sounds were tested bilaterally thus far due to limited attention span. Results of aided testing revealed that the child is receiving limited benefit from the BP110 aids as well. Aided Ling 6 sounds with the Baha BP110 aids with softband were in the moderate hearing loss range. At that time, the audiologist requested that the managing ENT order a CT scan. Results of the CT scan revealed "bilateral cochlear dysplasia with isolated left dysplastic cochlea." Additionally, canaloplasty was contraindicated bilaterally.

Table 28.1 Audiological testing

	250 Hz	500 Hz	1,000 Hz	2,000 Hz	4,000 Hz	8,000 Hz
Right AC	105 dB HL	95 dB HL	DNT	100 dB HL	105 dB HL	DNT
Left AC	NR	NR	NR	120 dB HL	120 dB HL	DNT
BC	55 dB HL	60 dB HL	NR	70 dB HL	60 dB HL	
SAT	75-right	100-left				

Abbreviations: AC, air conduction; BC, bone conduction; DNT, did not test; NR, no response; SAT, speech awareness threshold.

29 Middle Ear Trauma: 4-Year-Old Girl

Lindi Berry and Aubrey Chesner

29.1 Clinical History and Description

TS, a 4-year-old girl, was seen for an audiological evaluation. She came into the clinic for testing after being discharged from the emergency room. According to the mother's report, she experienced right ear hearing loss, middle ear bleeding, and vestibular problems after a small, plastic toy sword was inserted deeply into her right ear during play with her older brother. Her mother, who is a high-level medical professional, immediately removed the toy sword. Her mother noted instant onset of nystagmus after removal of the sword and brought her child to the hospital, where she remained for 2 to 3 days for observation. The child reported double vision while in the hospital. The child was seen in the hospital by the otologist, who recommended immediate exploratory middle ear surgery, but the parents elected to wait. The child was then discharged and brought to the clinic for evaluation.

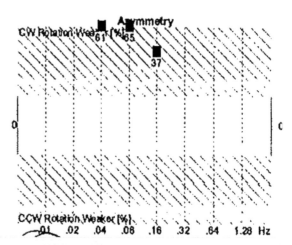

Fig. 29.1 Audiological results from TS's first visit following tympanic membrane (TM) trauma. The above figure displays the results of rotational chair testing.

29.2 Diagnostic Audiologic Evaluation Results

29.2.1 Visit 1

The child was initially seen for audiological testing the same day after being discharged from the hospital. She was frightened and still slightly sedated from her hospital stay. Testing was modified on this date to accommodate for her state of mind. Behaviorally, TS was able to complete tympanometry, speech reception thresholds (SRT), and rotational chair testing at this visit.

Tympanometry and SRT results for the left ear were well within normal limits, with a type A tympanogram and an SRT at 10 dB HL. Tympanometry in the right ear showed a large ear canal volume, which is consistent with right tympanic membrane perforation. SRTs of the right ear were found at 55 dB HL via masked air conduction and 10 dB HL via masked bone conduction. Results for the right ear indicated a moderate conductive hearing loss in the speech frequencies, at least. TS was also able to sit in the rotary chair with her mother at this visit. Rotational chair results demonstrated right asymmetry, which is consistent with an uncompensated right peripheral vestibular abnormality.[1] All results could be correlated to her recent right ear trauma. ▶ Fig. 29.1 shows all test results from this visit.

29.2.2 Visit 2

TS returned for further evaluation 2 days after the initial visit. She was in much better spirits and was able to perform more functional testing on this date. Pure tone audiometry was added to the test battery on this date. Because of the child's age and the complexity of masking, pure tone audiometry was only attempted for the right ear. Masking levels were assumed to mask the left ear by using the left SRT as a guideline. At only 4 years old, she was a reliable responder throughout behavioral testing.

Tympanometry and SRT results on this date remained within normal limits for the left ear. TS continued to have a large ear canal volume on the right ear tympanometry. SRTs of the right ear on this day were found at 40 dB HL via masked air conduction and 10 dB HL via masked bone conduction. Pure tone testing in the right ear revealed masked air-conduction thresholds between 35 and 65 dB HL at 500 to 4,000 Hz, with a sloping configuration. Pure tone masked bone-conduction thresholds were found between 5 and 10 dB HL at 500 to 4,000 Hz. Results from this visit indicated a mild to moderate conductive hearing loss and was again consistent with her right ear trauma and tympanic membrane perforation. Her rotary chair that day actually showed variable symmetry, which may have indicated the beginnings of compensation in her peripheral vestibular system.[1] ▶ Fig. 29.2 shows all test results from this visit.

29.2.3 Visit 3

TS returned for further evaluation 5 days after the initial visit. She began to report fluctuating right-sided tinnitus at this visit. Again, at 4 years of age, she was an excellent responder and reporter.

Tympanometry and SRT results on this date remained within normal limits for the left ear. She continued to have a large ear canal volume on the right ear tympanometry. Right ear SRTs were found at 35 dB HL via masked air conduction and 5 dB HL via masked bone conduction. Pure tone audiometry at this visit found right ear masked air-conduction thresholds at 30 to 85 dB HL. Masked bone-conduction thresholds were found between 10 and 20 dB HL. Results from this visit showed air-conduction threshold improvement at 500 to 2,000 Hz but deterioration at 4,000 Hz. Her rotational chair on the third visit continued to show improvement and compensation, with slight right asymmetry but mostly normal symmetry overall. ▶ Fig. 29.3 shows the test results from this visit.

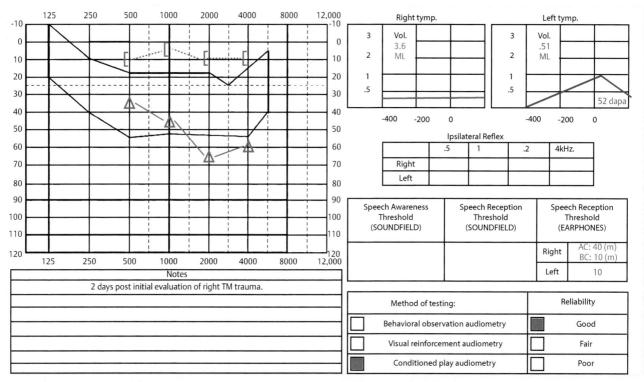

Fig. 29.2 Audiological results from TS's second visit following tympanic membrane (TM) trauma. The above figure displays the following test results: tympanometry, speech reception threshold (SRT), and pure tone audiometry of the right ear. △, right ear air conduction masked; [, right ear bone conduction masked.

29.2.4 Visit 4

Fourteen days later, TS returned for further monitoring. She reported complete resolution of her dizziness and double vision. However, she was still experiencing intermittent tinnitus. She was able to complete a comprehensive audiological evaluation in both ears on this day.

All audiological results for the left ear were within normal limits, with pure tone thresholds at 10 dB HL from 500 to 4,000 Hz, an SRT at 5 dB HL, 100% word recognition, and a type "A" tympanogram. Unfortunately, her right ear showed overall hearing deterioration at this visit. She continued to have a large ear canal volume on right tympanometry. Pure tone audiometry in the right ear now showed masked air-conduction thresholds at 50 to 100 dB HL from 500 to 6,000 Hz, with no response at 8,000 Hz. Masked bone-conduction thresholds were at 30 to 35 dB HL in the right ear. She now showed a right moderate to profound mixed hearing loss. Her masked air-conduction SRT was now 50 dB HL in the right ear. Even more alarming was her right ear word recognition score (WRS), which was first evaluated at this fourth visit. Her masked WRS (tested at 35 dB SL) was 20% in the right ear. ▶ Fig. 29.4 shows all test results from this visit.

29.2.5 Visit 5

At her last evaluation, her symptom complex had not changed. She was again able to reliably perform a full audiological evaluation.

This evaluation demonstrated consistent normal hearing sensitivity on the left ear, with 100% word understanding and a type "A" tympanogram. Her right ear showed continued deterioration at this visit. She still had a large ear canal volume on tympanometry in the right ear. Pure tone audiometry for the right ear now showed masked air-conduction thresholds at 50 to 100 dB HL and masked bone-conduction SRT at 60 dB HL and a WRS of 0%. She sat in her mother's lap during testing, so her mom could hear her responses. At the presentation level of 90 dB HL, her mother could plainly hear the words and hear how her daughter was responding incorrectly in the right ear. ▶ Fig. 29.5 shows all test results from this visit.

29.3 Outcome

Unfortunately, the patient did not return after her fifth visit and evaluation. Her mother's status in the medical field led her to seek a second opinion with colleagues in another city.

29.4 Questions for the Reader

1. Hindsight is 20/20. Looking back, what were some early signs that this may not be a typical tympanic membrane perforation trauma with a spontaneous healing and resolution of the hearing loss?
2. What etiologies could account for TS's hearing loss progression, and could these be a result of the trauma?

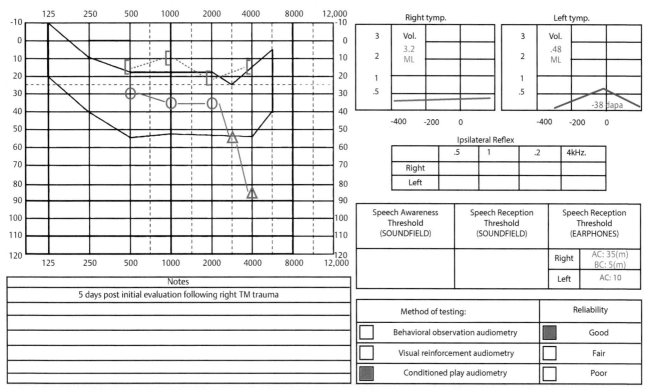

Fig. 29.3 Audiological results from TS's third visit following tympanic membrane (TM) trauma. The above figure displays the following test results: tympanometry, speech reception threshold (SRT), pure tone audiometry of the right ear, and rotational chair testing. O, right ear air conduction; △, right ear air conduction masked; [, right ear bone conduction masked.

3. Are there any additional tests that may have been useful during diagnosis and monitoring of this patient?

4. Why do you think the audiologist had the mother sit in the booth with her daughter during testing on the last visit?

5. Let us try to think ahead. If TS does not seek further medical care for her tympanic membrane perforation and the perforation fails to heal properly, what middle ear condition could develop?

6. With her change in hearing, what kind of difficulties would TS encounter on a daily basis?

7. What hearing device interventions would you recommend for this patient, assuming the right ear continues to progress and in consideration of her poor word understanding?

29.5 Discussion of Questions

1. **Hindsight is 20/20. Looking back, what were some early signs that this may not be a typical tympanic membrane perforation trauma with a spontaneous healing and resolution of the hearing loss?**

The child's onset of nystagmus upon removal of the sword was an indication that the labyrinth had been affected in the trauma.[2] Also, the sloping configuration of the hearing loss was opposite of what is typically seen with a tympanic membrane perforation that only affects the tympanic membrane. With a typical tympanic membrane perforation, a low-frequency conductive hearing loss is usually seen with the high

frequencies relatively intact.[3,4] The child's vertigo and high-frequency slope of hearing loss with continued deterioration could have been an early sign of inner ear involvement.[2,5] Also, the development of tinnitus at later appointments could also signal a sensorineural component.[6]

2. **What etiologies could account for TS's hearing loss progression, and could these be a result of the trauma?**

Since TS ceased care at this clinic, the exact site of lesion for her case remains unknown. However, penetrating trauma to the tympanic membrane can result in ossicular disarticulation and/or fracturing of the stapedial footplate.[5] Dislocated or fractured pieces of the ossicular chain can subsequently puncture the oval or round window, resulting in a perilymphatic fistula and leakage of perilymph into the middle ear space.[5] Ossification can also occur subsequently as a long-term effect of a penetrating injury to the tympanic membrane.[2]

3. **Are there any additional tests that may have been useful during diagnosis and monitoring of this patient?**

Earlier word recognition testing would have been beneficial to compare across evaluations. Given the low bone-conduction SRT along with normal bone-conduction thresholds, it was assumed by the clinician that the child's word recognition was good to excellent during her initial visits. However, it would have been interesting to compare WRS across all evaluations to determine whether the WRS declined simultaneously with the decline in bone-conduction thresholds or if the WRS was poor all along.

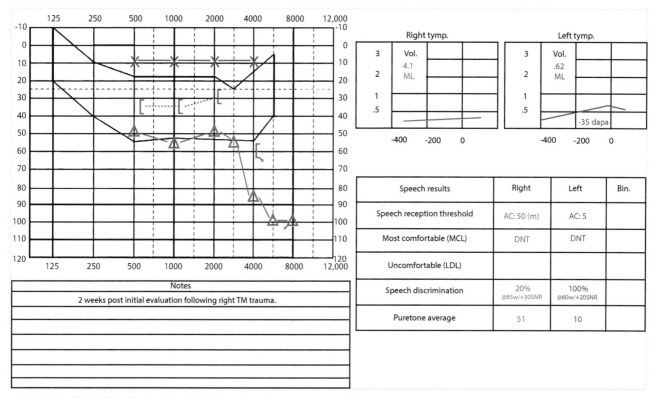

Fig. 29.4 Audiological results from TS's fourth visit following tympanic membrane (TM) trauma. The above figure displays the following test results: tympanometry, speech reception threshold (SRT), word recognition scores (WRS), and pure tone audiometry. X, left ear air conduction; △, right ear air conduction masked; [, right ear bone conduction masked; Arrows, no response.

4. **Why do you think the audiologist had the mother sit in the booth with her daughter during testing on the last visit?**

Given that the mother is in the medical field and had previously declined surgery, having the mother observe the difference in the child's responses between ears was used as a counseling opportunity.

5. **Let us try to think ahead. If TS does not seek further medical care for her tympanic membrane perforation and the perforation fails to heal properly, what middle ear condition could develop?**

An acquired secondary cholesteatoma can develop following tympanic membrane perforation. The perforation can allow squamous epithelium from the ear canal to migrate into the middle ear cavity. The squamous epithelium in the middle ear cavity can become trapped and can collect over time, causing a cholesteatoma to form.[6]

6. **With her change in hearing, what kind of difficulties would TS encounter on a daily basis?**

Patients with unilateral hearing loss may compensate in quiet, one-on-one environments, although the head shadow effect may result in some difficulty in quiet when the signal of interest arises from the side of the poor ear. However, in background noise, patients will struggle with clarity and word understanding. They also lose interaural timing and intensity cues, which leads to reduced ability to localize.[7]

7. **What hearing device interventions would you recommend for this patient, assuming the right ear continues to progress and in consideration of her poor word understanding?**

Given the poor word understanding score, a traditional monaural hearing may not provide benefit. The patient has one normal hearing ear as well. Treatment for single-sided deafness, such as an osseointegrated bone conduction implant system, would provide her the most benefit in quiet situations.[8] She may also be a candidate for a cochlear implant. Given her pediatric status and pending school enrollment, a device with wireless accessories and/or remote microphone technology should be a top consideration for noisy settings.[8] Other educational recommendations should also be part of the patient's educational plan, such as strategic seating or the teacher repeating and rephrasing as necessary.

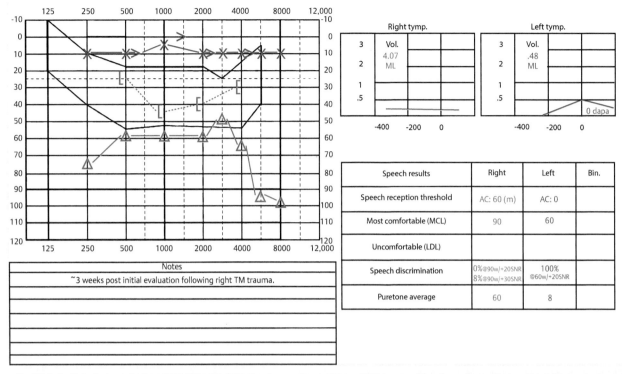

Speech results	Right	Left	Bin.
Speech reception threshold	AC: 60 (m)	AC: 0	
Most comfortable (MCL)	90	60	
Uncomfortable (LDL)			
Speech discrimination	0%@90w/+20SNR 8%@90w/+30SNR	100% @60w/+20SNR	
Puretone average	60	8	

Fig. 29.5 Audiological results from TS's fifth visit following tympanic membrane (TM) trauma. The above figure displays the following test results: tympanometry, speech reception threshold (SRT), word recognition scores (WRS), and pure tone audiometry. X, left ear air conduction; △, right ear air conduction masked; [, right ear bone conduction masked.

References

[1] Ahmed MF. Rotational chair testing in patients with unilateral peripheral vestibular disorders. Egypt J Otolaryngol. 2015; 31(2):115–121

[2] Adunka OF, Buchman CA. Surgical therapy of the temporal bone. In: Otology, Neurotology, and Lateral Skull Base Surgery. Stuttgart: Thieme; 2011: 287-289

[3] Mehta RP, Rosowski JJ, Voss SE, O'Neil E, Merchant SN. Determinants of hearing loss in perforations of the tympanic membrane. Otol Neurotol. 2006; 27 (2):136–143

[4] Nahata V, Patil CY, Patil RK, Gattani G, Disawal A, Roy A. Tympanic membrane perforation: Its correlation with hearing loss and frequency affected - An analytical study. Indian J Otol. 2014; 20:10–15

[5] Miyamoto R. Traumatic perforation of the tympanic membrane. MSD Manual Professional Edition. 2015. Available at: http://www.merckmanuals.com/professional/ear,-nose,-and-throat-disorders/middle-ear-and-tympanic-membrane-disorders/traumatic-perforation-of-the-tympanic-membrane#v944971. Accessed March 22, 2017

[6] Shanks J, Shohet J. Tympanometry in clinical practice. In: Katz J, Medwetsky L, Burkard R, Hood L, eds. Handbook of Clinical Audiology. 6th ed. Philadelphia, PA: Lippincott Williams & Wilkins; 2009:182

[7] Nishihata R, Vieira MR, Pereira LD, Chiari BM. Temporal processing, localization and auditory closure in individuals with unilateral hearing loss. Rev Soc Bras Fonoaudiol. 2012; 17(3):266–273

[8] Oyler R, McKay S. Unilateral hearing loss in children. ASHA Lead. 2008; 13 (1):12–15

30 Decreased Sound Tolerance (Misophonia)

Lori Zitelli and Catherine Palmer

30.1 Clinical History and Description

A 15-year-old adolescent girl presented with a primary complaint of decreased sound tolerance. Mary was initially seen with her mother in the otology clinic for medical clearance prior to an evaluation for tinnitus retraining therapy (TRT). She reported that she had suffered from decreased sound tolerance since she was approximately 7 years old and that she has had difficulty finding someone to help her with this condition. She had previously seen several ear, nose, and throat physicians as well as several psychologists without benefit. She had unsuccessfully tried cognitive behavioral therapy when she was younger. She reported occasional, very brief episodes of tinnitus that were not bothersome. She reported that certain sounds evoked a negative emotional and physical body response when she heard them. Sounds that were reported as especially bothersome included gum cracking, tongue clicking, keyboard tapping, coughing, sniffling, her dog drinking water from its bowl, birds chirping, candy wrappers being crinkled, and tapping sounds on desks. She did not specifically report that loud sounds were bothersome. When asked to rank the severity of her sound tolerance problem, annoyance level, and the overall effect on her life, each of those categories were rated as 10/10 problems (10 being the worst a problem could be).

She reported that she has a 504 plan at school, which provides accommodations (moving classes to a larger classroom so that she is not "trapped" by bothersome sounds, moving a triggering classmate to a seat behind her so that she does not see him typing or swinging his leg, changing her schedule so that the classes she likes most are at the end of the day when her coping resources are depleted). She reported that she tries to educate her classmates about her condition, although certain classmates are not cooperative when she asks them to stop making bothersome sounds.

When asked about depression, anxiety, or other relevant health issues, she reported that she experiences anxiety when she hears bothersome sounds and also in situations when she anticipates that sounds will bother her before they happen. She was encouraged to follow up with her pediatrician to discuss this issue and it was explained that many patients who are able to treat underlying anxiety or depression can experience a reduction in their negative reaction to sounds that are bothersome. She reported that she always carries earplugs and uses them frequently when *hearing* bothersome sounds and *in anticipation* of bothersome sounds. Her mother reported that Mary often isolates herself from her family and friends because she always believes that they will make sounds that she cannot tolerate.

30.2 Audiologic Testing

Otoscopy was completed and was consistent with normal external auditory canals and tympanic membranes. Pure-tone audiometric testing yielded normal hearing thresholds from 250 through 8,000 Hz (▶ Fig. 30.1). Speech understanding was tested using NU-6 (Northwestern University Auditory Test No. 6) recorded materials (25 word lists). This testing was completed in quiet at conversational levels and scores of 96% were obtained bilaterally. Mary was not hearing tinnitus at the time of testing, so pitch and loudness matching and masking could not be completed. Loudness discomfort levels (LDLs)

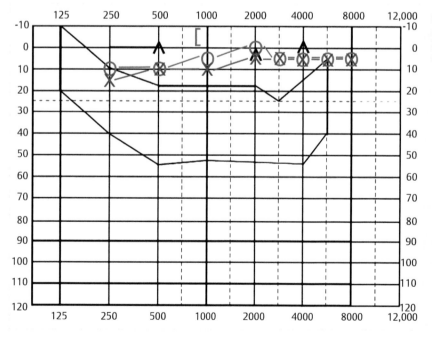

Fig. 30.1 Audiometric data. O, right ear air conduction; X, left ear air conduction; [, right ear bone conduction masked; Λ, unspecified bone conduction.

were assessed using pure tones and speech (▶ Fig. 30.2). In the right ear, LDLs for pure tones ranged from 75 to 105 dB HL and the LDL for speech was 95 dB HL. In the left ear, LDLs for pure tones ranged from 75 to 100 dB HL and LDL for speech was 90 dB HL. Distortion product otoacoustic emissions (DPOAEs) were assessed using a conventional protocol with 65-/55-dB intensities and a 10-point per octave recording (▶ Fig. 30.3). Results indicated largely present and robust DPOAEs from 1,000 through 8,000 Hz with some slightly reduced responses in the midfrequency range bilaterally.

30.3 Questions for the Reader

1. What is the difference between misophonia and hyperacusis?
2. Why complete LDL testing when she does not report that loud sounds are bothersome?
3. What are the services available for students with disabilities under Section 504 of the Rehabilitation Act of 1973?
4. Why do patients often find treatment of underlying anxiety and/or depression helpful when they also suffer from decreased sound tolerance?
5. Are earplugs an appropriate treatment option?

30.4 Discussion of Questions

1. **What is the difference between misophonia and hyperacusis?**
Hyperacusis occurs when there is an abnormally strong reaction to sound occurring within the auditory pathways. This reaction happens purely as a result of the physical characteristics of the sound (intensity, frequency, etc.). In contrast, misophonia occurs when a patient has abnormally strong reactions of the autonomic and limbic systems resulting from enhanced connections between the auditory and limbic systems. These reactions are dependent partially on the physical characteristics of the sound *and* the patient's previous experiences with that sound (i.e., the context in which they hear the sounds).

2. **Why complete LDL testing when she does not report that loud sounds are bothersome?**
Jastreboff and Jastreboff report that LDLs of 30 to 120 dB HL have been measured in individuals with misophonia.[1] Given this range, LDLs are insufficient to diagnose misophonia or separate it from hyperacusis, so a detailed interview is required in conjunction with testing. The LDL results are one more piece of the puzzle to consider when tailoring the treatment recommended for the individual.

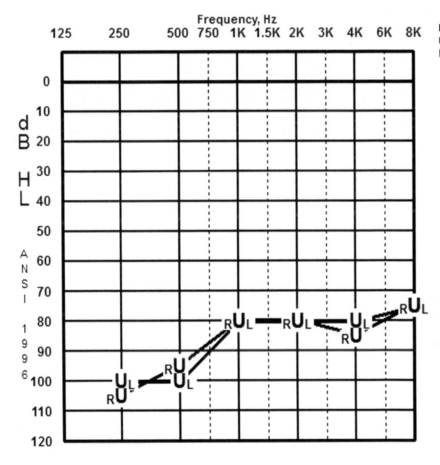

Fig. 30.2 Pure-tone loudness discomfort results. U, uncomfortable loudness level; R, right ear; L, left ear.

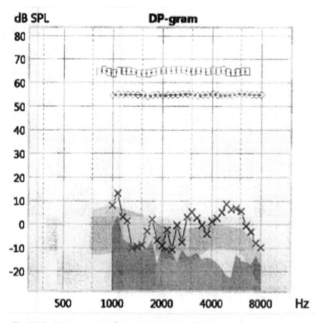 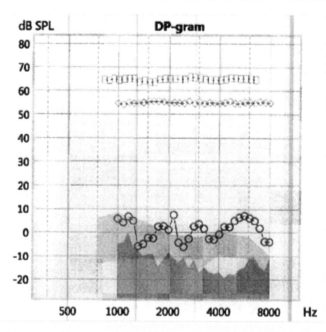

Fig. 30.3 Distortion product otoacoustic emission results.

3. What are the services available for students with disabilities under Section 504 of the Rehabilitation Act of 1973?

"Section 504 states that 'no qualified individual with a disability in the United States shall be excluded from, denied the benefits of, or be subjected to discrimination under' any program or activity that either receives Federal financial assistance or is conducted by any Executive agency or the United States Postal Service."

(https://www.ada.gov/cguide.htm)

"An appropriate education for a student with a disability under the Section 504 regulations could consist of education in regular classrooms, education in regular classes with supplementary services, and/or special education and related services."

(https://www.ed.gov/)

In Mary's case, a health care professional had to submit data to support her being considered an individual with a disability and the school had to accept this and therefore agree to have her services covered under Section 504 of the Rehabilitation Act of 1973.

4. Why do patients often find treatment of underlying anxiety and/or depression helpful when they also suffer from decreased sound tolerance?

Anxiety is often reported by patients with misophonia. This may be thought of as a consequence of misophonia and may be targeted in cognitive behavioral therapy to increase the individual's ability to manage their reactions to triggering sounds. If the patient is able to manage their reaction, anger outbursts may be reduced, which will assist the individual in participating in a variety of social situations. Wu et al support the notion that the maladaptive behaviors seen in misophonia are consistent with other cognitive behavioral models

of related constructs such as obsessive compulsive disorder (OCD) and anxiety and can be approached similarly in terms of treating the underlying anxiety caused by the condition.[2]

5. Are earplugs an appropriate treatment option?

Earplugs are not an appropriate treatment option because if patients are wearing earplugs, they are not hearing the offending sounds and consequently cannot extinguish their reaction to the sounds. Jastreboff and Jastreboff report that misophonia results from enhanced functional connections between the auditory, limbic, and autonomic nervous systems, which are governed by principles of conditioned reflexes.[3] The goal of the treatment used for misophonia is to weaken and then remove these connections by linking currently offensive sounds with something positive.

30.5 Diagnosis and Recommended Treatment

Despite Mary's reduced LDLs, she reported that loud sounds do not impact her functionally. She was diagnosed with misophonia in accordance with the proposed diagnostic criteria outlined by Schröder et al.[4] Enrollment in TRT was recommended. We discussed the specifics of the program in detail (counseling and sound therapy aspects, follow-up schedule, out-of-pocket costs, and realistic outcomes). She was made aware that the costs of TRT are typically not covered by insurance. She had previously tried behind-the-ear (BTE) hearing aids that had integrated sound therapy at a misophonia conference and found the sound included in these devices very pleasing, so these devices were eventually incorporated into her treatment protocol.

On the day of Mary's informational counseling session, we discussed her test results, hearing anatomy, concepts of auditory signal suppression and enhancement, conditioned reflexes, and sound therapy. We also discussed how sound therapy is incorporated into treatment for misophonia using devices. BTE hearing aids that she had previously tried were ordered, and she returned for the device fitting a few weeks later. Manual program sequence for these devices included three sound options with the volume control enabled in all programs via the on-board volume toggle. She had no difficulty inserting or removing the devices, changing the batteries, switching among programs, or operating the volume control toggle.

The four protocols for treatment of misophonia are outlined in detail in Jastreboff and Jastreboff.[1] These protocols begin with the type and intensity of sound that is used being totally under the patient's control and gradually removing control over time. The overarching goal is for the patient to be comfortable in any sound environment without having control over the sounds around them. In the beginning of therapy, this is partially achieved by the individual having sound therapy available to them through a personally worn device. Ideally, the sound therapy is finally entirely removed as the individual becomes tolerant of the world of sounds around them.

On the day of Mary's device delivery, protocol 1 was explained and recommended for use over the first few weeks of treatment. On the day of her 3-week follow-up, she reported that she had worn the devices consistently according to the assigned protocol 1. She requested some slight programming adjustments to the sound therapy sounds (slightly increasing default level) and was pleased with the results. At that time, we reviewed protocols 2 and 3, which she was instructed to implement in addition to continuing protocol 1 over the next 2 months. Mary and her mother reported a clear understanding of the protocols and associated goals. At that time, Mary also reported that she had seen a cognitive behavioral therapist at my recommendation and had a very positive experience. She also reported that she had begun pharmacologic treatment for her anxiety as recommended by her pediatrician.

On the day of her 3-month follow-up, Mary reported that she had difficulty completing protocol 2 (which requires her to watch television or listen to music with someone whom she trusted to control the level of sound) because she and her mother initially had difficulty finding things to watch or listen to for extended periods of time that they both enjoyed. They eventually did find that they liked watching animal shows together and completed that activity approximately four times per week. She also reported that they had implemented protocol 3 although not as diligently as they should have. She reported that she believed the devices were helping her and that she had been having easier days at school. Her mother reported that Mary sat down to eat Easter dinner with her family, which she had previously not done in years. She also reported three other occasions in recent weeks where Mary had joined a large group of people (a family cookout, Mary's own birthday party, and a regional choir festival) and was able to tolerate sounds much better than previously. Mary reported that she believed the combination of devices, therapy, and anxiety medication had all been helpful to her. She reported that

she really likes working with her therapist and was continuing to see her every 2 weeks. At this time, we discussed protocol 4, which Mary was instructed to implement over the next few weeks in addition to the other protocols when she could. She and her mother were both pleased with her progress at that time. Mary provided the following ranks when asked about the severity of her problem (9/10), her annoyance level (9/10), and the effect on her life (7/10), with 10 being the worst a problem could be.

Three months later, Mary reported that she has been doing very well. She reported working as a server in a restaurant where she says sounds typically do not bother her much although she does occasionally find the sound of plates clanking annoying. She reported that she was still seeing her cognitive behavioral therapist with benefit and was using coping strategies, which she believes are very effective for her. She also reported that she was continuing to use her antianxiety medications with benefit. At that time, she reported using the BTE hearing aids only when needed (e.g., when going to the mall with her friends or occasionally at work). Overall, she reported that she is still sometimes bothered by sounds but does not feel as though she reacts as strongly or stays bothered as long as she used to before beginning treatment. Mary applied the following ranks when asked about the severity of her problem (3/10), her annoyance level (3/10), and the effect on her life (2/10). Testing was repeated on this day and revealed essentially stable audiometric and tolerance results.

30.6 Outcome

Six months later, Mary reported that she was continuing to do very well. She reported that she still hears sounds that would have once been bothersome, but now feels that being bothered by them would be silly. She reported that school was not a problem and that her coping skills had dramatically improved. She reported that the restaurant she continued to work at often serves children (whose screaming she previously would not have been able to tolerate) and patrons who eat chips, which she also would not have tolerated well prior to treatment. She reported that misophonia no longer limited her participation in life. She reported rarely wearing the devices but still carried them in her purse in case she needed them in a challenging environment. Mary applied the following ranks when asked about the severity of her problem (1/10), her annoyance level (0/10), and the effect on her life (0/10). Mary was very pleased with her progress and expressed that she "owed her life to me." Her mother was also very grateful.

At that time, Mary was discharged from TRT and was encouraged to continue using the strategies that she had learned in addition to continuing cognitive behavioral therapy and antianxiety medications. She was asked to contact the audiology department as needed.

References

[1] Jastreboff PJ, Jastreboff MM. Decreased sound tolerance: hyperacusis, misophonia, diplacousis, and polyacousis. Handb Clin Neurol. 2015; 129:375–387

[2] Wu MS, Lewin AB, Murphy TK, Storch EA. Misophonia: incidence, phenomenology, and clinical correlates in an undergraduate student sample. J Clin Psychol. 2014; 70(10):994–1007

[3] Jastreboff PJ, Jastreboff MM. Treatments for decreased sound tolerance (hyperacusis and misophonia). Semin Hear. 2014; 35(02):105–120

[4] Schröder A, Vulink N, Denys D. Misophonia: diagnostic criteria for a new psychiatric disorder. PLoS One. 2013; 8(1):e54706

Suggested Readings

[1] Bernstein RE, Angell KL, Dehle CM. A brief course of cognitive behavioural therapy for the treatment of misophonia: a case example. Cogn Behav Ther. 2013; 6:e10

[2] Duddy DF, Oeding KA. Misophonia: an overview. Semin Hear. 2014; 35 (2):84–91

[3] U.S. Department of Justice. A Guide to Disability Rights Laws. U.S. Department of Justice. Available at: https://www.ada.gov/cguide.htm; 2017

[4] U.S. Department of Education. Home. U.S. Department of Education. Available at: https://www.ed.gov/; 2017

31 Congenital Profound Hearing Loss, Noonan's Syndrome, and Cochlear Implantation

Neil Sperling and Michelle Kraskin

31.1 Clinical History and Description

Michael is a baby boy with a history of premature birth, born at 30 weeks of gestation via C-section due to breech presentation. He is a fraternal twin. His birth weight is 2.4 lb (1,340 g)—normal birth weight is greater than 2,500 g.

Michael had an extended stay in the neonatal intensive care unit (NICU; 3 months) due to low birth weight and respiratory and feeding problems. He required intubation for respiratory support for several days and early placement of a gastrostomy feeding tube. He had multiple respiratory tract infections requiring antibiotics including aminoglycosides.

He did not pass the newborn hearing screening. Audiologic follow-up was delayed due to multiple medical problems.

There is no family history of hearing issues. His fraternal twin has no hearing issues.

31.2 Audiologic Testing

Examination of the external ear anatomy and tympanic membrane was normal.

Audiologic evaluation at 4 months of age revealed the following:
- Normal tympanograms using 1,000-Hz probe tone.
- Auditory brainstem response (ABR) results:
  - Right ear: moderate to profound mixed hearing loss.
  - Left ear: severe to profound hearing loss.

Michael was enrolled in early intervention that included physical therapy (PT), occupational therapy (OT), and speech/language interventions. He was referred to our institution.

Sedated ABR completed at 6 months was consistent with bilateral, profound hearing loss.

Air conduction: right and left ears—In response to tone bursts at 500, 2,000, and 4,000 Hz, a wave V was absent at the output limits of the equipment.

Bone conduction: right and left ears—In response to tone bursts at 500, 2,000, and 4,000 Hz, a wave V was absent at the output limits of the equipment.

Click ABR (to rule out auditory neuropathy) at 90 dB normal hearing level (nHL) showed no evidence of a present cochlear microphonic (CM). If a CM is present, then it will invert with a change in stimulus polarity. If the waveform does not invert, then the clinician can surmise that it is a neural response and not a CM.

Michael was provided amplification: Oticon Sensei Pro SP behind-the-ear (BTE) hearing aids coupled with full shell molds (▶ Fig. 31.1)

Genetic testing at 6 months: Whole exome sequencing revealed Noonan's syndrome, which is characterized by distinctive facial features, short stature, congenital heart defect, developmental delay, and platelet dysfunction. External ear anomalies and conductive and sensorineural hearing loss have been reported.

Otolaryngology evaluation at 6 months: Michael was alert but not responsive to auditory stimuli. Abundant verbalizations

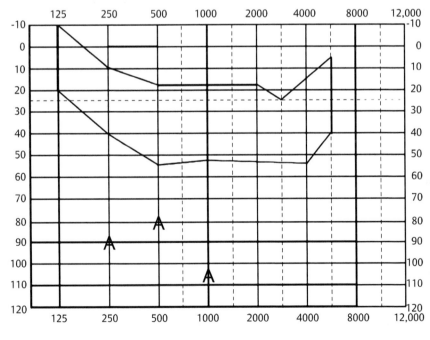

Fig. 31.1 Aided, binaural, behavioral testing at 12 months. A, binaural hearing aids behind the ear.

were noted. Ear examination was normal. On laryngoscopy, subglottic stenosis was diagnosed. Computed tomography (CT) and magnetic resonance imaging (MRI) were consistent with normal cochlea and cochlear nerve development.

Michael's mother reported no apparent benefit from or response to amplification. According to the audiometric results, the patient utilized his Oticon Sensei Pro SP BTE hearing aids coupled to full shell molds. In the binaural, aided condition, thresholds to narrow band noise (NBN) stimuli in the sound field obtained using visual reinforcement audiometry (VRA) were in the range of 80 to 90 dB HL between 250 and 500 Hz (marked in the figure as "A"). No responses could be obtained for tone burst at 750 to 6,000 Hz at the limits of the equipment.

Awareness thresholds to recorded Ling six sounds were obtained (▶ Table 31.1). No aided responses could be obtained for the right- or left-aided condition at limits of the equipment.

Speech/language evaluation at 12-month assessment was limited due to the absence of speech (▶ Table 31.2).

31.3 The Rossetti Infant-Toddler Language Scale

Interaction attachment: age appropriate.

Pragmatics: **DELAYED;** 0 to 3 months with emerging skills at 3 to 6 months.

Play: **DELAYED;** 3 to 6 months.

Language comprehension: **DELAYED;** developing skills at the 0- to 3-month level.

Language expression: **DELAYED;** 0 to 3 months with developing skills at the 3- to 6-month level.

31.4 Diagnosis and Recommended Treatment

Michael has a bilateral, profound sensorineural hearing loss with additional medical complications.

A plan for cochlear implantation (CI) by 12 months was not possible due to severe feeding problems and slow weight gain. At 12 months, height was 65 cm (< 1st percentile) and weight was 17.5 lb (7.95 kg; 10%). CI, therefore, was delayed until nutritional status improved, allowing for sufficient weight gain.

Unilateral CI was performed at 17 months and 20-lb body weight. A pediatric laryngologist was available for intubation. Full insertion of a left cochlear 522 slim straight electrode was obtained via a cochleostomy. Neural response telemetry revealed responses in 22 of 22 electrodes (▶ Fig. 31.1).

Table 31.1 Aided responses to the Ling six sounds

Ling	Right threshold	Left threshold	Bilateral
"m"	NR at 100 dB HL	NR at 100 dB HL	90 dB HL
"o"	NR at 100 dB HL	NR at 100 dB HL	NR at 100 dB HL
"a"	NR at 100 dB HL	NR at 100 dB HL	100 dB HL
"e"	NR at 100 dB HL	NR at 100 dB HL	NR at 100 dB HL
"sh"	NR at 100 dB HL	NR at 100 dB HL	NR at 100 dB HL
"s"	NR at 100 dB HL	NR at 100 dB HL	NR at 100 dB HL

NR, no response.

Table 31.2 Preschool Language Scales, Fifth Edition (PLS-5)

Auditory comprehension	
Standard score	50
Percentile rank	1st
Age equivalent	2 mo
Expressive communication	
Standard score	56
Percentile rank	1st
Age equivalent	5 mo
Total language score	
Standard score	50
Percentile rank	1st
Age equivalent	3 mo

Surgical blood loss was moderate (estimated at 30 mL). Modest hematoma occurred postoperatively due to thrombocytopenia and was contained with pressure dressing. Early resolution occurred over the first several days. Postoperative anemia occurred, and the patient was hospitalized for evaluation and support. Transfusion was not needed.

31.5 Outcome

Initial stimulation went well at 3 weeks postimplantation. Speech and language therapies were initiated. Testing was performed at 3 months post initial activation in the sound field, 0-degree azimuth, 4 feet from the speaker with the left N6 processor. The patient's father was standing with the patient in his arms as he had difficulty remaining seated. He was prone to fixating on assistant, light, ceiling, and VRA reward, and responses are likely suprathreshold as a result.

AutoNRT Threshold Chart

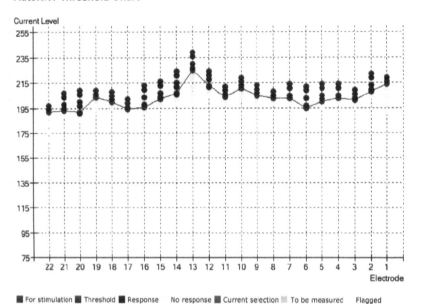

Fig. 31.2 Intraoperative neural response telemetry. Neural responses were present for all electrodes.

■ For stimulation ■ Threshold ■ Response   No response ■ Current selection ▨ To be measured   Flagged

Table 31.3 Implanted responses to the Ling six sounds

Ling	Left cochlear implantation
"m"	40 dB HL
"o"	35 dB HL
"a"	45 dB HL
"i"	40 dB HL
"sh"	40 dB HL
"s"	DNT

DNT, did not test.

Utilizing VRA in the booth, thresholds to NBN stimuli in sound field were in the range of 30 to 45 dB HL between 500 and 4,000 Hz with the left cochlear implant (see ▶ Fig. 31.2, plotted as "L"). Speech awareness threshold was obtained at 40 dB HL.

Awareness thresholds to recorded Ling six sounds obtained for six Ling sounds are listed in ▶ Table 31.3.

31.6 Questions for the Reader

1. What is the cause of hearing loss in this case?
2. What is the optimal time for CI in a child with a congenital, profound hearing loss?
3. Why was bilateral CI not done?

31.7 Discussion of Questions

1. **What is the cause of hearing loss in this case?**
   Although Noonan's syndrome is a recognized cause for hearing loss, there are many other risk factors in this case. These include prematurity, low birth weight, ventilator support,

and exposure to aminoglycosides. The exact cause and to what degree his hearing loss is multifactorial are unknown.

Noonan's syndrome is a genetic disorder with an incidence of approximately 1 in 1,000 to 2,500 live births. It can be inherited or spontaneous. It is characterized by craniofacial dysmorphic features, which include low set, posteriorly rotated ears, short stature, congenital heart defects, and coagulation defects. The phenotype is variable. Since 2001, the diagnosis can be obtained with genetic testing. Hearing loss is a variable feature of Noonan's syndrome, and has been reported in 40% of cases. Hearing loss varies in severity and type with reports of sensorineural, conductive, and mixed hearing loss types from mild to profound.

2. **What is the optimal time for CI in a child with a congenital, profound hearing loss?**
   There is universal agreement that early CI gives a congenitally deaf child the best chance for optimal speech and language development. The Food and Drug Administration indication for CI in children remains at 12 months of age, but many centers implant at earlier ages. Bilateral simultaneous or sequential implantation is optional.

3. **Why was bilateral CI not done?**
   This case presents the challenges of early implantation in the presence of mitigating medical conditions. There is a need for interdisciplinary planning. Engaging the multiple specialists involved in the care of Michael was required to determine the earliest time that the surgery can proceed safely. The relative fragile nature of a patient like Michael and the impact of even a limited amount of blood loss highlight some of the surgical challenges. Sequential implantation was deemed safer given the need for extended general anesthesia and increased blood loss from a simultaneous bilateral implantation. Sequential implantation is planned for Michael 3 to 6 months after the first implantation.

Suggested Readings

[1] van Nierop JWI, van Trier DC, van der Burgt I, et al. Cochlear implantation and clinical features in patients with Noonan syndrome and Noonan syndrome with multiple lentigines caused by a mutation in PTPN11. Int J Pediatr Otorhinolaryngol. 2017; 97:228–234

[2] Tokgoz-Yilmaz S, Turkyilmaz MD, Cengiz FB, Sjöstrand AP, Kose SK, Tekin M. Audiological findings in Noonan syndrome. Int J Pediatr Otorhinolaryngol. 2016; 89:50–54

[3] Kassebaum N, Kyu HH, Zoeckler L, et al. Global Burden of Disease Child and Adolescent Health Collaboration. Child and adolescent health from 1990 to 2015: findings from the global burden of diseases, injuries, and risk factors 2015 study. JAMA Pediatr. 2017; 171(6):573–592

32 Cytomegalovirus

Elizabeth Preston

32.1 Clinical History and Description

Amber, now 6 years old, received audiology services at a pediatric audiology clinic as a toddler after not passing a hearing evaluation at the otolaryngologist's office. Amber was born at 37 weeks' gestational age with no complications present. At 35 weeks' gestational age, an ultrasound was completed due to her mother suffering from cholestasis, a liver disease, during pregnancy, and results showed enlarged ventricles and a large fontanel. The day after she was born, a repeat ultrasound was completed, which showed a possible brain bleed. The next day, Amber underwent an MRI, which revealed germanic cysts consistent with a congenital toxoplasmosis, rubella, cytomegalovirus, herpes simplex, or HIV (TORCH) infection. At this time, no further recommendations were made regarding the MRI results and a definitive diagnosis of TORCH was not made.

Amber did not pass the newborn hearing screening in the hospital. An outpatient follow-up screening was completed at the hospital at 3 weeks of age, which is within the timeline recommended by the Joint Committee on Infant Hearing, and she had no response on the Automated Auditory Brainstem Response (A-ABR) screening for both ears.[1] A diagnostic ABR was done the same day by the audiologist. The report indicated thresholds obtained for a click stimulus were 30 dB normalized hearing level (nHL) in the right ear and 25 dB nHL for the left ear. The tone burst ABR was not able to be completed because Amber woke up. Based on these results, the audiologist diagnosed Amber with "essentially normal hearing sensitivity in the left ear for 500–4000 Hz." The right ear was "suspected" to have normal hearing; however, a mild hearing loss could not be ruled out. It was recommended Amber have a behavioral audiological evaluation at 9 months of age.

At 16 months of age, Amber was seen at the otolaryngologist (ear, nose, and throat [ENT]) due to recurrent ear infections over 4 months' time, which were all treated with antibiotics. Her parents reported she was only saying 3 to 4 single words. Her mother also reported noticing Amber does not always hear her mom approaching from behind. An audiometric evaluation was completed in the sound field using visual reinforcement audiometry (VRA) and responses were consistent with a moderate hearing loss in at least the better ear.

The American Academy of Otolaryngology-Head and Neck Surgery published *The Clinical Practice Guideline: Tympanostomy Tubes in Children*, which states that tympanostomy tubes should be offered as a treatment when a child has had otitis media with effusion (OME) in both ears for more than 3 months with a documented hearing loss.[2] Amber underwent surgery for pressure equalizer (PE) tube placement, and a hearing evaluation was attempted postoperatively. A speech detection threshold was obtained through the sound field at 50 dB, and no further responses could be obtained, so the recommendation was for a sedated ABR.

Results of the ABR were consistent with a moderate sensorineural hearing loss in the left ear, and a severe sensorineural hearing loss in the right ear. Hearing aids were recommended and a referral was made for early intervention (EI) services. Under the Individuals with Disabilities Education Act (IDEA) Part C regulation, it is required that a child be referred for Part C services "as soon as possible but in no case more than seven days" after a hearing loss has been diagnosed.[3]

Because of Amber's history of possible TORCH, she was suspected of having congenital cytomegalovirus (CMV). Blood work was completed and those results came back positive for the antibody. At this point, her blood spot from phenylketonuria (PKU) testing at birth was pulled and tested for CMV. It also came back positive, confirming congenital CMV.

CMV is the cause of 15 to 20% of moderate to profound sensorineural hearing loss and is the number one cause of hearing loss not associated with genetics.[4,5]

32.2 Audiologic Testing

Amber was 18 months of age at the time of her first visit to the pediatric audiology clinic, when she came for a diagnostic reevaluation.[6] Her test results were consistent with patent PE tubes, for each ear, when assessed using 226-Hz probe tone tympanometry. VRA with the use of insert earphones revealed hearing thresholds consistent with a profound hearing loss in the right ear and a severe rising to moderate hearing loss in the left ear.

32.3 Questions for the Reader

1. When a hearing loss is first diagnosed, what recommendations/referrals are appropriate?
2. Would you recommend a cochlear implant for Amber? Why/why not?
3. What type of follow-up testing is appropriate at this point?

32.4 Discussion of Questions

1. **When a hearing loss is first diagnosed, what recommendations/referrals are appropriate?**
- A referral to EI is a must, which in this case has already been initiated.[1]
- A referral to an otolaryngologist for a full medical evaluation (thorough case history, evaluation of head and neck, scans of ears to look for structural abnormalities, and possibly other blood work). Amber is established with an otolaryngologist, and a full medical evaluation has been completed.[1]
- A referral to an ophthalmologist for an assessment of vision.[1]
- Possible referral for genetic testing.[1]
- Resources should be given to the family for learning modules, family support groups, and organizations focused on families.

2. **Would you recommend a cochlear implant for Amber? Why/why not?**
- The Food and Drug Administration (FDA) has approved cochlear implantation for any child who is at least 12 months of

age and has a profound sensorineural hearing loss bilaterally (> 90 dB).[7]

- A lack of hearing aid benefit must be shown by proving inappropriate simple auditory skill development and/or less than or equal to 30% correct word recognition with the use of a simple open-set word list.[7]
- A hearing aid trial between 3 and 6 months should be completed.[7]

3. **What type of follow-up testing is appropriate at this point?**

- A follow-up hearing evaluation should be completed in 2 weeks to continue to monitor Amber's hearing. Due to her history of progressive hearing loss and the diagnosis of CMV, possibly congenital, it is important to aggressively follow this child.[10,11]
- Hearing aids would be an appropriate recommendation at this point. Earmold impressions were taken at this appointment and hearing aids will be fitted when they return in 2 weeks for follow-up testing.

32.5 Recommendations, Additional Testing, and Outcome

Amber returned for a reevaluation and hearing aid fitting in 2 weeks. The hearing aids were verified using simulated speech-mapping.[10] After the fitting, Amber was tired and uncooperative, so the hearing evaluation was postponed for a different day.

In a week, the hearing evaluation was completed and results were consistent with no measureable responses in the right ear and measureable responses at 2,000 and 4,000 Hz only in the left ear in the profound hearing range. Appropriate adjustments were made to the hearing aids and validation of the hearing aids was completed 2 days later with the use of aided thresholds. Validation of amplification is an important step in knowing the child is receiving sufficient auditory access for the reception of speech and language information.[11] Aided thresholds revealed auditory access to Amber's brain in the severe hearing loss range for her left ear, and in the profound hearing loss range for her right ear, showing virtually no benefit from hearing aids. As a result, cochlear implantation was pursued, immediately.

Amber underwent bilateral cochlear implantation at 21 months of age and was activated 2 weeks later. At her 1-month follow-up, validation of the cochlear implants was completed in the booth, and responses were obtained between 15 and 20 dB HL in both ears from 500 to 4,000 Hz.

Unfortunately for Amber, over the next year she made minimal progress with her receptive and expressive language. She continued to show good audibility with the cochlear implants as evidenced by her aided thresholds, but her word recognition was poor in both ears (40–45%).

At her cochlear implant mappings, the electrical stapedial reflex threshold (eSRT) was obtained to determine where loudness levels for each electrode should be set. The reflex is electrically stimulated through the cochlear implant software and measured through an immittance bridge. The threshold is the lowest electrical stimulus needed to produce a stapedial reflex response at the electrode being measured. Research has shown this objective measure correlates well with behavioral thresholds for upper limits of comfort for adults and children.[12,13,14]

Hodges et al also found maps created using eSRT reported sharper and clearer signals, and speech perception performance was comparable to maps created using loudness levels obtained behaviorally.[12]

Amber was beginning to require mapping almost every month due to declines in speech production and fluctuations in her eSRT thresholds, which typically are fairly stable over the course of a year. Her mother would report that her speech was becoming more "slushy" and she would confuse her Ling six sounds (m, ah, oo, ee, sh, s). It is currently recommended for children younger than 7 years for cochlear implant mapping to occur every 3 months to ensure the child has appropriate access to low-level sounds and typically very few changes need to be made at these appointments.[15] For Amber, significant fluctuations were occurring for the upper limits of her electrodes, while her impedences were remaining stable. An integrity test was completed by the cochlear implant company and nothing unusual was found. Amber also underwent a psychological evaluation to determine if the CMV was causing a cognitive delay, which could have been impeding her progress. It was determined there were no cognitive delays present. Due to Amber's lack of progress in speech and language, poor word recognition, and the need to remap every 4 to 6 weeks, a decision was made to reimplant her. Her parents chose to complete one ear at a time since there was no guarantee the implant was causing her lack of progress. Amber was reimplanted in the right ear 10 months after her first surgery. Within 2 months, her word recognition scores improved 20%, so a month later the left ear was reimplanted. Amber has improved from 10% intelligibility to 90%, and her word recognition scores are at 80% in each ear. She still receives intensive aural habilitation; however, she is currently mainstreamed and progressing on the same trajectory as her normal hearing peers.

References

[1] Muse C, Harrison J, Yoshinaga-Itano C, et al. Joint Committee on Infant Hearing of the American Academy of Pediatrics. Supplement to the JCIH 2007 position statement: principles and guidelines for early intervention after confirmation that a child is deaf or hard of hearing. Pediatrics. 2013; 131(4): e1324–e1349

[2] American Academy of Otolaryngology – Head and Neck Surgery. Clinical Practice Guideline: Tympanostomy Tubes in Children. Available at: http://www.entnet.org/content/clinical-practice-guideline-tympanostomy-tubes-children. Accessed May 12, 2017

[3] Office of Special Education and Rehabilitative Services, Department of Education. Early intervention program for infants and toddlers with disabilities. Federal Register: vol. 76; 188. Available at: https://www.federalregister.gov/documents/2011/09/28/2011 -22783/early-intervention-program-for-infants-and-toddlers-with-disabilities. Effective September 2011. Accessed May 2017.

[4] Grosse SD, Ross DS, Dollard SC. Congenital cytomegalovirus (CMV) infection as a cause of permanent bilateral hearing loss: a quantitative assessment. J Clin Virol. 2008; 41(2):57–62

[5] Fowler KB, Boppana SB. Congenital cytomegalovirs (CMV infection and hearing deficit. J Clin Virol. 2006; 35(2):226–231

[6] American Speech-Language-Hearing Association. The Practice Portal. Permanent Childhood Hearing Loss: Assessment. Available at: http://www.asha.org/Practice-Portal/Audiologists/. Accessed July 12, 2016

[7] US FDA/CDRH. Approved Cochlear Implants. Available at: http://www.fda.gov/MedicalDevices/ProductsandMedicalProcedures/ImplantsandProsthetics/CochlearImplants/default.htm. Accessed May 17, 2017

[8] Gravel JS, Seewald RC. Audiologic assessment for the fitting of Hearing Instruments: Big Challenges from Tiny Ears. Proceedings of an international conference on A Sound Foundation through Early Amplification; 2000: 33–46

[9] Williamson WD, Demmler GJ, Percy AK, Catlin FI. Progressive hearing loss in infants with asymptomatic congenital cytomegalovirus infection. Pediatrics. 1992; 90(6):862–866

[10] Scollie S, Seewald R. Hearing aid fitting and verification procedures for children. In: Katz J, eds. Handbook of Clinical Audiology. 5th ed. New York, NY: Lippincott/Williams and Wilkins; 2002:695–696

[11] The Pediatric Working Group. Amplification for infants and children with Hearing Loss. Nashville, TN: Bill Wilkerson Press; 1996

[12] Hodges AV, Balkany TJ, Ruth RA, Lambert PR, Dolan-Ash S, Schloffman JJ. Electrical middle ear muscle reflex: use in cochlear implant programming. Otolaryngol Head Neck Surg. 1997; 117(3, Pt 1):255–261

[13] Brickley G, Boyd P, Wyllie F, O'Driscoll M, Webster D, Nopp P. Investigations into electrically evoked stapedius reflex measures and subjective loudness percepts in the MED-EL COMBI 40 + cochlear implant. Cochlear Implants Int. 2005; 6(1):31–42

[14] Walkowiak A, Lorens A, Kostek B, Skarzynski H, Polak M. ESRT, ART, and MCL correlations in experienced paediatric cochlear implant users. Cochlear Implants Int. 2010; 11(1) Suppl 1:482–484

[15] Wolfe J, Schafer E. Clinical considerations: putting all of the pieces together. In Programming cochlear implants. 2nd ed. San Diego, CA: Plural Publishing Inc.; 2015:237–262

33 Congenital Ossicular Chain Anomalies and Hearing Loss

Darius Kohan

33.1 Clinical History and Description

Jason, a 4-year-old African American boy born at term via C-section, presented in April 2010 with increasing hearing loss, left ear more than the right ear. He had passed the otoacoustic emission (OAE) newborn screening before hospital discharge. Developmental milestones were normal except for speech delay that was successfully treated with speech therapy and early intervention. Jason rarely developed ear infections, and there was no history of trauma or high-level noise exposure. The child had no other otologic symptoms, and the family history was negative for hearing loss. Past medical history is negative, but the mother had been suspecting hearing loss for at least 1 year. On physical examination, everything was normal except Jason had narrow ear canals, bilaterally. There were no stigmata of any syndromes.

33.2 Audiologic Testing

On April 1, 2010, the audiogram (▶ Fig. 33.1) revealed a mild, mostly low-frequency conductive hearing loss (CHL) with 25-dB air–bone gap (ABG) in the right ear. The left ear had a moderate CHL at all frequencies, with about a 40-dB ABG. The speech discrimination scores (SDSs) were excellent bilaterally, at high presentation levels. The tympanograms were normal, and acoustic reflexes were absent on both sides. The child had good reliability on the tests.

33.3 Questions for the Reader

1. What further tests, if any, are needed?
2. What is your differential diagnosis?
3. How would you address the child's hearing loss?

33.4 Discussion of Questions

1. **What further tests, if any, are needed?**
   One should not make a diagnosis and formulate a treatment plan based only on one test, no matter who performed the audiogram. First, repeat the full audiogram, tympanogram, and reflex tests to determine accuracy. Repeat evaluation to confirm test results should be considered. Auditory brainstem response testing would not be helpful or required with a cooperative child presenting only with a CHL.

2. **What is your differential diagnosis?**
   Congenital otosclerosis is by far the most likely diagnosis. This disorder has an autosomal dominant inheritance with variable expressivity and penetrance. Ten percent of the Caucasian population (with a lot fewer in the Asian and African gene pool) has histologic evidence on temporal bones (TBs) of otosclerosis; however, only 1% of Caucasians are symptomatic. Although clinical otosclerosis is more frequent in women with a 2:1 ratio versus men, genetics and histology point to almost equal prevalence among sexes. The process is bilateral in 80% of symptomatic patients, but timing of presentation may vary. It has been thought in the past that hormonal storm associated with pregnancy may aggravate otosclerosis; however, recent studies negate this. Most often patients have a progressive CHL and tinnitus starting in their third decade of life. Relatively rarely, there is a sensorineural component of hearing loss or balance deficit.

   The pathophysiology involves multifocal remodeling of endochondral bone at the stapes and otic capsule with both resorption of bone and deposition of new sclerotic bone, especially at the anterior stapes footplate annulus junction at the oval window (OW). During the initial bone resorption, there is increased vascularity, which may be evident as a reddish tinge on the promontory as seen on otoscopy, known as

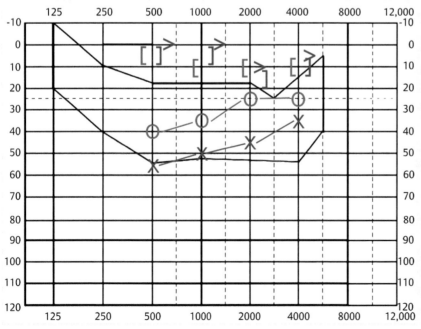

Fig. 33.1 Pre-op audiogram: AD—mild, mostly low-frequency conductive hearing loss (CHL) with 25-dB air–bone gap (ABG). AS—moderate CHL at all frequencies with about a 40-dB ABG. The speech discrimination scores (SDS) are excellent bilaterally, at high presentation levels. The tympanograms were normal, and acoustic reflexes (ARs) were absent on both sides. O, right ear air conduction; X, left ear air conduction; >, left ear bone conduction; [, right ear bone conduction masked;], left ear bone conduction masked.

the Schwartz sign. Later in the process, this disappears, and ossicular fixation occurs medially at the anterior footplate. Less frequently, a sensorineural hearing loss (SNHL) may develop with injury to the cochlea and spiral ligament from the lytic process or from release of proteolytic enzymes. Besides progressive CHL, one frequently notes an increase in bone conduction (BC) threshold on the average of about 15 dB at 2 kHz (known as a Carhart's notch), which is the resonant frequency of the ossicular chain. Otosclerotic stiffening of the ossicular chain raises the resonant frequency and presents a clinical marker for medial ossicular chain fixation. Surgery may restore the BC to baseline.

The more lateral malleus and incus are normally mobile in otosclerosis, resulting in tympanograms that are either normal or shallow (type As). Stapes fixation also affects the stapedius reflex. The stapedius muscle contraction is no longer able to stiffen the now fixed stapes and will no longer decrease admittance and protect from loud noise exposure. In unilateral otosclerosis, the reflex thresholds cannot be determined when the admittance probe is located on the affected side and may result in elevated or absent reflexes when the stimulus is presented in the affected ear and the admittance probe is placed in the opposite ear.

There are other congenital ossicular abnormalities. Multiple syndromes may result in a fixed ossicular chain and CHL. Relatively often, there is a bone bridge formation between the head of the malleus and the scutum, leading to malleolus fixation, also a surgically correctable condition. Tympanosclerosis, a very common condition resulting from frequent ear infections, may also result in progressive CHL and may involve any ossicle in multiple areas of the middle ear cleft. Infections and trauma may also lead to ossicular discontinuity usually involving the long process of the incus, which has a poor blood supply and is relatively fragile. A dehiscent superior semicircular canal (SSC), either congenital or traumatic, may result in a third window phenomenon with a CHL, tinnitus, and echolalia. This anatomy is frequently noted on TB CT as an incidental finding, and few of these individuals actually are symptomatic. Other rare anomalies of the middle ear, such as an aberrant internal carotid artery in the middle ear, may affect ossicular mobility.

3. **How would you address the child's hearing loss?**
A high-quality fine-resolution TB CT may be very helpful in distinguishing among the above differential diagnosis. In our case, the pre-op CT revealed left fusion of the malleus and incus but did not identify an otosclerosis focus. The right side was normal. A cVEMP test may help identify a dehiscent SSC. TB and brain MRI does not show bone and are more useful in conditions involving SNHL.

The child should continue speech-language-listening treatment services. Amplification options should be provided including hearing aids, remote microphone systems, preferential school seating when appropriate, preview and review of academic materials, etc.

33.5 Outcome

The family opted for surgical intervention for the worse hearing ear, the left side. On an ambulatory basis, a canalplasty to widen the meatus and a middle ear exploration with ossicular reconstruction was performed on September 6, 2010. At surgery, the child had multiple ossicular abnormalities. The malleus and incus were fused as one unit, but they were freely mobile. The stapes was fixed at the OW. A stapedotomy was performed with a 5.5-mm Scheer piston prosthesis inserted. The surgery and postoperative course were uneventful. The audiogram at 6 weeks postsurgery (▶ Fig. 33.2) revealed borderline normal hearing in the left ear where the SRT improved from 40 dB pre-op to 20 dB post-op. The SDS was still 100%. At that time, the patient relocated and was lost to follow-up until March 9, 2016, when he presented with progressive right CHL and tinnitus (▶ Fig. 33.3). He had borderline normal hearing levels on the

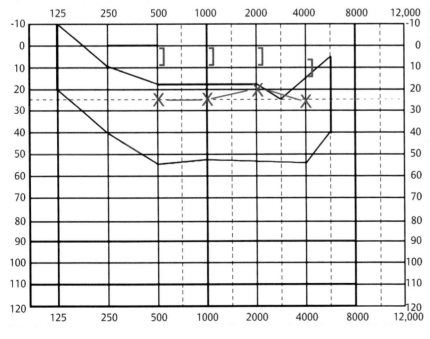

Fig. 33.2 Post-op audiogram at 6 weeks: AS—borderline normal hearing where the SRT improved from 40 dB pre-op to 20 dB post-op. The SDS was still 100% with normal tympanogram. AD—no changes. X, left ear air conduction;], left ear bone conduction masked.

left ear with a 15-dB ABG, and a moderate CHL on the right ear with a 40-dB ABG. He was doing well in school and had a normal ENT exam including microtoscopy. His local ENT and pediatrician recommended conservative management, amplification, FM system, etc. The child and parents were informed that surgery would be of no benefit.

33.6 Additional Questions for the Reader

1. What would you do now? Was the local ENT wrong to recommend against surgery?

33.7 Discussion of Additional Questions

1. **What would you do now? Was the local ENT wrong to recommend against surgery?**

   Conservative management as noted above is a viable option. The child would have to be monitored frequently to determine progression of his hearing loss, language, and academic performance. In this instance, it was the child who convinced the parents to allow him to have surgery to fix his new hearing loss. There was no need to repeat the earlier TB CT since the prior operated left ear has preserved the benefits of the stapedotomy, and one can assume that the right ear has similar pathology. On May 26, 2016, he underwent surgery on an ambulatory basis, consisting of a transcanal middle ear exploration and ossicular reconstruction. At surgery, the long process of the incus was attenuated and the stapes fixed. A laser stapedotomy was performed with a Scheer 5.5-mm piston prosthesis insertion, and OtoMimix cement was used to buttress and strengthen the long process of the incus.

The post-op course was uneventful, and ▶ Fig. 33.4 shows his last audiogram. There is now bilateral borderline normal hearing with an ABG less than 15 dB. The patient and his parents are satisfied with the outcome. Jason will avoid contact sports and will have biannual audiologic follow-up at his local ENT office.

The reluctance of the local otologist to perform the surgery was a valid opinion. The medical literature generally indicated poorer surgical outcome of stapedotomy for children versus adults, with ABG closure under 10 dB in only about 80% of procedures. However, more recent literature involving up-to-date surgical techniques reveal a 90 to 95% ABG closure to under 10 dB. The complication rate of about 1% of severe SNHL with stapes surgery is now reported to be similar in children as in adults. It has been well documented that the experience of the surgeon performing the stapes surgery has a direct correlation to good outcomes. It is appropriate for even well-experienced and talented otologists to refer patients to colleagues with special expertise in stapes surgery. Of note, the average life expectancy of a successful stapes surgery is thought to be about 20 years, at which time the surgery may be revised with almost equal success rates by modifying the technique.

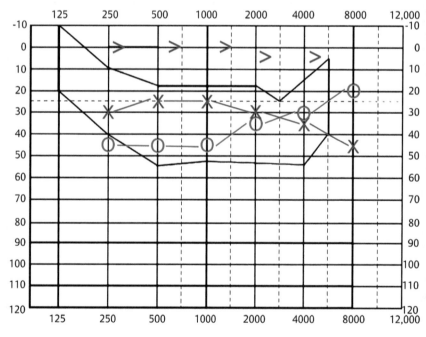

Fig. 33.3 Audiogram 5.5 years post-op: AS—borderline normal hearing levels with a 15-dB ABG. AD—moderate CHL with a 40-dB ABG, and AU normal discrimination and tympanograms. O, right ear air conduction; X, left ear air conduction; >, left ear bone conduction.

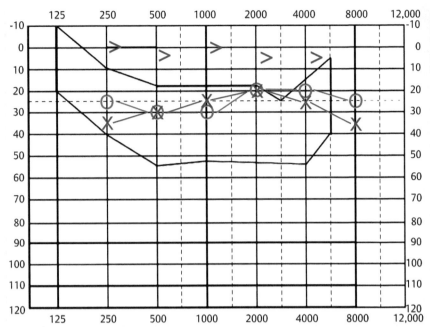

Fig. 33.4 Post-op audiogram at 6 weeks: AU—borderline normal hearing with an ABG less than 15 dB. AU—normal discrimination and tympanograms. O, right ear air conduction; X, left ear air conduction;>, left ear bone conduction.

Suggested Readings

[1] Kisilevsky VE, Bailie NA, Dutt SN, Halik JJ. Hearing results of stapedotomy and malleo-vestibulopexy in congenital hearing loss. Int J Pediatr Otorhinolaryngol. 2009; 73(12):1712–1717

[2] Massey BL, Hillman TA, Shelton C. Stapedectomy in congenital stapes fixation: are hearing outcomes poorer? Otolaryngol Head Neck Surg. 2006; 134 (5):816–818

[3] Carlson ML, Van Abel KM, Pelosi S, et al. Outcomes comparing primary pediatric stapedectomy for congenital stapes footplate fixation and juvenile otosclerosis. Otol Neurotol. 2013; 34(5):816–820

[4] Vincent R, Wegner I, Vonck BM, Bittermann AJ, Kamalski DM, Grolman W. Primary stapedotomy in children with otosclerosis: A prospective study of 41 consecutive cases. Laryngoscope. 2016; 126(2):442–446

[5] Benedict PA, Zhou L, Peng R, Kohan D. The malleus to oval window revision stapedotomy: Efficacy and longitudinal study outcome. Laryngoscope. 2018; 128(2):461–467

34 Auditory Neuropathy Spectrum Disorder

Megan Kuhlmey

34.1 Clinical History and Description

EM was born at full term. At birth, it was discovered that she was positive for group B streptococcal (GBS) and was intubated shortly after birth for 4 to 5 days due to respiratory distress. EM was treated with IV antibiotics. She remained in the neonatal intensive care unit (NICU) for 5 weeks. Parents report that cognition and motor function are normal.

34.2 Audiologic Testing

Her parents report that during her hospital stay, EM was tested using otoacoustic emissions (OAE) and was referred for an auditory brainstem response (ABR) test. She passed a follow-up OAE at her pediatrician's office bilaterally. A follow-up ABR was performed at the hospital where she did not pass the first OAE test, which indicated bilateral auditory neuropathy spectrum disorder (ANSD). It was recommended that EM receive follow-up with further testing when she could be tested behaviorally. EM was behaviorally evaluated around 6 months of age. Responses were obtained in the normal range and the parents were told not to be concerned. Her parents report that EM was not developing babbling skills or consistent detection to sounds in her environment. They decided to seek a second opinion at another center that also diagnosed ANSD on a repeat ABR. Behavioral thresholds demonstrated moderate to severe hearing loss, and the center fitted her with binaural hearing aids. Parents and therapists noticed that upon initial fitting, EM was responsive and demonstrated increased vocalizations. After 7 months of amplification, EM had made little progress in her speech and language development. Parents report that EM fluctuates in her responsiveness and mainly grunts to express herself. Her speech therapists felt that she plateaued and at 22 months old, her parents sought out a cochlear implant (CI) evaluation. Reliable behavioral thresholds were obtained (via visual reinforcement audiometry [VRA] and conditioned play audiometry [CPA]) at moderate to severe hearing loss levels. Her present hearing aids were not providing enough high-frequency gain. It was recommended to try stronger aids to see if better detection could be obtained and if so, what would be the outcome expressively. Upon initial fitting, EM was more responsive and detecting more, but after 8 weeks of use and intensive auditory-based therapy, she plateaued again, was inconsistent in responsiveness, and did not make further progress. Her parents report that her better days were better, but there were not more of them than before (▶ Table 34.1).

34.3 Questions for the Reader

1. What is significant in EM's history that suggests ANSD?
2. Do you think the patient is a CI candidate?
3. If so, do you think she should be implanted bilaterally (simultaneously or sequentially) or unilaterally?

Table 34.1 Pre-op testing

Unaided results				
	500 Hz	1,000 Hz	2,000 Hz	4,000 Hz
Right ear	45	50	60	70
Left ear	50	55	65	70
Aided results				
Warble tones	500 Hz	2,000 Hz	4,000 Hz	
Aided right	20 dB HL	20 dB HL	20 dB HL	
Aided left	25 dB HL	25 dB HL	25 dB HL	
Speech awareness	"ba"	"sh"	"s"	
Aided right	10 dB HL	15 dB HL	15 dB HL	
Aided left	15 dB HL	20 dB HL	15 dB HL	

4. If implanted, how would you counsel the parents regarding expected outcomes with the CI?

34.4 Discussion of Questions

1. **What is significant in EM's history that suggests ANSD?**
   EM's birth history is positive for NICU stay and mechanical ventilation, which are clinical indicators for possible ANSD. EMs demonstrated abnormal ABR and absent acoustic reflexes. Functionally, EM demonstrated inconsistent behavioral test results. Initial behavioral testing indicated normal hearing, but second testing indicated a hearing loss. Parents reported inconsistent responses to sound with EM hearing better at some times than at other times. Although it seemed EM was receiving good benefit from technology and was using the technology on a regular basis, she was not making progress. This kind of inconsistency is typical of children diagnosed with ANSD.

2. **Do you think the patient is a CI candidate?**
   EM is not making progress in speech and language development even though she is receiving sufficient gain from her technology. This would indicate that the signal she is receiving from the hearing aids is not sufficient. She appears to be a good candidate for CIs.

3. **Do you think the patient is a CI candidate?**
   Children with ANSD who do not do well with hearing aids may benefit from CIs.
   If EM has ANSD bilaterally, bilateral CI should be considered. There is a chance that implanting only one ear will leave the other ear open and continue to receive a distorted signal, which can continue to interfere with language development. The decision about simultaneous or sequential implantation may be left to the parents. They may be uncomfortable implanting both ears at the same time or may prefer not to have two surgeries. They need

to be counseled about what to expect from CIs and what may happen if implanting only one ear.

4. **If implanted, how would you counsel the parents regarding expected outcomes with the CI?**
Parents need to be counseled about what to expect from a CI. While a CI will improve auditory access, it is not possible to predict how much benefit EM will receive. Children with deafness not caused by ANSD often have a more predictable course of development. Counseling needs to include discussion about the possibilities that one implant will still leave an ear with ANSD open and that this may continue to interfere with auditory, speech and language development. If parents choose one implant, they need to be instructed to monitor performance carefully to observe listening and language development.

34.5 Conclusion

After working closely with her speech therapist (who is experienced in working with children with hearing disorders), it was decided that due to her lack of progress that she receive a CI. Her parents decided to implant one ear at time out of concern that the outcome may not be successful due to the ANSD (▶ Table 34.2).

Table 34.2 EM's post-op results (3 months postactivation)

Tone thresholds with cochlear implant (CI)			
Warble tones	500 Hz	2,000 Hz	4,000 Hz
Implant right	25 dB HL	25 dB HL	20 dB HL
Recorded Ling sounds with CI			
	"oo"	"ah"	"s"
Implant right	20	25	25

At the time of testing, EM was getting good access with her CI and her vocal intent increased. She began to develop words (*up, mama, papa*) and was also consistent in her responses compared to her performance with hearing aids.

Suggested Readings

[1] National Institutes of Health. Auditory Neuropathy. Available at: https://www.nidcd.nih.gov/health/auditory-neuropathy#a. Accessed February 28, 2018
[2] Rance G, Barker EJ. Speech perception in children with auditory neuropathy/dyssynchrony managed with either hearing AIDS or cochlear implants. Otol Neurotol. 2008; 29(2):179–182
[3] Walton J, Gibson WPR, Sanli H, Prelog K. Predicting cochlear implant outcomes in children with auditory neuropathy. Otol Neurotol. 2008; 29(3):302–309

35 A Complex Audiologic Case Demonstrating Professional Collaboration

Amy McConkey Robbins and Cathryn A. Luckoski

35.1 Clinical History and Description

Owen, a child with bilateral hearing loss (HL) diagnosed at the age of 21 months, had an eventful early history. His mother was found to have intrauterine growth restriction (IUGR) in her third trimester of pregnancy, necessitating a C-section delivery at 37 weeks of gestation. Owen's neonatal growth rate was very slow and he had difficulty feeding. At 9 weeks, a cleft of the soft palate and uvula was identified; surgical repair took place at 1 year of age. Low muscle tone was identified and treatment was provided by an occupational therapist (OT) and a physical therapist (PT) from the age of 1 year through the present. Concerns for delayed communication, including limited engagement with peers and key aspects of Owen's environment, led to multiple assessments for hearing. Following the diagnosis of HL, genetic testing at the age of 2-8 revealed the presence of Pendred's syndrome. Owen received intensive intervention, including emersion into a listening and spoken language (LSL) preschool; however, he remained severely delayed in communication by the age of 4 years. The first author met Owen at approximately this time. This case describes the 2 years that followed in which collaboration between specialties, and the family, became key to opening the door for Owen to learning and communication.

35.2 Speech and Language History

Owen had demonstrated severe delays in communication development throughout early childhood. Even during his first 2 years, when hearing was deemed to be normal, he used few words, and those he said were only understood by his parents. When he turned 3, he had been placed in a full-day LSL preschool. As the school year progressed, staff were concerned about restricted advancements in spoken language and Owen's "limited attention and increasing noncompliant behaviors during therapy and class instruction." This resulted in a team recommendation to move him into a classroom that included visual cues and to have him seen by the first author for a communication assessment, which took place when Owen was 3-11. Owen's language comprehension and expression fell at the 18-month level on the Reynell Developmental Language Scales, a finding corroborated by his mother's report on the MacArthur-Bates Communicative Development Inventories. His speech was judged to be 0% intelligible to all listeners except his family. A very restricted speech sound repertoire was documented that was not typical of children with HL. For example, while many children with HL use visually salient "p," "b," or "m" sounds as substitutes for other consonants, Owen used "g" or "h." Almost all vowels were produced as a centralized "uh," so his word attempts were undifferentiated and sounded like "guh guh" or "huh huh." Visual cues did not help his speech accuracy, as they would for most children with HL. Rather, Owen struggled to imitate articulatory postures for vowels and consonants even when he could see the adult's mouth.

Speech prosody was normal, though, and suprasegmental patterns (intensity, duration, and vocal pitch) sounded much like a child with typical hearing. Lacking effective ways to express his needs and wants, Owen used behaviors, often negative and disruptive, rather than language, to communicate. Based on the assessment, the first author's primary recommendations were the following: (1) a diagnostic teaching period of sign exposure (signing exact English) to determine if sign support could increase his spoken language learning rate; (2) use of visual schedules in therapy to increase compliance; and (3) referral to a speech-language pathologist (SLP) with expertise in childhood apraxia of speech (CAS), a condition characterized by difficulty in achieving and maintaining articulatory configurations; presence of vowel distortions; limited consonant and vowel repertoire; use of simple syllable shapes; ability to produce a sound correctly in a simple context ("ba" imitated correctly) but not in a longer one ("bababa" becomes "guhguhguh"). A diagnosis of CAS was confirmed and he began twice-weekly treatment with his CAS SLP in addition to his weekly sessions with the first author. As part of her sessions, the first author often reviewed Owen's Ling six-sound results, aided audiogram, functional auditory responses, and informal speech perception information with the parents to explore whether he was getting adequate benefit from his hearing aids. The possibility of pursuing cochlear implant (CI) candidacy was discussed. The parents were reluctant to pursue CI candidacy for two reasons. First, their level of confidence with audiological test results was not high, largely as a result of the many conflicting reports they had received about Owen's hearing during the first 2 years of life. Second, they had seen a substantial increase in his auditory responsiveness after his recent fitting with Phonak SoundRecover technology and wanted to give him more time to adjust to these new hearing aids before pursuing other options. With effective interventions, Owen began to make progress in spoken language for about 8 months and then a noted drop in auditory responsiveness was seen at home and school and progress slowed. In fact, at the age of 4-10, a significant drop in left ear hearing was recorded. At this point, Owen was referred to the second author for a CI candidacy evaluation.

35.3 Hearing and Amplification History

The early hearing history was provided by the parent's and a collection of professional reports. ▶ Table 35.1, ▶ Table 35.2, ▶ Table 35.3, and ▶ Table 35.4 summarize the course of testing and diagnoses provided to the parents. His hearing history started with a fail on the newborn hearing screen. Multiple hearing tests followed over the course of his first years of life, often with contradictory findings. At 1 month of age, follow-up auditory brainstem response (ABR) measures suggested normal hearing in the left ear and possible low-frequency HL in the right ear, consistent with middle ear pathology. ABR results at 4 months of age were read as "repeatable responses obtained down to 30 dB normal hearing level (nHL) in the right ear and 25 to 30 dB nHL in the left ear with a diagnosis of mild hearing loss." This was deemed consistent with the recently diagnosed soft palate/uvular cleft. At 5 months, ABR testing revealed "repeatable responses down to 20 dB nHL in both ears, suggestive of normal hearing." Behavioral evaluations beyond this time were challenging, as Owen often worked for only 10 minutes in a session, and then refused to cooperate (shut his eyes, turned away, or threw a tantrum), effectively ending the session. Often the results were noted to be consistent with either past testing or current medical history. Sound field testing at 13 and 17 months showed normal hearing in at least one ear. Throughout this time period, the parents often reported continued concern for speech and language development. Their concern elevated after the age of 17 months prompting a sedated ABR at 21 months of age.

Table 35.1 Right ear assessments: ABR and sound field (SF), 0 to 2–2

Age	ABR/click	ABR/0.5 k	ABR/1.0 k	ABR/4.0 k	DPOAE	SF	Test reliability	Dx given to parents
1 mo	30–40	a	a	a	a	a	a	Conductive
4 mo	30	a	a	a	a	a	Unknown	Mild
5 mo	20	a	a	a	a	a	Unknown	Normal
9 mo	a	a	a	a	a	CNT	Unknown	Unknown
13 mo	a	a	a	a	a	Normal	Unknown	Normal/*Better Ear*
17 mo	a	a	a	a	a	Normal	Unknown	Normal/*better ear*
21 mo	90	NR	NR	NR	Present	a	Good	ANSD
2–2	95	80	85	90	Absent	a	Good	Severe/profound

Abbreviations: ABR, auditory brainstem response; ANSD, auditory neuropathy spectrum disorder; CNT, could not test; DPOAE, distortion product otoacoustic emission; Dx, Diagnosis; NR, No Response.
Note: Frequency in Hz. Results given in dB HL or dB nHL.
[a]Data not reported.

Table 35.2 Left ear assessments: ABR and sound field (SF), 0 to 2–2

Age	ABR/click	ABR/500	ABR/1,000	ABR/4,000	DPOAE	SF	Test reliability	Dx given to parents
1 mo	25/30	a	a	a	a	a	a	Normal
4 mo	30	a	a	a	a	a	Unknown	Mild
5 mo	20	a	a	a	a	a	Unknown	Normal
9 mo	a	a	a	a	a	CNT	Unknown	Unknown
13 mo	a	a	a	a	a	Normal	Unknown	Normal/*better ear*
17 mo	a	a	a	a	a	Normal	Unknown	Normal/*better ear*
21 mo	36	20	30	CNT	Absent	a	Fair	Normal/mild
2–2	50	20	40	75	Absent	a	Good	Mild/moderate

Abbreviations: ABR, auditory brainstem response; CNT, could not test; DPOAE, distortion product otoacoustic emission; Dx, diagnosis.
Note: Frequency in Hz. Results given in dB HL or dB nHL.
[a]Data not reported.

Table 35.3 Right ear behavioral assessments with earphones

Age	250	500	1,000	2,000	3,000	4000	6,000	8,000	Speech	Test reliability	Dx given to parents
23 mo	a	60	90	a	a	a	a	a	85	Good	Moderate/severe
24 mo	a	CNT	a	105	a	a	a	a	DNT	Good/fair	Profound
2–2	a	60	90	105	a	105	a	a	DNT	Good/fair	Moderate/profound
3–6	50	75	85	85	95	100	105	NR	55	Good	Moderate/profound
4–10	55	70	80	100	a	105	NR	NR	DNT	Good	Moderate/profound

Abbreviation: CNT, could not test; DNT, did not test; Dx, diagnosis; NR, no response.
Note: Frequency in Hz. Results given in dB HL or dB nHL.
[a]Data not reported.

Table 35.4 Left ear behavioral assessments with earphones

Age	250	500	1,000	2,000	3,000	4,000	6,000	8,000	Speech	Test reliability	Dx given to parents
23 mo	a	30	40	a	a	a	a	a	35	Good	Mild
24 mo	a	a	a	35	a	30	a	a	DNT	Good/fair	Mild
2–1	a	a	a	55	70	75	80	75	35	Good	Moderate/severe
2–2	a	35	a	40	a	35	a	a	DNT	Good/fair	Mild/moderate
3–6	25	20	20	40	70	80	105	90	15	Good	Mild/profound
4–10	35	20	50	70	85	95	95	NR	DNT	Good	Mild/profound

Abbreviation: CNT, could not test; DNT, did not test; Dx, diagnosis; NR, no response.
Note: Frequency in Hz. Results given in dB HL or dB nHL.
aData not reported.

The ABR at 21 months showed a response to click stimulation in the right ear at 90 dB nHL and in the left ear at 35 dB nHL. A fully detailed ABR was not completed due to sedation complications; however, sufficient information was found to provide a tentative diagnosis of auditory neuropathy spectrum disorder (ANSD) in the right ear and mild sensorineural HL in the left ear. Amplification was recommended for the left ear only.

Between 23 and 24 months of age, the first of two behavioral individual ear tests was completed, both in agreement with the ABR. They suggested mild HL in the left ear and moderate to severe HL in the right ear. The composite audiogram is shown in ▶ Fig. 35.1.

At this point, amplification, recommended 2 months earlier, had still not been fitted and Owen's mother expressed frustration with the slow process and a desire to binaurally aid him. Shortly thereafter, at age 24 months, he was fitted with Oticon Safari 600 power hearing aids. He adapted well and quickly became a full-time user who never resisted wearing amplification. At the age of 2–2, a repeat sedated ABR indicated "mild-to-severe loss in the left ear and severe-to-profound loss in the right." Distortion product otoacoustic emissions (DPOAEs) were absent in both ears, essentially ruling out ANSD. Aided testing was completed potentially for the first time at the age of 2–3, but only in sound field by the report. These results were interpreted as auditory responses being present between 25 and 30 dB from 500 Hz to 6,000 Hz.

Hearing was reported stable from this point until around age 3–6 when a significant drop in the left (better) ear thresholds was documented at 4,000 Hz and above, as shown in ▶ Fig. 35.2.

After the drop in hearing was confirmed at age 3–6, his audiologist discussed options for giving Owen better access to sound. The family opted to purchase Phonak Sky Q90 behind-the-ear hearing aids with SoundRecover, and Owen was fitted with these instruments at the age of 3–11. This is also the time period when Owen met the first author. Sound Recover technology is a nonlinear frequency compression algorithm designed to enhance audibility in cochlear regions impacted by severe/profound HL.[1] ▶ Fig. 35.3 shows the aided results with this technology at the age of 3–11. This was also the aided hearing assumed at the time that the first author began seeing Owen for evaluation and speech-language therapy.

At this time, the parents reported that with the Phonak Sky Q90 hearing aids, Owen's responsiveness to sound at home improved; however, Owen's binaurally aided audiogram indicated thresholds at 250 Hz, 3,000 Hz and 6,000 Hz that were outside the range of audibility for soft conversational speech. In therapy, the first author noted several important auditory and behavioral indicators. Owen developed consistent responses to both "s" and "sh" in his left (better) ear during Ling six-sound checks at speech-language sessions, even at a distance of 10 ft at conversational levels. However, he produced both consonants as undifferentiated frication or blowing. He did not respond to these sounds in his right ear. As with other activities, Owen's degree of cooperation on the Ling six-sound check was variable and considerably below that expected for his age. He would sometimes put his head on the table or say, "No" and refuse to participate in the task. A pointing format was also tried with this task so that Owen could indicate what he heard without producing anything, as this would eliminate the confounding factor of his poor speech production accuracy. Owen refused to select an answer, asking, "This one?" over and over again while pointing to various alternatives. A therapy goal was added by the first author to address Owen's ability to select items in a closed set using a pointing response, although this took considerable time to accomplish.

Another significant drop in hearing was documented when Owen was 4–10 (▶ Fig. 35.4). The first author discussed options with the parents who determined they would like to pursue CI candidacy. A referral was made to the CI center where Owen and his family met the second author.

35.4 Questions for the Reader

1. What impact did the relatively late (at age 2–8) diagnosis of Pendred's syndrome have on Owen's audiological management and treatment planning?
2. What concerns should be raised regarding Owen's failure to develop any intelligible spoken language, as seen at the initial SLP evaluation. What diagnoses would the clinician want to rule out?
3. What are the significant challenges facing the audiologist at the CI center?
4. What can be done in preparation for the CI evaluation to assure an effective session with Owen and his parents?

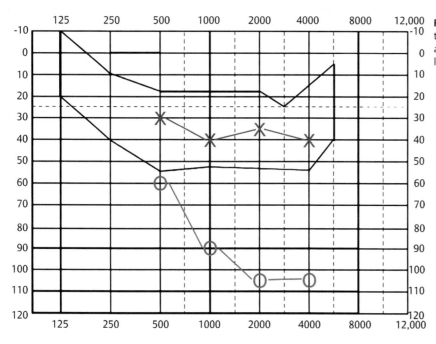

Fig. 35.1 Composite audiogram at the age of 23 to 24 months, approximately 2 months after the age of diagnosis. O, right ear air conduction; X, left ear air conduction.

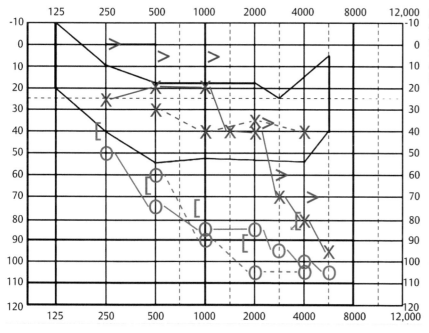

Fig. 35.2 Behavioral play audiogram at age 3–6. Good reliability reported. Audiologic information from 23 to 24 months superimposed for comparison. O, right ear air conduction; X, left ear air conduction; >, left ear bone conduction; [, right ear bone conduction masked; Arrows, no response.

35.5 Discussion of Questions

1. **What impact did the relatively late (at age 2–8) diagnosis of Pendred's syndrome have on Owen's audiological management and treatment planning?**

   Pendred's syndrome is a complex disorder in which the following conditions commonly are present at birth or develop over time: progressive sensorineural HL secondary to enlarged vestibular aqueduct (EVA) syndrome and cochlear malformation (Mondini), vestibular dysfunction, and thyroid gland enlargement (goiter).[2] An earlier referral for genetic testing would have identified the potential for these associated conditions. Most importantly, a hallmark symptom of this disorder is fluctuating, progressive HL. Children with

these conditions can have persistent fluctuation of hearing levels, even presenting at times with normal to near-normal assessment results. It is crucial to understand that EVA with Mondini malformation can be an expected contributor to slower-than-predicted progress in speech and language therapy, as well as behavioral noncompliance in daily activities, both structured and unstructured. The diagnosis of Pendred's syndrome earlier in Owen's life would have informed the assessment and treatment plan for this child. In addition, the parents would have been counseled that these inconsistencies, and subsequent loss of residual hearing, were largely expected. This counseling might have allowed the parents to view variable test results through the lens of a genetic syndrome, rather than to question the accuracy of audiological

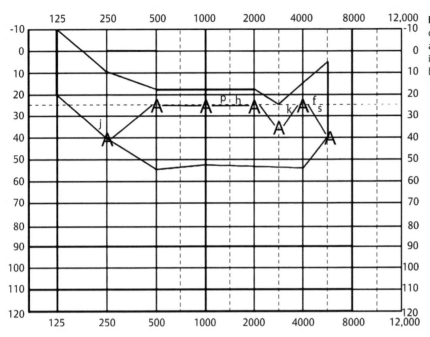

Fig. 35.3 Binaurally aided test results at the age of 3–11. Note: the speech sounds that potentially are missed in everyday listening are superimposed for reference. A, binaural hearing aids behind the ear.

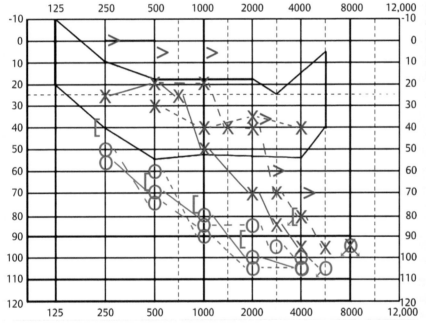

Fig. 35.4 The audiogram captured at the age of 4–10. Good reliability reported. Audiogram from 23 to 24 months and age 3-6 superimposed for comparison. O, right ear air conduction; X, left ear air conduction; >, left ear bone conduction; [, right ear bone conduction masked; Arrows, no response.

findings. The parents and early hearing professionals failed to develop a *therapeutic alliance* whose characteristics include the following: agreement on the goals of treatment, agreement on the tasks to achieve those goals, and a personal bond made up of reciprocal positive feelings. *The establishment of a therapeutic alliance is considered essential to successful intervention in any approach.*

2. **What concerns should be raised regarding Owen's failure to develop any intelligible spoken language, as seen at the initial SLP evaluation. What diagnoses would the clinician want to rule out?**

Although he was aided at a late age, Owen wore his technology full time and had been enrolled in a high-quality LSL program; however, he made very limited progress in devel-

oping spoken language, and his speech was completely undifferentiated. It would be important to (1) demonstrate that he had good auditory access with his hearing aids and (2) determine if an underlying issue was present, such as CAS. This would require specialized therapy for Owen to make progress. Regarding the first point, it would be critical to evaluate aided and unaided detection levels, Ling six-sound results, and speech discrimination abilities. Assessing speech discrimination was a formidable task, given Owen's limited language, undifferentiated speech, and challenging test behaviors. Establishing a corpus of vocabulary words with accompanying signs greatly widened the information that could be obtained. Based on the audiograms, the question should be asked if a CI should have been recommended sooner.

3. **What are the significant challenges facing the audiologist at the CI center?**

Owen's history implied that he was noncompliant or that he was limited in his ability to stay on task, but this should not be the primary focus during an audiologic assessment. In this respect, Owen is like many children who will be anxious or reluctant when they walk into a potentially stress-infused situation, such as a new place, new task, or new people. The true challenge existed in the following: (1) development of Owen's trust and (2) establishment of an effective method to document his aided hearing (detection and discrimination). To the first point, Owen had seen many specialists in his short 5 years of life. In general, children are perceptive to situations in which they are challenged and unsuccessful. A new person (meaning the second author) would need to be patient and creative in establishing a relationship in which Owen would be able to participate with success. This should be the primary objective of the first test session. To the second point, the capture of meaningful data would be imperative to develop a treatment plan. To this end, a strategy to assess Owen's hearing with and without hearing aids was needed that bypassed the confounding issues of severe language delay and CAS.

4. **What can be done in preparation for the CI evaluation to assure an effective session with Owen and his parents?**

A key element to this first session would be information that was already known. Owen had an extensive history of audiologic and speech records with key data to inform the pending evaluation. These records would be needed prior to the session as possible and utilized to not only validate the session findings, but also inform the treatment plan. In addition, the SLP should be contacted. As noted earlier, within the previous year, CAS had been diagnosed and the audiologist would need to understand the implications of this on testing, as well as on the long-term impact on expectations related to spoken language development. This last point would inform the discussion with the parents on the realistic expectations should a CI be pursued. A primary question that parents have in a CI evaluation is "if the cochlear implant surgery is done, will this help my child learn to talk?" This is a complex question requiring input from all specialists involved in case management. The text box below highlights features of a collaborative model in the assessment and treatment process.

Features of a Collaborative Model between Audiologist and SLP

- Exchanged goals needed to be accomplished (e.g., the audiologist needs Owen to attend longer to complete testing, so the SLP shares strategies for doing so).
- Similar visual schedules used in both settings (a successful template for visual schedule in SLP sessions was used by the audiologist and Owen's mother during testing).
- The SLP provided word lists of known vocabulary for the audiologist to use in testing.
- The audiologist asked the SLP to monitor the child's Ling six-sound test results and functional listening.
- Parent engagement is encouraged. Mother served as liaison.

35.6 Diagnostic Assessment for a Cochlear Implant

The second author met Owen at the age of 5-0. He was accompanied by his mother at the first visit, but joined by both parents at later visits. Preceding the evaluation, the first author contacted the CI center, as well as the neurotologist. Significant, but brief, details of Owen's case history were shared, such as his HL, maturity, language level, and expressive motor issues. The diagnosis of apraxia (CAS) was referenced in terms of the potential impact on the test session. To address these challenges, the first author offered nontraditional tools for the assessment to improve the chance of capturing reliable data representative of speech discrimination abilities. In addition, a model of behavior management was described with the use of a visual schedule and parent involvement during testing. This information, as it turned out, was essential to the first session's success.

During the parent interview, Owen's mother stated that the right ear was thought to be very poor, aided or unaided. The left ear had been dominant and generally responded well to the current amplification, bilateral Phonak Sky Q90 behind-the-ear hearing aids. This being said, a recent drop in left ear hearing had resulted in inconsistent responses to softer high-frequency speech sounds, like /s/ or /sh/. In addition, Owen had a limited repertoire of expressive language even though he had been aided and closely followed by specialists since the age of 24 months. Owen's mother came to the session prepared. She had researched CI technology resulting in several intuitive questions, including device reliability and the potential to restore hearing in an ear with EVA/Mondini malformation. She also brought records of the recent audiograms and hearing aid verification measures. The reports indicated that Owen was frequently evaluated with varied results utilizing play techniques, nearly every 2 months, sometimes more often. Notations indicated that Owen fatigued to task quickly and required frequent changes in games. This being said, many of the reports included good reliability. The most recent was dated within the previous 2 months. This is the audiogram with test results from approximately age 2 to age 3-5 superimposed is shown in ▶ Fig. 35.4.

With a 120-minute session scheduled and a dense history to interpret, selecting the proper assessment tools was imperative to collecting substantial information. The decision was made to combine the most recent audiologic measures with aided detection and discrimination captured at this session. In addition, parent reporting was refined by utilizing an age-appropriate scale to determine the extent to which Owen used meaningful auditory information to understand his world. The Meaningful Auditory Integration Scale (MAIS) was given to Owen's mother. This structured interview schedule, with a maximum score of 40 points, allows the clinician to probe areas of listening and development. Owen scored 22/40 points. A summary of the information collected included the following details:

- Owen wore his technology without resistance, but was described as "passive" in his alerting to sounds that occurred at home and did not show curiosity about new sounds.

- Owen failed to report when his hearing aids were malfunctioning.
- On multiple occasions, Owen had been found to be watching a cartoon without the hearing aid(s) turned on.
- Owen did not appear to recognize speech and nonspeech sounds as different categories.
- Owen could not hear/understand in the presence of background noise.
- Owen was unable to spontaneously learn by listening alone and was only responsive to new sounds when highlighted for him.

This information was extremely informative in that the team now had a method to separate Owen's auditory abilities from his spoken language abilities. A review of the audiologic records indicated that Owen had been appropriately fitted with amplification. No other traditional hearing aids would have provided better benefit than those prescribed. With nearly 3 years of full-time hearing aid use and intensive intervention, Owen should have scored 40/40 on this scale. The questions remaining were the following:

- If Owen had an optimal hearing aid fitting, then why was a persistent delay in auditory development present?
- Would an alternative treatment, such as a CI, be more effective?

A review of records provided indicated that Owen had been seen 13 times between the ages of 3–6 and 4–10. The decision was made to focus on the missing pieces, as well as give Owen time to acclimatize to the new environment. To this end, ear-specific aided testing was attempted with measures of aided discrimination.

35.6.1 Ear-Specific Aided Detection

Aided right ear detection levels are shown in ▶ Fig. 35.5. These were obtained with fair to good reliability due to the presence of false positives. This being said, all recorded responses were repeated and represented the softest level of audibility on this day. Owen's mother assisted and the visual schedule was developed by the first author. Results indicated audibility well below the targeted 20 dB HL for each test frequency, 250 to 8,000 Hz. The left ear was attempted, but Owen remained true to form and would not continue with the play task regardless of game. The total time for this test was approximately 30 minutes. We could not have expected Owen to sit longer; therefore, speech discrimination became the next target.

35.6.2 Ear-Specific Speech Discrimination

Aided speech discrimination was captured with a set of modified word lists provided by the SLP (see ▶ Table 35.5). These words were randomly presented at 50 dB HL utilizing monitored live speech in both an open set and closed set format. If Owen had not fatigued to task, then additional words would have been added and scores at 35 dB HL would have also been elicited. Testing was started with a closed set of 10 prompts for two-syllable words and 6 prompts for single-syllable words, utilizing objects in the office. For instance, when Owen heard "airplane," he selected the airplane from the set of toys on the table. This was very effective. It is important to note here that the SLP had previously set a goal and worked extensively on developing Owen's ability to take a risk and point to a target in a closed-set task. Once the closed-set task was completed, the test session was reconfigured for an open-set task. The objects were removed from the table and the room and testing was completed in an aided auditory only configuration with the benefit of visual/tactile cue.

Closed set:
- Right ear: two-syllable words = 54%; one-syllable words = 45%.
- Left ear: two-syllable words = 90%; one-syllable words = 100%.

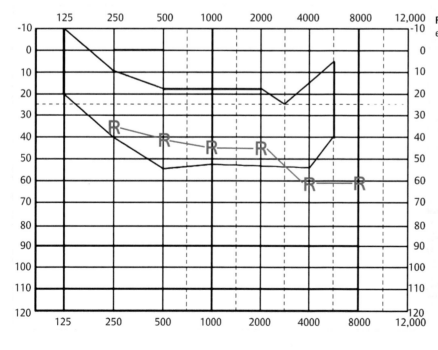

Fig. 35.5 Aided right ear detection levels. R, right ear hearing aid.

Open set:
- Right ear: 0%.
- Left ear: 100%.

This evaluation highlighted the significant differences in aided sound clarity between ears. Although the audibility of the left ear remained unknown, the score on modified aided speech discrimination implied significant, although not sufficient, access to speech information. With the corroborating evidence of the MAIS, extensive reports from outside specialists, and failure of progress in auditory development, the recommendation was made to proceed with a right ear CI. Staying on the current course of amplification would not lead to spoken language competence through hearing. Although the SLP, audiologist, and parents were in agreement, the family had reservations. There had been several varied results on past tests and the change in hearing was thought to be recent. The decision was made to monitor hearing levels and revisit the option for a CI at a future date. Owen returned two more times to the clinic over a 6-month period. The elements of ▸ Table 35.5 were implemented to validate and expand on information during this period. The time period also benefited the development of a therapeutic alliance between the family and specialists. In the interim, Owen was seen one time by an outside clinic for assessment with an alternative amplification system. At the age of 5–4, a repeat audiogram indicated stable left ear hearing and a further drop of 20 dB in the right ear at 1,000 Hz. At the age of 5–6, the parents and team decided to proceed with the right ear CI.

35.7 Diagnosis and Treatment

At the age of 5–9, Owen was implanted with an Advanced Bionics CI in the right ear. This device was activated at the age of 5–10. Owen immediately accepted bimodal device use and by 5 weeks postactivation provided a reliable detection audiogram. By the age of 6–0, Owen had become very comfortable with the test situation and was able to sit for bilateral verification measures in the sound booth. He continues to be managed by the second author for hearing loss. ▸ Fig. 35.6 shows the aided detection levels captured for both ears at 9 weeks post activation of the right ear cochlear implant. At this test session, aided discrimination in the right ear with the CI was 83% for closed-set words and 100% for open-set words. The left ear discrimination was stable. Owen was reported to be learning new words and phrases each day, he could take turns in an oral conversation, and he had started back at the LSL preschool. Owen's mother said that he was fully participating in the classroom and making friends.

35.8 Additional Questions for the Reader

1. Should Owen have been considered for a CI earlier than the age of 5?

Table 35.5 Modified word list (developed by first author for audiologic evaluation).

Two-syllable Words	Single-syllable words
School bus	Bed
French fries	Milk
Bath tub	Chair
Apple	Boat
Airplane	Bird
Birthday	Book
Bunny	
Ice cream	
Toothbrush	
Cookie	

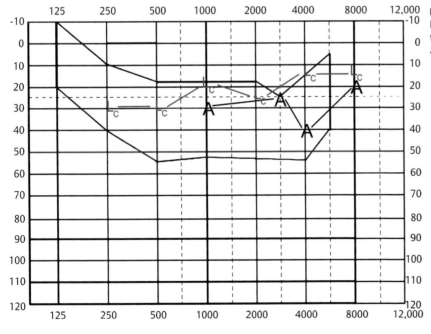

Fig. 35.6 Aided detection levels for the right and left ears. Recorded at 9 weeks postactivation of the right ear cochlear implant. A, binaural hearing aids behind the ear; LC, left cochlear implant.

35.9 Discussion of Additional Questions

1. **Should Owen have been considered for a CI earlier than the age of 5?**

   It is likely that Owen would have benefited from receiving a CI—and thus having greater access to sound—at an earlier age. However, clinicians interact with families within the broader context of parents' past experiences with professionals, as well as the information they have received about their child. Owen's parents had been told of the possibility of "dead regions" in his cochlea and had been counseled that his Mondini dysplasia made him high risk for reduced benefit from a CI. From their vantage point, a CI was not a promising technology for Owen based on what they had been told in the past, particularly because it required a surgical procedure. This case study illustrates the importance of establishing a therapeutic alliance with families so that as updated information is gathered and a child's status changes, parents may trust clinicians to help them navigate through new and uncertain waters.

35.10 Summary

Professional collaboration is beneficial for patient management, but essential in pediatric audiology. Case complexities and subsequent opportunities to improve treatment rise out of the fog during collaboration. In Owen's case, that collaboration now includes his LSL school staff, as well. They share valuable information with his audiologist and SLPs and, in turn, benefit from the input they receive. This broader collaboration has benefited Owen and his parents, contributing to a strong therapeutic alliance with the professionals who serve them. It is imperative that audiologists think outside of the test box when working with children.

35.11 Definitions

- Pendred's syndrome: a complex disorder in which the following conditions are commonly present at birth or develop over time: sensorineural HL secondary to EVA syndrome and cochlear malformation (Mondini), vestibular dysfunction, and thyroid gland enlargement (goiter).[2]
- CAS: a motor speech disorder resulting in difficulty with production of sounds, syllables, and words. The source has been identified to be an oral motor central processing issue. In other words, the brain has difficulty planning the movements needed to produce speech. The child receptively understands and formulates the expressive intent, but cannot produce the words or sentences to communicate the thoughts.[3]

References

[1] Audiology Online. Sound recover: a breakthrough in enhancing intelligibility. 2008. Available at: http://www.audiologyonline.com/releases/soundrecover-breakthrough-in-enhancing-intelligibility-3719. Accessed August 19, 2017

[2] Genetics Home Reference. Pendred syndrome. Available at: https://ghr.nlm.nih.gov/condition/pendred-syndrome. Accessed July 27, 2017

[3] American Speech Language Hearing Association. Childhood apraxia of speech. Available at: http://www.asha.org/public/speech/disorders/ChildhoodApraxia/. Accessed July 27, 2017

36 Multidisciplinary Assessment and Management of a Complex Case

Jeffrey Simmons and Catherine Carotta

36.1 Clinical History and Description

Linus was born at 39 weeks' gestational age via C-section delivery. His mother took insulin, metformin, methyldopa, aspirin, and other medications during the pregnancy. Apgar scores were 8 and 9, and birth weight was 9.10 lb. His family history included an older sister with profound hearing loss and bilateral cochlear implants (CI). She utilized primarily spoken communication, but despite getting her first implant by the age of 13 months, she experienced early and continued delays in language and academic development. Linus did not pass his newborn hearing screen, and follow-up testing at 1 month of age yielded high-frequency tympanograms within normal limits, absent distortion product otoacoustic emissions (DPOAEs), and auditory brainstem responses for clicks and for tone burst at 250, 1,000, 2,000, and 4,000 Hz consistent with bilateral profound sensorineural hearing loss.

At approximately 7 weeks of age, Linus was fitted with bilateral amplification using Desired Sensation Level (DSL) 5.0a child prescriptive targets and real-ear-to-coupler difference (RECD) measurements with his earmolds. No consistent responses to sound were observed even with amplification in use. There were some challenges in establishing consistent use of amplification due to recurrent middle ear infections. Linus had two different sets of pressure equalization (PE) tubes placed in the first year of life.

Linus began assessment for CI candidacy at 8 months of age. As part of the evaluation, rotary chair testing was conducted, and there were no indications of peripheral vestibular system involvement noted.

A pediatric ophthalmological evaluation at the age of 9 months revealed early evidence of myopia and astigmatism with a likelihood of eventual need for eyeglasses.

Just short of his first birthday, genetic testing was conducted. Results led to the conclusion that Linus's hearing loss was likely associated with Usher's syndrome type 2C. This diagnosis was based on discovery of two novel variants (c.13345G > T and c.17992G > A) in the *GPR98* gene, which is a locus for Usher's syndrome type 2C.

Linus was enrolled in early intervention services at 1 month of age. Home-based services were provided weekly by a parent–infant provider who specialized in working with children who are deaf or hard of hearing. Linus's family chose to use spoken language with support from sign language as their communication approach. At 8 months of age, Linus's development was assessed using the Developmental Profile-3 (DP-3).[1] Results of the DP-3 indicated that Linus's overall development was within normal limits for his chronological age. Expected age-level performance was noted in the following domains: physical, adaptive behavior, social-emotional, and cognitive. However, Linus's communication skills were found to be delayed for his chronological age. Linus presented as an alert, attentive, interactive child who was easy to engage in play and turn taking. During the assessment, he produced the sounds "ah," "uh," "m," and he was reported to use the signs for "milk" and "eat."

36.2 Questions for the Reader

1. Was the timeline for identification and early intervention appropriate?
2. Are there "red flags" in the case history of which an audiologist should take note?
3. What types of issues might arise in this child?

36.3 Discussion of Questions

1. **Was the timeline for identification and early intervention appropriate?**
   The 1–3-6 guidelines from the Joint Committee on Infant Hearing recommend that all children have a hearing screen by 1 month of age, that hearing loss be identified by 3 months of age, and that intervention services, including fitting of amplification, be initiated by 6 months of age.[2] In Linus's case, these three milestones occurred even earlier than the recommended times. Identification of the hearing loss, fitting of amplification, and enrollment in early intervention services all took place within the first two months after birth.

2. **Are there "red flags" in the case history of which an audiologist should take note?**
   It is noteworthy that Linus's older sister was experiencing progress with her CI that was slower or more limited than might be expected. Exploration of reasons for her slow progress would be warranted. Was it due to inconsistent device use, overall developmental delays, language stimulation from parents, or some other factors? Whatever the reasons might be, is there a possibility that Linus may experience additional learning challenges?

3. **What types of issues might arise in this child?**
   Although Usher's syndrome type 2C is not a form of the syndrome that involves vestibular function, progressive degeneration of the retinas (retinitis pigmentosa) is associated with this genetic condition. Rate of progression and ultimate degree of vision loss are both variable, but the visual field can become quite limited by the time of the fourth decade.[3] Referral to a pediatric ophthalmologist is an important early step in management of a child diagnosed with Usher's syndrome. Given Linus's sister's language and learning challenges, it will be important to carefully monitor Linus's language acquisition.

36.3.1 Audiologic Testing and Additional History

Linus had surgery for a CI on the right side at 12 months of age. He received a second CI on the left side 2 weeks later. A measure of hearing sensitivity with the CI in use was obtained with fair reliability about 4 months following surgery (▶ Fig. 36.1).

Unfortunately, a pocket of fluid developed over the right implant at approximately 4 to 5 months postsurgery. Repeated treatment efforts to resolve the issue were unsuccessful, and surgery for removal of the right implant and granulation tissue was performed at approximately 6 months postimplant. After an additional 5 months, the right side was reimplanted, and reactivation of the right side implant occurred at age 23 months.

During the interim period without an implant on the right side, a tonsillectomy was performed due to continued issues with ear infections and with sleep apnea. There were also indications that medical issues and other factors contributed to less-than-consistent use of the left implant during the months that the right device was explanted.

After reinitiating bilateral implant use following the second CI surgery for the right ear, progress in development of auditory skills was slower than expected. For example, at 16 months postimplant, Linus's score of 50% on the Infant Toddler Meaningful Auditory Integration Scale (IT-MAIS) was at an age equivalent of 5 to 6 months compared to children with normal hearing.[4,5]

Shortly after the time Linus first received his implants, he began frequently producing continuous vocalizations. The vocalizations consisted of basically monotonic "humming" or neutral vowels that did not appear to be intentional communication. These vocalizations made it difficult to obtain information from tests or procedures that require the child to be quiet while measures are being performed (e.g., threshold testing for speech and nonspeech stimuli, electrically evoked stapedial reflex threshold [ESRT], etc.). The programming audiologist was consequently limited to setting CI stimulation by using electrically evoked compound action potential (ECAP) measures and subjective observation of responses to sound as guides. The limited audiogram in ▶ Fig. 36.2 was obtained at age 2 years, 4 months, and more than a year postimplant surgery. Thresholds with the CI were improved over the preimplant unaided hearing sensitivity in the profound range, but Linus was not consistently responding in the 20- to 30-dB HL range typically seen with children who are implanted at an early age. It was not clear if these response levels were truly the lowest that Linus could detect or if they were more representative of minimum response levels. Regardless, in the test environment, Linus was not responding to narrowband noise sounds or speech at levels as low as what generally would be seen in a child with his history of early identification and early implantation. Also at around this time, parent report of Linus's auditory behaviors was not appreciably changed from what had been recorded 1 year earlier, and his score on the IT-MAIS remained at the age equivalent level of 5 months, despite the fact that he was nearly one and a half years postimplant.

Not surprisingly, Linus's speech and language development was also showing limited progress in development. As a part of the parent–infant home intervention process, Linus's developmental skills were assessed using the DP-3 when he was 26 months of age. Assessment revealed appropriate age standard scores in the physical (97) and adaptive (101) domains, low average performance in the social-emotional domain (85), and below average performance in the cognitive (67) and communication (71) domains. The MacArthur-Bates Communicative Development Inventory (MCDI) was used to document Linus's words/signs and gesture usage in the home.[6] At 25 months of age, Linus was reported to understand 192 words/signs, use 95 signs, and say 6 words. Production of two-word/sign combinations was not observed. When compared to other children of his age, Linus' word production was determined to be at less than the 1st percentile.

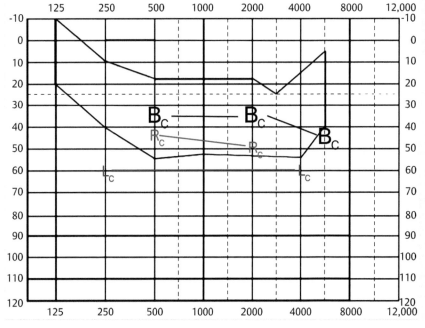

Fig. 36.1 Behavioral thresholds measured with cochlear implants at approximately 4 months postsurgery. RC, right cochlear implant; LC, left cochlear implant; BC, binaural cochlear implants.

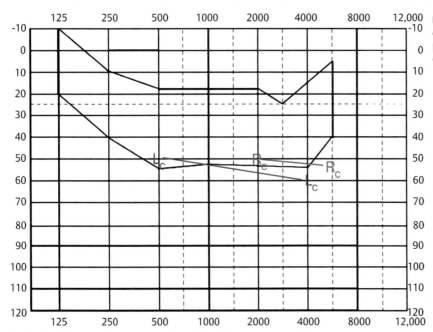

Fig. 36.2 Behavioral thresholds measured with cochlear implants at slightly beyond 1 year postsurgery. RC, right cochlear implant; LC, left cochlear implant.

At 25 months of age, a speech-language therapist was asked to assess vocal and speech development through a speech sampling procedure during a home visit. Linus's vocal output was mostly characterized by prolonged vowels (e.g., "ee" or "ah"), a prolonged consonant (e.g., /m/), and vocal play (e.g., gurgling, raspberries, glottal sounds). On occasion, Linus attempted to imitate the vocal play of his parent–infant provider. This speech sample indicated that Linus's vocal development was similar to the vocal output of a child with normal hearing between the ages of 2 and 8 months (i.e., reflexive sounds, 0–2 months; cooing and laughter, 2–4 months; vocal play, 4–8 months). No true words or sign language was used during the speech assessment. Linus used vocalizations and gestures to communicate such communication functions as requesting, refusing, protesting, and commenting. Linus's Individual Family Service Plan (IFSP) and outpatient speech-language services focused on developing his speech, language, and listening skills using routine and play-based approaches. Parent involvement during this time was consistent, and throughout the early intervention period his mother reported concern for lack of speech development and difficulty managing Linus's behavior.

In preparation for the transition from parent–infant home visit services to school-based services, a broad range of developmental assessments were conducted. Physical therapy and occupational therapy evaluations were conducted when Linus was 34 months of age. Linus achieved an average Gross Motor Quotient of 94 and a Fine Motor Quotient of 100 on the Peabody Developmental Motor Scales-2. Given age-level motor performance, physical therapy services were not recommended. The occupational therapy evaluation revealed sensory seeking behaviors impacting Linus's ability to attend to tasks, and educationally based occupational therapy services were recommended.

Developmental assessment using the DP-3 was again conducted at 37 months of age, prior to Linus's entry into preschool. Results indicated age-level performance in the physical (105) and adaptive (97) domains, and below average perform-

ance in the social-emotional (78), cognitive (81), and communication (61) domains. Speech sampling conducted in the home at 37 months of age revealed no oral motor concerns, prolonged vocalizations consisting primary of vowels, and use of the following consonants in noncommunicative vocalizations: /m, n, b, g, f, w, y/. No true words or sign language was observed during the sampling process in the home. However, Linus's clinical speech therapist reported use of such single-word signs as "listen," "think," "more," "fish," "bird," "TV," "bye," "bath," and "stop." The therapist reported that Linus was able to say the following words: "mom," "mama," and "papa," and that he attempted word approximations for "stop," "dog," "up," and "out." Upon transition into preschool, Linus's parent–infant specialist expressed continued concerns regarding his slow rate of vocal development and acquisition of formal language (sign or spoken), and she reported that Linus preferred to use gestural communication strategies to express himself.

At 39 months of age, his mother sought a second opinion regarding Linus's sensory seeking behaviors. The parent completed the Sensory Processing Measure (SPM).[7] Results of the measure indicated definite dysfunction in the following areas: social participation (e.g., joins in activities), vision (e.g., easily distracted), and body awareness (e.g., exerts too much pressure, chews on nonfood objects, seeks movement such as pushing, pulling, dragging, or jumping). Additional difficulties were also noted in the areas of touch (e.g., dislikes teeth brushing) and balance/motions (e.g., poor coordination, clumsy, leans on other people).

Throughout this period, there were challenges with determining Linus's auditory status and development of auditory skills. It was necessary to continue use of visual reinforcement audiometry (VRA) with Linus until he was close to 3 years old, because he could not be reliably conditioned to do a conditioned play audiometry (CPA) activity. Even after CPA could be used with Linus, it continued to be difficult to obtain reliable results because of challenges keeping him attending to the task at hand. He routinely displayed high levels of activity and was very distractible, difficult to keep on task, and impulsive.

Upon entrance into a preschool program for children who are deaf and hard of hearing, Linus's classroom teacher conducted preacademic skill assessment. At 3 years, 7 months of age, this curriculum-embedded assessment was conducted using the Creative Curriculum Gold Child Assessment Portfolio and revealed below age–level performance in the social-emotional, language, literacy, mathematics, and cognitive domains.[8] Age-level performance was noted in the physical domain. Linus was noted to enjoy block- and train-building activities. He reportedly became upset when there was a change of expectations or activities. He demonstrated frequent tantrums, seemed to bump into other children's play, and had difficulty expressing his basic wants and needs using sign or spoken language. A picture schedule was used to establish understanding of the preschool routine and the Picture Exchange Communication approach was used to help Linus understand how to express his wants and needs. A school-based sensory reassessment revealed limited body awareness as noted by his bumping into children or using excessive force. He was observed to seek extra sensory input as noted by his constant movement and touching everything in his environment. He was observed to sit for up to 3 minutes, but his typical engagement time in most activities was 1 minute. School and clinically based occupational therapy services recommended sensory techniques and tools, a weighted compression vest, visual teaching strategies, and a variety of heavy work sensory strategies (e.g., pushing and pulling heavy objects) to calm Linus and increase his attention.

It was not until Linus was age 3 years, 9 months that a complete audiogram was finally recorded for him (▶ Fig. 36.3). This was about 4 months after he began attending preschool. The weighted compression vest he had been using in the preschool setting also helped with managing Linus's attention and activity level during audiometric testing in the clinic.

Shortly after this audiogram was recorded, some limited speech perception testing was completed with fair reliability for the first time with Linus. On the Pattern Perception subtest

of the Early Speech Perception (ESP) Test–Low Verbal Version, Linus correctly identified 12 targets presented from a four-item closed set with 100% accuracy.[9] This would suggest development of detection and discrimination skills in terms of Erber's hierarchy of development.[10]

At age 4 years, the variants of the *GPR98* gene that had been identified in Linus following his genetic testing were reclassified as variants of uncertain clinical significance and were no longer deemed to be pathogenic or associated with Usher's syndrome type 2C. This was based on findings from genetic testing completed for Linus's older sister, who also has bilateral profound hearing loss. Her testing revealed the fact that she does not have either of the variants in the *GPR98* gene described in Linus.

Fine motor skills were reassessed at 4 years of age. Results of the Peabody Developmental Motor Scales-2 revealed a below-average Fine Motor Quotient of 79 with specific difficulty noted in Linus's ability to use his hands to grasp objects and low average ability in his ability to perform visual perceptual skills involving complex eye–hand coordination tasks.

Speech and language testing at 4 years of age revealed below-average receptive vocabulary knowledge as measured by the Peabody Picture Vocabulary Test-4 (standard score = 66, percentile = 1, age equivalent = 2 years 2 months).[11] Formal broad-based language and articulation assessments using the Preschool Language Scale-5 and the Goldman–Fristoe-3 were attempted, but could not be completed due to Linus's developmental level of readiness to comply with the assessment procedures.[12,13] He was reportedly able to follow such one-step directions as "go pack your back pack" when sign and spoken language was used. Limited understanding was noted when directions were presented in the auditory condition only. He demonstrated inconsistent understanding of "what," "who," and "where" questions. According to a vocabulary list collected at school, Linus was noted to use 45 words/signs spontaneously. Linus continued to imitate two-word sign constructions but was not noted to independently produce two- to three-word

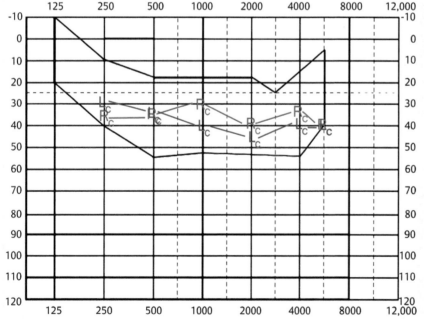

Fig. 36.3 Behavioral thresholds measured with cochlear implants at 2 years, 9 months postsurgery. RC, right cochlear implant; LC, left cochlear implant.

signed or spoken language combinations. Pictures and visual sentence strips were used to support his communication development. Linus frequently engaged in random vocalizations consisting of consonant–vowel and vowel–consonant vocalizations.

A speech sound inventory was obtained and revealed he was able to produce a range of vowel sounds and the following consonant sounds: /m, n, b, f, g, w, y/. Inconsistent imitation of consonant–vowel–consonant syllables was noted. His Individual Education Program (IEP) targeted production of the following word productions: consonant–vowel (e.g., me, go, no), vowel–consonant (e.g., on, eat), consonant–vowel–consonant–vowel (e.g., mama, papa), and consonant–vowel–consonant (e.g., mom, cup, more). Review of IEP progress updates indicated limited progress in spontaneously producing or imitating a variety of simple words. At 4 years, 1 month, a language sample revealed a mean length of utterance (MLU) of 1.21 words/signs, which is the expected performance of a 12- to 26-month-old child. He was observed to produce frequent noncommunicative vocalizations throughout his play, work, and social interactions. Linus's vocal quality was noted to be harsh and strained. At 4 years, 7 months of age, Linus was referred for counseling and behavior consultation due to his unpredictable aggressive behaviors that quickly escalated into such behaviors as kicking, hitting, biting, and spitting. At 4 years, 8 months of age, Linus transitioned from using the Picture Exchange Communication approach to spontaneously using single words/signs, word/sign combinations, and short phrases (e.g., "I want ____").

Linus's preschool teacher conducted curriculum-embedded assessment using the Creative Curriculum Gold Child Assessment Portfolio again at 4 years, 10 months of age and revealed continued below-age-level performance for social-emotional, language, literacy, and mathematics domains. However, age-level performance was noted in the physical domain and most aspects of the cognitive domain.

At 4 years, 11 months of age an assessment of Linus's social-relatedness, communication, and sensory behaviors was requested by his mother, who specifically wanted to know if Linus had autism. Results of the Vineland-II, Autism Screening Instrument for Educational Planning-3, Social Responsiveness Scale-2, Autism Diagnostic Observation Schedule-2, and classroom observation yielded an autism spectrum diagnosis due to Linus's significant difficulties with social relationships, significant impairment in expressive and receptive communication, a narrow range of interests, and sensory regulation issues. These behaviors and limited communication development were viewed to be outside of what would be expected for a child who was implanted at an early age and who received consistent and strong intervention.

36.4 Additional Questions for the Reader

1. What are potential effects of the temporary explantation of the right-side CI?
2. How did Linus's development trajectory compare with what is typically expected in children implanted at around the age of 12 months?
3. What types of collaboration or referral should be pursued in a case like Linus's?

36.5 Discussion of Additional Questions

1. **What are potential effects of the temporary explantation of the right-side CI?**
Because Linus's brain would potentially still have had access to auditory input from the implant on the left ear, removal of the right implant, even for a period of several months, would not likely have had significant negative effects. In Linus's case, though, recurrent ear infections and a tonsillectomy contributed to some periods of nonuse of the external equipment for the left implant during the time in which the right implant was explanted. The resulting lack of regular auditory input to the brain could easily slow or even halt progress in development of listening and spoken language skills, for a time. Linus's persistent and significant delays in development over time, however, would not be attributable primarily to the period when the right device was explanted, even if inconsistent use of the left implant occurred during that time as well.

2. **How did Linus's development trajectory compare with what is typically expected in children implanted at around the age of 12 months?**
By 1 year post CI, a child implanted at age 1 year would typically be expected to be consistently responding to his name and many environmental sounds, to be deriving meaning from a number of speech and environmental sounds, and to be exhibiting a major improvement in language.[14] Linus was not showing these behaviors and measures of speech perception ability could not be reliably obtained. Similarly, at 16 months postimplant, his score of 20 out of 40 on the IT-MAIS was at an age equivalency of a 5- to 6-month-old child with normal hearing.[4] At a point 1 year later, just short of 2.5 years postimplant, Linus's reported auditory behaviors had not appreciably changed, and his score on the IT-MAIS was still at the age-equivalent level of 5 months. Shortly after this, speech perception scores were obtained on Linus for the first time and suggested that he was at least developing pattern perception (discrimination) skills. Speech and language development similarly showed delayed or limited progress. Just after his fourth birthday and 3 years of CI use, differences between Linus's chronological age and language age were in the range of 2 years or greater. Because of issues with behavior and compliance, formal testing results may have underestimated the actual development of Linus's auditory skills to some degree. Nevertheless, all signs suggested that Linus's rate of progress in development of auditory, speech, and language skills was much slower than would be typically seen in a child implanted at 1 year of age.

3. **What types of collaboration or referral should be pursued in a case like Linus's?**
Because between 20 and 40% of children with hearing loss are reported to have additional disabilities outside of their hearing loss, it is important for all providers to engage in developmental surveillance.[15] Monitoring children's development over time and across the social-emotional, cognition, auditory, speech, language, fine motor, and gross motor domains is an essential function of individuals working with children who are deaf or hard of hearing. Collecting informa-

tion about the child's interactions in the home, speech therapy sessions, audiology appointments, day care settings, and classroom environments using a variety of assessment methods (e.g., parent inventories, interviews, classroom/home observations, standardized tests, criterion-referenced instruments, curriculum-embedded assessment, etc.) will ensure that a holistic and authentic ecological approach has been used to obtain a thorough view of the child.[16] When a child appears to be delayed in any of these domains, it is appropriate to consider bringing in professionals who specialize in the specific domains (e.g., physical therapists, occupational therapists, psychologists, counselors, vision specialists, speech-language specialists, etc.). Further, referral to the various medical experts, when appropriate, is essential when children are displaying additional challenges impacting their learning (e.g., neurologists, developmental pediatricians,

vestibular specialists, otolaryngologists, psychiatrists, etc.). A careful and ongoing multidisciplinary case review is necessary in order to ensure the child who is deaf or hard of hearing receives the care that is needed in a timely fashion.

36.6 Outcome

Linus's most recent audiometric testing, completed at age 4 years, 11 months, finally showed sensitivity thresholds with the CI in the target range of what is typically observed in pediatric implant recipients (▶ Fig. 36.4).

Some measures of Linus's auditory-only speech perception abilities also have recently been successfully obtained. ▶ Fig. 36.5 shows results for speech perception testing at ages 4 years, 2 months; 5 years, 1 month; and 5 years, 2 months. With the smaller, four-item closed sets of the low verbal version

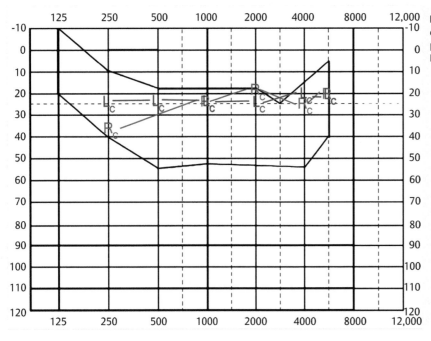
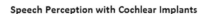

Fig. 36.4 Behavioral thresholds measured with cochlear implants at a point nearly 4 years postimplant surgery. RC, right cochlear implant; LC, left cochlear implant.

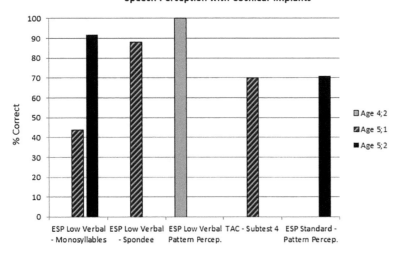

Fig. 36.5 Speech perception test findings with cochlear implants in use.

of the ESP, Linus is able to consistently identify monosyllables (e.g., boat, bird, ball, bed) and spondees (e.g., hotdog, airplane, French fries, ice cream) that are in his vocabulary. He also does fairly well at accurately identifying target words in the 12-item closed set from the Pattern Perception subtest of the ESP—Standard Version. These results suggest that Linus is beginning to develop skills that are at least in the identification stage of Erber's hierarchy of auditory development.

Comprehensive speech-language testing was conducted when Linus was 5 years of age prior to his transition to kindergarten (▶ Table 36.1). Receptive vocabulary (standard score: 68; percentile: 2) and expressive vocabulary (standard score: 57; percentile: 0.2) scores were in the below-average range on the Peabody Picture Vocabulary Test-4 and the Expressive Vocabulary Test-2.[11,17] Board-based language testing using the Preschool Language Scale-5 revealed auditory comprehension to be in the below-average range (standard score: 62; percentile: 2) and expressive language to be in the below-average range (standard score: 61; percentile: 1).[13] Spontaneous language sampling revealed an MLU of 1.57. Assessment of Linus's ability to attend to increasing lengths of information in the listening condition only revealed that he was able to attend to single words with 60% accuracy, two critical elements with 70% accuracy, and three critical elements with 20% accuracy. He was able to follow one-step routine directions such as "go get your back pack," "wash your hands," and "sit down" when presented in an auditory-only condition. He needed sign support for such directions as "line up" or "put that away." Depending on his motivation and temperament, he reportedly needed adult guidance and multiple repetitions. He did not consistently follow one-step nonroutine directions or two-step directions. He was able to answer simple "what's that," "who," "where," and "yes/no" questions. He was not yet able to answer "why," "when," or "how" questions. Linus was noted to put two to three signs together to convey his wants. He engaged in multiple conversational turns on topics he initiated. He displayed limited eye contact and would not typically attend to adult initiated conversations. He told visual stories through drawing or use of gestural actions. Assessment of Linus's nonspeech oral movements revealed that Linus was able to execute all nonspeech oral movements (e.g., lateralizing his tongue, puckering his lips, protruding his tongue, etc.). He was noted to be inconsistent with early developing speech sounds (/m, p, b, t, d, n/) in syllables and words. Linus relied on signs to communicate his message to adults and peers, marking each sign he produced with a vocalization, although vocalizations were not intelligible.

Linus's case history and these test results were reviewed by a multidisciplinary educational and clinical team who met with his mother to discuss his kindergarten IEP. Linus was placed in a neighborhood school where he was enrolled in a classroom for children who are deaf and hard of hearing. He was mainstreamed for some activities and received speech-language therapy, occupational therapy, and audiology services. Specific behavior and sensory strategies were provided to support Linus's sensory and autism-related needs. Linus will continue to be followed by his CI team who will work with his school team to ensure optimal success.

Table 36.1 Language results at 5 years of age

Test	Standard score	Percentile	Age equivalent
Peabody Picture Vocabulary Test 4	68	2	2;9
Expressive Vocabulary Test 2	57	.2	2;3
Preschool Language Scale 5	62		
Auditory Comprehension	62	1	2;9
Expressive Communication	61	1	2;7
Total Language	59	1	2;8

36.7 Acknowledgments

The authors would like to acknowledge the contributions of Elizabeth Baruch, speech-language pathologist; Debbie Smith, parent–infant communication specialist; and Shelly Carney, teacher of the deaf/hard of hearing.

References

[1] Alpern GD. Developmental Profile. 3rd ed. Los Angeles, CA: Western Psychological Services; 2007

[2] American Academy of Pediatrics, Joint Committee on Infant Hearing. Year 2007 position statement: Principles and guidelines for early hearing detection and intervention programs. Pediatrics. 2007; 120(4):898–921

[3] Lentz J, Keats B. Usher Syndrome Type II. Available at:https://www.ncbi.nlm.nih.gov/books/NBK1341/#usher2.Management; 2016. Accessed March 23, 2018

[4] Kishon-Rabin L, Taitelbaum R, Elichai O, Maimon D, Debyiat D, Chazan N. Developmental aspects of the IT-MAIS in normal-hearing babies. Israeli Journal of Speech and Hearing. 2001; 23:12–22

[5] Zimmerman-Phillips S, Osberger MJ, Robbins AM. Infant-Toddler Meaningful Auditory Integration Scale. Sylmar, CA: Advanced Bionics Corp; 1997

[6] Fenson L, Marchman VA, Thal D, Dale PS, Reznick JS, Bates E. MacArthur-Bates Communicative Development Inventories: User Guide and Technical Manual. 2nd ed. Baltimore, MD: Paul H. Brookes Publishing Co; 2007

[7] Parham LD, Ecker C. Sensory Processing Measure (SPM). Los Angeles, CA: Western Psychological Services; 2007

[8] Dodge DT, Colker LJ, Heroman C, Bickart T. The Creative Curriculum for Preschool. 5th ed. Washington, DC: Teaching Strategies; 2010

[9] Moog JS, Geers AE. Early Speech Perception Test for Profoundly Deaf Children. St. Louis, MO: Central Institute for the Deaf; 1990

[10] Erber NP. Auditory Training. Washington, DC: AG Bell Association for the Deaf; 1982

[11] Dunn LM, Dunn DM. Peabody Picture Vocabulary Test. 4th ed. Minneapolis, MN: NCS Pearson, Inc; 2007

[12] Goldman R, Fristoe M. Goldman-Fristoe Test of Articulation. 3rd ed. San Antonio, TX: Pearson PsychCorp; 2015

[13] Zimmerman IL, Steiner VG, Pond RE. Preschool Language Scales. 5th ed. San Antonio, TX: Pearson; 2011

[14] Robbins AM. Clinical Red Flags for Slow Progress in Children with Cochlear Implants. Loud and Clear, Issue 1. Boston, MA: Advanced Bionics Corp; 2005

[15] Gallaudet Research Institute. Regional and National Survey Report of the data from the 2007–08 Annual Survey of deaf and hard of Hearing Children and youth. Washington, DC: Gallaudet Research Institute; 2008

[16] Ganguly D, Ambrose S, Carotta C. The assessment role of the speech-language specialist on the clinical cochlear implant team. In: Eisenberg L, ed. Clinical management of children with Cochlear Implants. 2nd ed. San Diego, CA: Plural Publishing; 2017:273–372

[17] Williams KT. EVT-2: Expressive Vocabulary Test. Circle Pines, MN: AGS Publishing; 2007

37 Sudden-Onset Hearing Loss with Bilateral Enlarged Vestibular Aqueducts

Hilary Gazeley

37.1 Clinical History and Description

Eme, a nearly 4-year-old girl, presents with a parent report of a sudden change in hearing and speech production. Case history reveals a normal birth history with a bilateral "pass" for newborn hearing screening, as well as a recent "pass" for preschool hearing screening. Parents report that Eme has periodically appeared to not hear well but that at other times she appears to hear very well, thus causing them to believe the instances of poorer responding were due to age, inattention, or activity level. Eme recently experienced a sudden significant change in the way she responds to voices and environmental sounds, prompting parents to have her seen by her primary care physician who referred Eme immediately to ear, nose, and throat (ENT).

37.2 Audiologic Testing

Audiological evaluation was completed with good reliability and revealed an asymmetric, bilateral sensorineural hearing loss. Both ears presented a mild to profound degree of hearing loss with the left ear pure-tone average (PTA) of 77 dB HL, and the right ear PTA of 88 dB HL. At the time of initial diagnosis, Eme also reported "screaming" in both ears.

Eme completed a course of oral prednisone as an anti-inflammatory treatment, and hearing was retested 1 week later. At that time, both ears presented with a further progression of hearing loss with the left ear PTA now at 87 dB HL and the right ear PTA at 98 dB HL. Eme was fit with hearing aids, and an evaluation for cochlear implantation was initiated with close audiological monitoring. Fluctuation of the hearing loss continued with dramatic recovery of the right ear occurring approximately 2 months after the initial drop in hearing sensitivity. PTAs at that time were 90 dB HL for the left ear and 65 dB HL for the right ear. The hearing loss remained stable for an additional 2 months at which time aided speech perception testing, completed at a 60 dB sound pressure level (SPL) presentation level, revealed 0% understanding for the left ear and 72% understanding for the right ear on the Lexical Neighborhood Test (LNT).

37.3 Questions for the Reader

1. What evidence is there that Eme has had a fluctuating and progressive hearing loss even prior to the initial audiological evaluation?
2. What are some considerations for the management of fluctuating hearing loss?

37.4 Discussion of Questions

1. **What evidence is there that Eme has had a fluctuating and progressive hearing loss even prior to the initial audiological evaluation?**
Eme passed both her newborn hearing screening and follow-up preschool screening (▶ Table 37.1; ▶ Table 37.2). She has also developed spoken language and then demonstrated a sudden and significant change in her speech production. The parent-raised concern of Eme's inconsistent hearing is also in line with a potentially fluctuating hearing loss.

2. **What are some considerations for the management of fluctuating hearing loss?**
Counseling parents, caregivers, educators, and therapists regarding the need for close monitoring of changes in hearing as well as the impact of fluctuating hearing loss (e.g., delayed speech and language development, poor attention, and difficulty following directions particularly when background noise is present) is critical. Monitoring is even more important when the child is fit with hearing aids because amplification will need to be adjusted with changes in hearing sensitivity.

Table 37.1 Unaided audiograms left ear (dB HL)

	250 Hz	500 Hz	1,000 Hz	2,000 Hz	4,000 Hz	8,000 Hz
Initial diagnosis	35	55	75	100	80	75
Following prednisone course	35	65	90	105	150	NR
2 mo after initial diagnosis	45	70	90	110	115	DNT

DNT, did not test; NR, no response.

Table 37.2 Unaided audiograms right ear (dB HL)

	250 Hz	500 Hz	1,000 Hz	2,000 Hz	4,000 Hz	8,000 Hz
Initial diagnosis	35	60	95	110	110	NR
Following prednisone course	50	85	100	110	110	NR
2 mo after initial diagnosis	45	40	80	75	65	DNT

DNT, did not test; NR, no response.

37.5 Diagnosis and Recommended Treatment

Computed tomography (CT) of the temporal bones was completed and a diagnosis of bilateral enlarged vestibular aqueducts (EVA) was confirmed. Approximately 4 months after the initial diagnosis of hearing loss, Eme underwent left ear cochlear implantation of a MED-EL Sonata ti[100] device with a fully inserted standard electrode array (▶ Table 37.3). Acoustic hearing was measured at 2 months postoperatively for each ear and was stable compared to thresholds obtained immediately prior to implantation, with the exception of 250 and 500 Hz for the left ear, which demonstrated a further progression in hearing loss. At 6 months post-implant, the left ear cochlear implant thresholds were 25 to 30 dB HL for all frequencies, and speech perception testing for that ear improved to 92% correct LNT from 0% pre-implant (▶ Table 37.4). Eme also scored 80% correct using Phonetically Balanced Kindergarten (PB-K) words in the same condition, presented at 60 dB SPL.

At 18 months post-implant, Eme experienced another sudden drop in hearing for the right ear with a resulting PTA of 103 dB HL (▶ Table 37.5). The left ear cochlear implant thresholds remained stable during that time. Prednisone was not administered with this episode. Hearing began to recover in the right ear after 2 weeks, and stabilized again to a moderate to severe degree of hearing loss within 6 weeks.

37.6 Outcome

Eme is now approximately 8 years post-implant. She communicates via listening and spoken language and receives a mainstream education in her neighborhood public school. She continues to receive services under an individualized education program (IEP) to include consultative deaf and hard of hearing teacher and educational audiology services and FM system use in all classroom settings. Eme prefers to wear the FM system with her hearing aid only. Cochlear implant thresholds and performance have been stable for several years (▶ Table 37.6). The hearing aid for the right ear has required frequent reprogramming with fluctuations in hearing sensitivity.

Table 37.3 Unaided audiogram and aided speech perception testing 4 months after initial diagnosis immediately prior to left cochlear implantation

	250 Hz	500 Hz	1,000 Hz	2,000 Hz	4,000 Hz	8,000 Hz	Aided LNT @ 60 dB SPL
Right (dB HL)	45	40	75	75	60	75	72%
Left (dB HL)	45	65	80	110	115	NR	0%

Abbreviations: LNT, lexical neighborhood test; NR, no response; SPL, sound pressure level.

Table 37.4 Cochlear implant thresholds and speech perception scores at 6 months post-implant

	250 Hz	500 Hz	1,000 Hz	2,000 Hz	4,000 Hz	Aided LNT @ 60 dB SPL	Aided PB-K @ 60 dB SPL
Left (dB HL)	30	30	30	30	25	92%	80%

Abbreviations: LNT, lexical neighborhood test; PB-K, phonetically balanced kindergarten; SPL, sound pressure level.

Table 37.5 Unaided audiogram for right ear fluctuation 18 months after initial diagnosis and subsequent recovery

	250 Hz	500 Hz	1,000 Hz	2,000 Hz	4,000 Hz	8,000 Hz
Right (dB HL) fluctuation	55	85	110	115	115	NR
Right (dB HL) recovery	45	45	75	70	65	65

NR, no response.

Table 37.6 Five years post-implant: aided speech perception scores and cochlear implant (CI) thresholds remain stable

	250 Hz	500 Hz	1,000 Hz	2,000 Hz	4,000 Hz	6,000 Hz	Aided CNC @ 60 dB SPL
Left CI (dB HL)	25	30	30	25	30	25	82%
Left CI + right HA							88%
Right HA							50%

Abbreviations: CNC, consonant–nucleus vowel–consonant; HA, hearing aid; SPL, sound pressure level.

37.7 Additional Questions for the Reader

1. What are some specific considerations for auditory training and auditory learning when a patient has a cochlear implant in one ear and significant residual hearing in the contralateral ear?
2. What role should the known etiology of EVA play in the decision-making process for implanting a patient with a significantly asymmetric hearing loss, when the better ear is not meeting traditional cochlear implant candidacy criteria?
3. At what point could there be consideration of a cochlear implant in the right ear for this patient?

37.8 Discussion of Additional Questions

1. **What are some specific considerations for auditory training and auditory learning when a patient has a cochlear implant in one ear and significant residual hearing in the contralateral ear?**

   While the aim of auditory training post-implant is generally to develop auditory skills with the cochlear implant, the habilitation of listening with both ears together is also critical, particularly for those children in the early stages of their speech and language development. During training, patients may find it helpful to practice cochlear implant listening by turning off the contralateral hearing aid or plugging that ear or, when possible, streaming directly to the cochlear implant processor alone. These patients often have difficulty reporting on the status of their cochlear implant, particularly when they are younger children. For example, they may not initially be able to report if their battery has depleted with the implant because they are still hearing with the non-implant ear.

2. **What role should the known etiology of EVA play in the decision-making process for implanting a patient with a significantly asymmetric hearing loss, when the better ear is not meeting traditional cochlear implant candidacy criteria?**

   Knowing that a patient has an etiology that increases the likelihood of progressive hearing loss in the better ear impacts counseling and recommendations for cochlear implantation of the poorer ear sooner rather than later. In Eme's case, the stable aided hearing from the cochlear implant proved invaluable during periods of fluctuation with her non-implant ear. This stability allowed her to participate fully in her education during these periods of fluctuation.

3. **At what point could there be consideration of a cochlear implant in the right ear for this patient?**

   Implantation of the right ear was considered at the time of the large fluctuation 18 months post left implant. However, with the recovery in hearing, Eme was able to use both the implant and hearing aid together for several years, and that continues to be her preference. Speech perception in the hearing aid alone, implant alone, and implant and hearing aid together conditions continue to be monitored closely to ensure that any further fluctuations in hearing are quickly addressed to maintain audibility and speech understanding.

Suggested Readings

[1] Cadieux JH, Firszt JB, Reeder RM. Cochlear implantation in nontraditional candidates: preliminary results in adolescents with asymmetric hearing loss. Otol Neurotol. 2013; 34(3):408–415

[2] Dewan K, Wippold FJ, II, Lieu JE. Enlarged vestibular aqueduct in pediatric sensorineural hearing loss. Otolaryngol Head Neck Surg. 2009; 140 (4):552–558

[3] Mok M, Galvin KL, Dowell RC, McKay CM. Speech perception benefit for children with a cochlear implant and a hearing aid in opposite ears and children with bilateral cochlear implants. Audiol Neurootol. 2010; 15(1):44–56

[4] Sweetow RW, Rosbe KW, Philliposian C, Miller MT. Considerations for cochlear implantation of children with sudden, fluctuating hearing loss. J Am Acad Audiol. 2005; 16(10):770–780

38 Living in the Genome Generation: Biparental *GJB2* Pathogenic Variants Detected by Expanded Carrier Screening—Outcome from Newborn Screening and Management of Child Following Audiologic Testing

Juan Shen, Cui Song, Marie Tan, Margaret A. Kenna, and Cynthia C. Morton

38.1 Clinical History and Description

Baby John was born to a 30-year-old G2P1 mother at 36 weeks and 5 days of gestational age by spontaneous vaginal delivery. The father was 42 years old. The baby weighed 3,060 g at birth and had Apgar scores of 8 and 9 at 1 and 5 minutes, respectively. John passed the state mandatory newborn hearing screening for both ears in the birth hospital at 1 day of age.

John's parents had undergone expanded carrier screening tests for greater than 175 serious inherited disorders, including hearing loss, during the second trimester of the pregnancy. Both parents were reported to have normal hearing. The couple had a healthy 3-year-old daughter at that time, and there was no significant family history of hereditary diseases. Peripheral whole blood was collected for expanded carrier screening tests at a gestational age of 16 weeks. Carrier screening results were received 2 weeks later and revealed that both parents have different heterozygous pathogenic variants in the *GJB2* gene (NM_004004.5) encoding connexin-26 (Cx26). The father carries the c.235delC/p.(Leu79fs) variant in *GJB2* and the mother carries the c.109G > A/p.(V37I) variant. Because these two variants, if present *in trans* (in different copies of the gene) in the compound heterozygous state, will result in hearing loss, the couple's offspring have a 25% risk of developing *GJB2*-related hearing loss, which is much higher than the prevalence of congenital hearing loss in the general population.

A 3 ml aliquot of umbilical cord blood was collected immediately after John's birth and then submitted to a certified clinical genetic testing laboratory on the same day to determine the genotype of the two variants in John. Genetic test results on the DNA extracted from the cord blood sample became available after 4 weeks, which revealed that John is a compound heterozygote for both of the parental variant alleles, *GJB2* (NM_004004.5):[c.235delC/p.(Leu79fs)];[c.109G > A/p.(Val37Ile)]. The presence of pathogenic variants in both paternal and maternal copies of the *GJB2* gene indicates that John is at high risk for congenital hearing loss.

Although John passed his newborn hearing screening for both ears shortly after birth, he was still referred to a local pediatric hospital audiology clinic because of the parental genetic testing results. The referral was made based on increased risk for hearing loss indicated by parental carrier screening results, before the genetic test results on John's cord blood were known.

38.2 Audiologic Testing

John underwent an initial auditory brainstem response (ABR) evaluation during natural sleep when he was about 7 weeks old. The ABR evaluation showed that his hearing was in the normal range on the right ear from 1,000 to 8,000 Hz (▶ Fig. 38.1). On the left ear, ABR evoked potential waveforms were obtained in the normal hearing range from 1,000 to 4,000 Hz and in the mild hearing loss range at 8,000 Hz. John's initial ABR evaluation suggested a possible mild high-frequency hearing loss on the left. His tympanometry was normal in both ears. Because John does not have a normal copy of the *GJB2* gene, follow-up audiology evaluation was recommended in about 3 months.

John was followed regularly at the same hospital to monitor his hearing status. He was re-evaluated at 4.5 months of age. Tympanometry showed normal middle ear function, bilaterally. Distortion product otoacoustic emissions and ABR evaluations showed normal hearing thresholds on both ears from 2,000 to 4,000 Hz, but mild hearing loss at 8,000 Hz bilaterally, which indicated that his hearing decreased from unilateral (left-side) to bilateral mild hearing loss affecting 8,000 Hz. The audiogram presented is based on the ABR results. John's hearing was still considered adequate for speech and language acquisition for normal developmental purposes given the type and degree of his loss. An appointment was scheduled to monitor his hearing again in 6 months.

38.3 Questions for the Reader

1. Why is it that individuals with pathogenic variants in the *GJB2* gene, which are associated with hearing loss, may have audiologic findings consistent with normal hearing?
2. Was it necessary to perform invasive procedures for the prenatal genetic testing in this case?
3. Why was it necessary to perform audiologic evaluation of the baby who passed the newborn hearing screening?
4. Why are genetic testing results important, even though a baby passes newborn hearing screening?
5. What should be considered when combining genetic screening and newborn hearing screening results to evaluate babies' hearing condition?
6. Why was a decision made to recommend regular hearing evaluations, every 3 to 6 months, of the infant with no normal copy of the *GJB2* gene?

38.4 Discussion of Questions

1. **Why is it that individuals with pathogenic variants in the *GJB2* gene, which are associated with hearing loss, may have audiologic findings consistent with normal hearing?**
   Loss of the *GJB2* gene function is the most frequent cause of congenital nonsyndromic hearing loss, which is inherited in an autosomal recessive manner.[1,2] Autosomal recessive

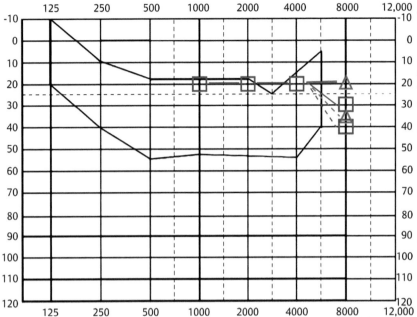

Fig. 38.1 Baby John's audiograms of both ears at 7 and 20 weeks based on auditory brainstem response results. Solid lines, 7 weeks; dashed lines, 20 weeks. Hearing thresholds were within normal range at 20 dB at 1, 2, and 4 kHz at 7 weeks and at 2 and 4 kHz at 20 weeks for both ears. Overlapping symbols and lines were masked. △, right ear air conduction masked; □ left ear air conduction masked.

hearing loss is caused by homozygous or compound heterozygous pathogenic variants in the same gene. The *GJB2* gene on chromosome 13q12 encodes the gap junction protein Cx26. When both copies of the *GJB2* gene are defective, an individual will have hearing loss. Both of c.235delC/p.(Leu76fs) and c.109G > A/p.(V37I) are common pathogenic variants in *GJB2* in people with East Asian origin.[2,3,4] The c.235delC variant causes a frameshift of the coding sequence, which alters the protein's amino acid sequence beginning at codon 79 and leads to a premature termination codon three amino acids downstream. This alteration is then predicted to lead to a truncated product of Cx26. It is associated with a more severe audiologic phenotype. People who are homozygous for the c.235delC variant are usually born with severe to profound hearing loss. The c.109G > A is predicted to alter the amino acid residue at position 37 of Cx26 from a valine (V) to an isoleucine (I). In vitro biochemical and electrophysiological studies of cell lines showed that p.V37I reduces the oligomerization efficiency of Cx26 and significantly compromises the channel function of gap junctions.[5] This variant is more prevalent in individuals with hearing loss than in those with normal hearing.[6] People who are homozygous for the c.109G > A variant may have congenital or later-onset mild to moderate hearing loss. People who are compound heterozygous with c.109G > A and another premature truncating variant such as c.235delC are expected to have mild to moderate hearing loss. Population studies indicate that the penetrance of the c.109G > A variant for the hearing loss phenotype is incomplete and age-dependent.

Individuals with pathogenic variants in *GJB2* may appear to have normal hearing for several reasons. First, heterozygous carriers of pathogenic variants in *GJB2* are expected to have normal hearing, because *GJB2*-related nonsyndromic hearing loss is largely inherited in an autosomal recessive manner. Heterozygous carriers have a functional copy of the *GJB2* gene. Second, different pathogenic variants in *GBJ2* are associated with a wide spectrum of hearing loss severity and

age of onset; some patients with biallelic pathogenic variants may have mild hearing loss that is limited to certain frequency ranges. In the case presented here, the child with compound heterozygous pathogenic variants only showed mild hearing loss at 8,000 Hz in one ear at 7 weeks of age. Should his hearing not be tested at 8,000 Hz, his audiologic findings would appear normal. Third, c.109G > A is a pathogenic variant in *GJB2* known to have incomplete penetrance. The penetrance is age dependent, as hearing thresholds in c.109G > A homozygotes progress at approximately 1 dB/year and the baseline hearing varies among different individuals with the same genotype.[7] When tested at a young age, many individuals with biallelic mild pathogenic *GJB2* alleles may still retain normal hearing.

2. **Was it necessary to perform invasive procedures for the prenatal genetic testing in this case?**
Prenatal genetic diagnostic testing is available to determine the fetus' genotype and to predict the outcome of monogenic conditions. Genetic testing can be performed using DNA extracted from a fetal sample. Fetal samples may be obtained by chorionic villus sampling at gestational age of 10 to 13 weeks, amniocentesis at 14 to 20 weeks, and cordocentesis, also known as percutaneous umbilical blood sampling, at 18 or more weeks.[8] All of these procedures are invasive. Although generally safe, they are associated with a small increased risk of damaging the fetus, miscarriage, and infection.

John's parents declined invasive procedures for prenatal genetic testing. They made the decision based on the following considerations.

First, the hearing loss caused by the loss of *GJB2* function is inherited in an autosomal recessive manner; therefore, the risk of having a compound heterozygous baby is only 25%. Fifty percent of pregnancies in which both parents carry a heterozygous pathogenic *GJB2* variant will result in heterozygous offspring with a single *GJB2* pathogenic variant, in this specific situation a c.235delC or c. 109G > A. A baby inheriting one or the other variant will still have a normal copy of the *GJB2* gene, and therefore is expected to have normal hearing like the parents as discussed above. Another 25% of the pregnancies will end up with two normal copies of the *GJB2* gene. Therefore, the likelihood of having a baby with normal hearing (75%) is three times that of one with hearing loss. Second, prenatal genetic testing results are most likely not to influence the couple's decision on whether to continue or terminate the pregnancy in this case. The hearing loss in compound heterozygous individuals with [c.235delC]; [c.109G > A] is typically mild to moderate with variable onset. Termination of such pregnancies is neither clinically indicated nor ethically acceptable for many people. However, knowing the results may bring emotional and financial burden to the family. Prenatal genetic testing results of this family also do not change the prognosis of the fetus. Although an active area of research and development, no known prenatal procedures have been approved for treating or managing hearing loss. Furthermore, postnatal management and effective early intervention programs are available for infants with hearing loss. Postnatal genetic testing using cord blood is noninvasive and yields results within the time frame to inform management.

Because of these considerations, invasive prenatal genetic testing was deemed not only unnecessary but also a potential risk factor for this family.[9] Nonetheless, had the family desired such testing, it is likely that their insurance would have covered the cost of the procedure and testing even in the setting of a woman not of advanced maternal age.

3. **Why was it necessary to perform audiologic evaluation of the baby who passed the newborn hearing screening?**
Because of the importance of early identification and management of congenital hearing loss, newborn hearing screening occurs in all 50 states and most territories in the United States. It involves use of objective physiologic measures.

Currently, otoacoustic emission and automated ABR tests are most often used to detect hearing loss. Both technologies are noninvasive measurements of physiologic activity that is easily recorded in newborns and is highly correlated with the degree of peripheral hearing sensitivity. However, there are many factors that may influence newborn hearing screening results (such as the testing environment, the newborn's medical status, and the presence of cerumen or middle ear fluid), which could cause false-positive results. According to statistics of some studies, including those of the birth hospital in this case, about 60 to 80% of infants referred for further audiologic testing are found to have normal hearing.

Newborn hearing screening is only considered to be a screening test. A definitive diagnosis of permanent hearing loss requires a more extensive evaluation by physical examination and diagnostic audiologic testing. Current clinical practice standards in the United States were set by the Joint Committee on Infant Hearing (JCIH) in their 2000 and 2007 position statements.[10] In those statements, the JCIH endorsed integrated, interdisciplinary state and national systems of universal newborn hearing screening, evaluation, and

family-centered intervention. The JCIH recommended that all infants have access to universal newborn hearing screening and be screened before 1 month of age. Infants who do not pass the screening test should undergo audiologic and medical evaluations before the age of 3 months, and infants with confirmed hearing loss should receive appropriate intervention before the age of 6 months. In addition, all infants with risk indicators should undergo periodic monitoring for 3 years. Per current clinical practice, infants with any known risk factors should undergo audiologic evaluation even if they pass their newborn hearing screening.

Risk indicators are used because newborn hearing screening may miss some children with permanent hearing loss, especially those with unilateral mild or progressive hearing loss. False-negative results may be due to the high hearing threshold used to identify babies with moderate hearing loss in newborn hearing screening; thus, many babies with mild hearing loss that is still educationally relevant may be missed. Some babies may have progressive or late-onset hearing loss that was normal at birth but may have gradual loss of hearing at an older age. Many known genetic conditions including some pathogenic variants in *GJB2*, such as in the case presented here, are reported to present as late-childhood-onset hearing loss. Early audiologic evaluation of babies who pass newborn hearing screening, but who have other risk indicators for hearing loss, especially a genetic diagnosis of high risk, will ensure early detection and intervention.

4. **Why are genetic testing results important, even though a baby passes newborn hearing screening?**
Without genetic testing on John, John's parents had a 75% of chance to have a baby with normal hearing due to the presence of at least one functional copy of the *GJB2* gene, and a 25% of chance to have a baby like John who is a compound heterozygote for [c. 235delC];[c.109G > A] in *GJB2*. However, children like John may pass newborn hearing screening and experience progressive hearing loss as they grow up.[7] It is important to perform genetic testing to differentiate these two possibilities because of different management implications.

Knowing the genotype of the child is helpful in developing a follow-up monitoring and surveillance strategy. If John were tested and found to be a heterozygous carrier or homozygous for the wild-type *GJB2* allele, follow-up auditory evaluation would not be necessary. Because John was found to be compound heterozygous for both parental pathogenic alleles in *GJB2*, the genetic test results alerted parents and care providers to monitor his development and to pay close attention to his hearing status. Diagnostic audiologic evaluation is more sensitive to detect mild hearing loss in specific frequency ranges. In the case presented here, John passed his newborn hearing screening, but had mild hearing loss at 8,000 Hz in the left ear at the initial hearing evaluation. Regular monitoring of his hearing was recommended based on the genetic diagnosis, which showed progression of the hearing loss in both ears at the 4.5-month evaluation. Continued monitoring will ensure access to rehabilitation services at the earliest indication of hearing loss. Furthermore, newborn genetic testing results can compensate for inherent limitations of conventional newborn hearing screening by detecting babies with mild hearing loss and those at risk for later-onset hearing loss. A definitive genetic diagnosis will qualify a child who passes newborn hearing screening to receive insurance coverage for audiologic evaluation and early intervention services.

In addition, genetic testing results not only guide the care for the affected baby, but also have profound implications for other family members, because they share genetic materials. Although not applicable in this case where both parents knew their risk of having children with hearing loss from the carrier screening results, identification of pathogenic variants associated with hearing loss will allow targeted genetic testing and precise calculation of disease risk for other family members including future offspring.

5. **What should be considered when combining genetic screening and newborn hearing screening results to evaluate babies' hearing condition?**
Conventional newborn hearing screening relies on phenotypic evaluation. However, there may be false-positive and false-negative results as explained above. Incorporating genetic screening into the universal newborn hearing screening scheme will greatly enhance the sensitivity and specificity of the screening to identify children affected with and at risk for permanent hearing loss.

However, careful considerations in many aspects should be given to ensure proper implementation. First, there are ethical issues involved. Newborn genetic screening for hearing loss may introduce risks of discrimination or stigmatization and undue parental anxiety. As mentioned previously, genotype–phenotype correlations are not clear-cut for many genetic variants. Genetic counseling is necessary to help parents understand implications of genetic findings. Second, there are socioeconomic consequences, which may include the necessity to modify or expand the infrastructure and human resources of the health care system to support testing, interpretation, counseling, education, treatment, and follow-up.

6. **Why was a decision made to recommend regular hearing evaluations, every 3 to 6 months, of the infant with no normal copy of the *GJB2* gene?**
Clinical manifestation varies significantly among individuals with pathogenic variants in *GJB2* because of the heterogeneity in the frequencies and types of pathogenic variants in Cx26 within populations and among ethnicities. Studies have shown that some babies with compound heterozygous pathogenic variants in *GJB2* passed newborn hearing screening; however, they were found to have mild hearing loss in follow-up evaluations. While hearing loss exerts a

negative effect on speech, language, and cognitive development, early identification and management are of paramount importance to optimize language, communication, mental health, and employment prospects of children with hearing loss. This case demonstrates that John, with biallelic pathogenic variants in *GJB2*, is predicted to have congenital hearing loss, yet he passed his newborn hearing screening. Regular hearing evaluations are needed to detect the change of hearing status of babies with a genetic diagnosis of high risk for permanent hearing loss. By doing so, children with progressive or later-onset hearing loss can receive presymptomatic diagnosis, and can benefit from better monitoring to allow early clinical diagnosis and early intervention prior to onset of disabling hearing impairment. In this case, follow-up evaluations every 3 to 6 months can help monitor potential progression of the hearing loss and initiate interventions as soon as deemed necessary.

38.5 Diagnosis

Genetic testing indicated that baby John had a high risk for permanent hearing loss based on the compound heterozygosity of biallelic pathogenic variants [c.235delC];[c.109G > A] in the *GJB2* gene *in trans*.

Audiologic evaluation at 7 weeks of age revealed that baby John has mild high-frequency hearing loss in the left ear, and at 4.5 months of age showed progression to bilateral mild high-frequency hearing loss.

Baby John was diagnosed with *GJB2*-related autosomal recessive nonsyndromic hearing loss.

38.6 Outcome

Baby John's general health has been excellent since his birth. He lives at home with both of his parents. His parents believe that he hears well. They do not describe any recent ear pain, ear drainage, ear infection, or any other clinical symptoms regarding his ears. Moreover, John has been regularly monitored for his hearing status both behaviorally at home and through regular follow-up audiologic evaluations. Baby John's parents were informed of the importance of creating a language-rich listening environment to facilitate his auditory brain development.

38.7 Note

Identifiable information such as the baby's name was changed to protect the family's privacy.

References

[1] Kelsell DP, Dunlop J, Stevens HP, et al. Connexin 26 mutations in hereditary non-syndromic sensorineural deafness. Nature. 1997; 387(6628):80–83

[2] Kenna MA, Wu BL, Cotanche DA, Korf BR, Rehm HL. Connexin 26 studies in patients with sensorineural hearing loss. Arch Otolaryngol Head Neck Surg. 2001; 127(9):1037–1042

[3] Abe S, Usami S, Shinkawa H, Kelley PM, Kimberling WJ. Prevalent connexin 26 gene (GJB2) mutations in Japanese. J Med Genet. 2000; 37(1):41–43

[4] Wattanasirichaigoon D, Limwongse C, Jariengprasert C, et al. High prevalence of V37I genetic variant in the connexin-26 (GJB2) gene among non-syndromic hearing-impaired and control Thai individuals. Clin Genet. 2004; 66 (5):452–460

[5] Bruzzone R, Veronesi V, Gomès D, et al. Loss-of-function and residual channel activity of connexin26 mutations associated with non-syndromic deafness. FEBS Lett. 2003; 533(1–3):79–88

[6] Chai Y, Chen D, Sun L, et al. The homozygous p.V37I variant of GJB2 is associated with diverse hearing phenotypes. Clin Genet. 2015; 87(4):350–355

[7] Wu CC, Tsai CH, Hung CC, et al. Newborn genetic screening for hearing impairment: a population-based longitudinal study. Genet Med. 2017; 19 (1):6–12

[8] Ralston SJ, Craigo SD. Ultrasound-guided procedures for prenatal diagnosis and therapy. Obstet Gynecol Clin North Am. 2004; 31(1):101–123

[9] Ghiossi CE, Goldberg JD, Haque IS, Lazarin GA, Wong KK. Clinical utility of expanded carrier screening: reproductive behaviors of at-risk couples. J Genet Couns. 2017 Sep 27:(e-pub ahead of print)

[10] American Academy of Pediatrics, Joint Committee on Infant Hearing. Year 2007 position statement: Principles and guidelines for early hearing detection and intervention programs. Pediatrics. 2007; 120(4):898–921

39 Monitoring Performance for a Child with Hearing Loss

Jane R. Madell

39.1 Clinical History and Description

The patient, Molly, is 6-years-old and in first grade at her local elementary school. Molly has a moderately-severe bilateral hearing loss and wears digital hearing aids. Her hearing loss has been stable since it was identified at birth. Molly received auditory-verbal therapy until age five and has received check-ups with her auditory-verbal therapist twice yearly. The speech-language evaluation indicates that language is at age level. With her hearing aids, she easily follows conversation when she is near the talker and there is no competing noise. However, she is having difficulty hearing soft speech and when background noise is present.

The classroom teacher uses a remote microphone system, and Molly has receivers attached to her hearing aids. However, Molly reports that the remote microphone system does not always work well. Molly's classroom teacher is concerned that Molly appears confused in the classroom much of the time. If Molly understands what is required of her, and if it is a task she can accomplish on her own, she does well. Because of classroom concerns, Molly is referred back to the audiologist.

39.2 Audiologic Testing

Audiological testing reveals no change in hearing with thresholds stable at moderately-severe hearing loss levels. Aided testing was accomplished binaurally and indicated aided thresholds at mild hearing loss levels through 2000 Hz with thresholds at moderate hearing loss levels above 2000 Hz. Speech perception testing was accomplished at 50 dB HL and indicated good speech perception (84%) in quiet binaurally. ▶ Fig. 39.1

39.3 Questions for the Reader

1. Was the testing the audiologist performed sufficient to determine why Molly is having problems in school?
2. Is Molly receiving sufficient benefit from her hearing aids?
3. Do you have enough speech perception information to understand Molly's hearing problems in the classroom?

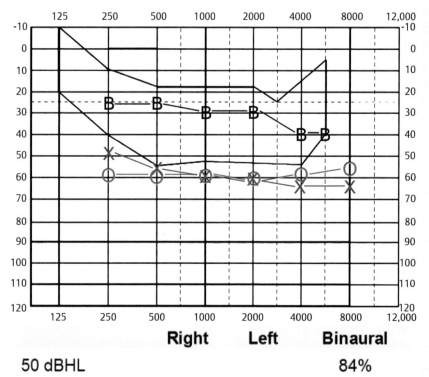

Fig. 39.1 Audiologic evaluation. O, right ear air conduction; X, left ear air conduction; B, hearing aids with bone conduction device.

Right   Left   Binaural

50 dBHL   84%

35 dBHL

50 dBHL+5SNR

4. If additional testing is warranted, describe the testing needed.

5. What other recommendations would you offer?

39.4 Discussion of Questions

1. **Was the testing the audiologist performed sufficient to determine why Molly is having problems in school?**

Because testing was only accomplished binaurally, we do not know what is happening with each hearing aid.

2. **Is Molly receiving sufficient benefit from her hearing aids?**

Molly is not receiving sufficient auditory information from her hearing aids. Ideally, we would like her to be hearing at the top of the speech banana in each ear (at the level of the speech bean).

3. **Do you have enough speech perception information to understand Molly's hearing problems in the classroom?**

Speech perception testing was only accomplished at a normal conversational level, so we do not know how Molly is hearing soft speech or receiving speech at a distance. Without that information, we do not know how Molly will hear comments of other children in the classroom. Without information about hearing in background noise, we do not know what Molly might be hearing in a typical classroom situation.

4. **If additional testing is warranted, describe the testing needed.**

Additional testing should include
- Aided thresholds for each ear separately.
- Speech perception testing.
  - Normal conversational levels (50 dB HL) with technology using right hearing aid alone, left hearing aid alone, and binaurally.
  - Soft conversational levels (35 dB HL) with technology binaurally.
  - Normal conversational levels in noise.

5. **What other recommendations would you offer?**
- Testing indicates that Molly is not hearing well with the right hearing aid. The hearing aid needs to be adjusted to permit Molly to hear at softer levels.
- Aided testing for both ears indicates insufficient high-frequency gain. If a change in hearing aid settings cannot improve high frequency hearing, a change in hearing aids and/or earmolds should be considered.
- Speech perception testing indicates that Molly does not have good access to soft speech. This indicates that she will have reduced incidental learning, will have difficulty hearing when she is not close to the talker, and will have difficulty hearing her peers in the classroom.
- Molly would benefit from the use of a pass-around microphone in the classroom to enable her to hear her classmates. ▶ Fig. 39.2

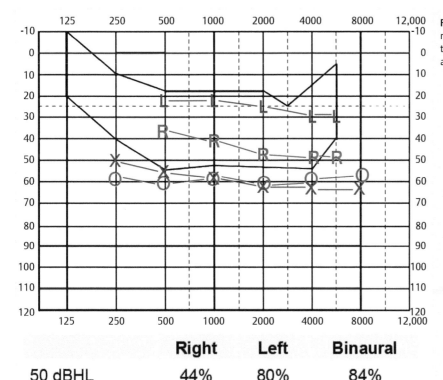

Fig. 39.2 Additional audiological evaluation. O, right ear air conduction; X, left ear air conduction; R, right ear hearing aid; L, left ear hearing aid.

	Right	Left	Binaural
50 dBHL	44%	80%	84%
35 dBHL			64%
50 dBHL+5SNR			72%

39.5 Additional Questions

1. What does testing indicate about Molly's ability to hear with each hearing aid separately?
2. What measures can be implemented to improve Molly's auditory access?
3. What can we conclude from the additional speech perception testing?
4. What additional recommendations would you make for the classroom?

39.6 Discussion of Additional Questions

1. **What does testing indicate about Molly's ability to hear with each hearing aid separately?**
   Testing indicates that Molly is not hearing well with the right hearing aid. The hearing aid needs to be adjusted to permit Molly to hear at softer levels.
2. **What measures can be implemented to improve Molly's auditory access?**
   Aided testing for both ears indicates insufficient high-frequency gain. If a change in hearing aid settings cannot improve high-frequency hearing, a change in hearing aids and/or earmolds should be considered.
3. **What can we conclude from the additional speech perception testing?**
   Speech perception testing indicates that Molly does not have good access to soft speech. This indicates that she will have reduced incidental learning, will have difficulty hearing when she is not close to the talker, and will have difficulty hearing her peers in the classroom.
4. **What additional recommendations would you make for the classroom?**
   Molly would benefit from the use of a pass-around microphone in the classroom to enable her to hear her classmates.

Suggested Readings

[1] Madell JR. Evaluation of Speech Perception in Infants and Children. In: Madell, JR and Flexer, C, eds. Pediatric Audiology: Diagnosis, Technology, and Management, 2nd ed. New York, NY: Thieme; 2014.

[2] Wolfe J, Morais M, Neumann S, et al. Evaluation of speech recognition with personal FM and classroom audio distribution systems. J Educ Audiol. 2013; 19:65–79

40 Borderline Cochlear Implant Candidate with EVA

Carol Flexer

40.1 Clinical History and Description

The patient, Alan, now 10 years old, was first seen at a university clinic at age 3 years, 6 months for a second opinion about technology management.

Alan was diagnosed at 2 years 8 months of age with an asymmetrical, mild dropping to a profound sensorineural hearing loss in his right ear, and a moderately-severe sloping to a profound sensorineural hearing loss in his left ear. The hearing loss was believed to be progressive, secondary to bilateral enlarged vestibular aqueducts (EVA), as observed in a CT scan.

Screening for genetic mutations indicated that Alan carries a single mutation of the *SLC26A4* gene, the most common cause of EVA–associated with Pendred syndrome.[1] Testing for Connexin 26 and 30 mutations was negative.

Alan passed newborn hearing screening at birth in the right ear, and was "referred" in the left ear. At one month of age, auditory brainstem response (ABR) testing showed the right ear was fine, but the left ear had a possible moderate hearing loss. A second ABR at 2 months of age found both ears to be within normal limits.

At about two and a half years of age, Alan's parents became concerned about his hearing because he did not respond consistently when people called his name, without visual cues. His asymmetrical hearing loss was subsequently diagnosed at 2 years 8 months of age.

Alan received bilateral hearing aids at 2 years 9 months of age, and began auditory-verbal, parent-focused early intervention at that time. He was making good progress in the acquisition of spoken communication, but he was not producing or even detecting high frequency speech sounds. Alan's parents were concerned, and wanted information about possibly changing his technology. Their desired outcome for Alan continues to be listening and spoken language, and also mainstream school placement with hearing peers.

40.2 Audiologic Testing

At the time of the visit to this clinic, at age 3 years 6 months, Alan's hearing loss had progressed since his initial diagnosis, to an asymmetrical, moderate dropping to a profound sensorineural hearing loss in his right ear, and a severe sloping to a profound sensorineural hearing loss in his left ear (▶ Fig. 40.1). Tympanometry indicated normal middle ear systems on the day of the test. He wore his hearing aids every waking moment, and was receiving consistent, parent-focused auditory-verbal therapy.

40.3 Questions for the Reader

1. What is EVA, and how could it impact hearing loss diagnosis and technology management?
2. Would you recommend a cochlear implant? And if so, would you recommend a unilateral implant, bilateral implants, bimodal fitting, or electroacoustic stimulation (EAS), if possible? Why?
3. If you were to advocate for a cochlear implant for this child, what might you say?
4. What expectations might you have for a successful listening and spoken language outcome? Why?

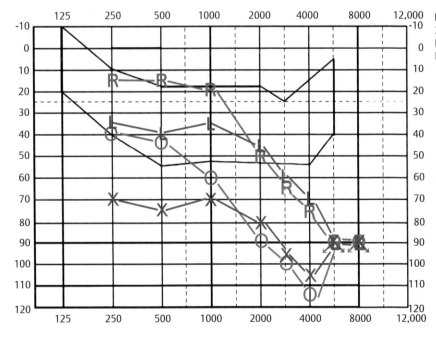

Fig. 40.1 Unaided and aided testing at age 3 years, 6 months. O, right ear air conduction; X, left ear air conduction; R, right ear hearing aid; L, left ear hearing aid; Arrows, no response.

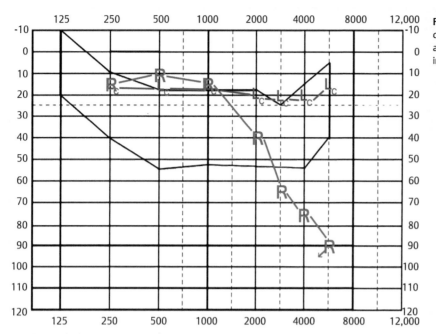

Fig. 40.2 Right ear aided (R-HA), and left ear cochlear implant (L-CI) thresholds at 10 years of age. R, right ear hearing aid; L$_c$, left ear cochlear implant; Arrows, no response.

40.4 Discussion of Questions

1. **What is EVA and how could it impact hearing loss diagnosis and technology management?**

   Enlarged vestibular aqueduct (EVA), also known as large vestibular aqueduct syndrome (LVAS), is a malformation of the temporal bone where the vestibular aqueduct, the bony channel that houses the endolymphatic duct, is abnormally enlarged.[2] EVA is the most common inner ear abnormality found on CT scans with an incidence of between 4 and 10% in children with sensorineural hearing loss.[3]

   Because the hearing loss caused by EVA is typically early onset, fluctuating and progressive, confusion may exist as to the nature and extent of the hearing loss, causing diagnosis and management to be delayed—as transpired in this case. In addition, technology recommendations may vary over time. That is, a child may begin wearing hearing aids, but as hearing loss progresses, a change to more powerful hearing aids or to a cochlear implant should be considered to allow the child better brain access of auditory information.

2. **Would you recommend a cochlear implant? And if so, would you recommend a unilateral implant, bilateral implants, bimodal fitting, or electroacoustic stimulation (EAS), if possible? Why?**

   Yes, the audiologist should absolutely recommend a cochlear implant.[4] Even when aided (▶ Fig. 40.1), Alan's brain has virtually no access to critical high frequency speech sounds. Specific reasons are detailed in the 3rd question.

   At this point in time, it seems prudent to start with a bimodal fitting; a cochlear implant in the left ear that has a severe to profound hearing loss across frequencies, and a hearing aid in the right ear that has good low frequency residual hearing (▶ Fig. 40.1).[5] If the hearing loss in the right ear continues to worsen due to the EVA, a second cochlear implant would most certainly be recommended. Following cochlear implantation, if residual hearing is preserved in the low frequencies, EAS should be considered because it may result in better speech recognition in quiet and in noise, localization, and sound quality when compared to electric-only stimulation.[6,7]

3. **If you were to advocate for a cochlear implant for this child, what might you say?**

   To advocate for the value-added benefits of a cochlear implant for a child, the audiologist could detail the limitations posed by the severe to profound degree of hearing loss and subsequent hearing aid fitting, rather than emphasizing what the child can detect. That is, identifying what the child cannot hear, and how this would likely change with a cochlear implant would be discussed. One could start by saying that Alan's future progress likely will be severely compromised without better auditory access of information to his brain provided by a cochlear implant—for the following reasons[8]:

   - A significant amount of what children learn, they learn by overhearing conversations around them, and by hearing from a distance. The inability to hear soft speech will make it difficult to follow classroom discussion and to hear the comments of peers.
   - Alan cannot distinguish soft, high frequency speech sounds unless they are spoken within inches of his hearing aid.
   - Alan has substantial difficulty hearing unstressed words when spoken in a typical conversational exchange, which will interfere with his language development.
   - Alan is exhibiting consonant deletions in his speech; problems that can be most efficiently addressed by having better auditory (brain) access of soft, high frequency speech sounds.
   - Alan cannot distinguish soft speech that is spoken more than 6 feet from him—putting him at an enormous disadvantage when competing in a typical educational and social environment. To date, Alan has functioned in a much protected and appropriate environment where most communicators are closer to him than 6 feet. This will change as he moves into larger classrooms.

- As Alan progresses in school, academic and social demands will escalate and will likely exceed the capabilities of his current auditory brain access. This will cause him to expend a substantial "level of effort" and experience unnecessary communicative stress.
- Alan would have been identified as an "excellent hearing aid user" in 1990. However, at this current point in time, our expectations for brain access of soft speech (including voiceless consonants such as "s") at distances and with rapid tracking of incidental conversational exchanges, have expanded tremendously. With appropriate auditory therapy, the electrical input from the cochlear implant in his left ear could integrate, in Alan's brain, with the acoustical input from the hearing aid on his right ear, giving him bimodal hearing.[5]

4. **What expectations might you have for a successful listening and spoken language outcome? Why?**

Based on audiometric reports and observation and conversations with Alan and his family, it is highly likely that the enhanced brain access provided by a cochlear implant could add substantial value to Alan's linguistic, phonologic, academic, social, and family life.[4,9] Of course, Alan would require appropriate and intensive family-based auditory therapy/education to assist his brain in organizing, integrating, and using this enhanced bimodal input of auditory information to his brain.[8]

40.5 Recommended Treatment

Alan received the Nucleus Freedom Contour Advance CI24RE (CA) cochlear implant for his left ear at 3 years, 9 months of age. He continues to wear a hearing aid on his right ear—Phonak Naida SII UP (bimodal fitting)—and both devices are coupled to a remote microphone system in school. Alan should continue auditory-verbal enrichment in a parent-focused program, and attend preschool with typically hearing peers.

40.6 Outcome

Now at 10 years of age, Alan continues to receive excellent auditory brain access with his cochlear implant. Implant thresholds, obtained with warble tones in the sound-field, are 15–20 dB HL across the frequency range (▶ Fig. 40.2). He reports that he likes wearing the hearing aid and cochlear implant together, with added use of the Roger remote microphone system coupled to both devices in school.[10]

Alan's hearing continues to fluctuate by 10–15 dB in his right ear, but he still obtains substantial benefit from his hearing aid, especially in the low frequencies (speech recognition is 76% at 45 dB HL). A cochlear implant will be obtained for the right ear, should hearing continue to fluctuate or should speech scores decline.[4]

Currently, Alan is completely mainstreamed in the 4th grade, and is doing well academically. Results from the CELF-5 (Clinical Evaluation of Language Fundamentals - 5th Edition) indicate well above average skills (in comparison to same age hearing peers) for all subtests. The CELF-5 is designed for use with hearing children, ages 5–21 years, to assess receptive and expressive language skills.[8]

Even though Alan has attained and surpassed age and grade-level skills, he has an IEP (Individualized Education Plan) for the purposes of monitoring and sustaining his academic progress. As part of his IEP, Alan receives 30 minutes per week of speech-language therapy (pull-out), and 30 minutes per week of literacy enrichment, both for language and literacy advancement and practice. In addition to this, Alan receives consults from a program specializing in children with hearing loss. This allows his audiologist to monitor his progress and to make sure he does not slip behind as academic demands escalate.

It is important to remember that the skills Alan has developed are the result of a great deal of time, effort, thought, and planning. Alan's family has worked diligently to provide him with an optimal auditory-language environment, and Alan has a long history of consistent technology management, and parent-focused auditory-verbal therapy.

References

[1] Lafferty KA, Hodges R, Rehm HL. Genetics of hearing loss. In: Madell, JR and Flexer, C, eds. Pediatric Audiology: Diagnosis, Technology, and Management, 2nd ed. New York, NY: Thieme; 2014:22–35

[2] Alexiades G, Hoffman RA. Medical evaluation and medical management of hearing loss in children. In: Madell, JR and Flexer, C, eds. Pediatric Audiology: Diagnosis, Technology, and Management, 2nd ed. New York, NY: Thieme; 2014:36–43

[3] Lai CC, Shiao AS. Chronological changes of hearing in pediatric patients with large vestibular aqueduct syndrome. Laryngoscope. 2004; 114(5):832–838

[4] Gifford RH. Cochlear implants for infants and children. In: Madell, JR and Flexer, C, eds. Pediatric Audiology: Diagnosis, Technology, and Management, 2nd ed. New York, NY: Thieme; 2014:238–254

[5] Shpak T, Most T, Luntz M. Fundamental frequency information for speech recognition via bimodal stimulation: cochlear implant in one ear and hearing aid in the other. Ear Hear. 2014; 35(1):97–109

[6] Adunka OF, Dillon MT, Adunka MC, King ER, Pillsbury HC, Buchman CA. Hearing preservation and speech perception outcomes with electric-acoustic stimulation after 12 months of listening experience. Laryngoscope. 2013; 123(10):2509–2515

[7] Incerti PV, Ching TYC, Cowan R. A systematic review of electric-acoustic stimulation: device fitting ranges, outcomes, and clinical fitting practices. Trends Amplif. 2013; 17(1):3–26

[8] Cole EB, Flexer C. Children with hearing loss: Developing listening and talking birth to six. 3rd ed. San Diego, CA: Plural Publishing; 2016

[9] Wolfe J, Schafer E. Programming cochlear implants, 2nd ed. San Diego, CA: Plural Publishing;2015

[10] Wolfe J, Morais M, Schafer E, et al. Evaluation of speech recognition of cochlear implant recipients using a personal digital adaptive radio frequency system. J Am Acad Audiol. 2013; 24(8):714–724

Suggested Readings

[1] Madell JR, Flexer C. Pediatric audiology: Diagnosis, technology and management, 2nd ed. New York, NY: Thieme; 2014

[2] Madell JR, Flexer C. Pediatric audiology casebook. New York, NY: Thieme; 2011

[3] Robertson L. Literacy and deafness: Listening and spoken language (2nd edition). San Diego, CA: Plural Publishing; 2014

[4] Thibodeau LM, Schaper L. Benefits of digital wireless technology for persons with hearing aids. Semin Hear. 2014; 35(3):168–176

41 Determination of Bimodal/Bilateral Cochlear Implant Candidacy

Jace Wolfe

41.1 Clinical History and Description

The patient, Harper, now 10 years old, was seen at a pediatric audiology clinic at 9 years of age for an audiologic evaluation to determine the optimal hearing technology required to best meet her diverse needs.

Harper was diagnosed via visual reinforcement audiometry (VRA) using insert earphones with a moderate to moderately severe, bilateral, sensorineural hearing loss (see audiogram in ▶ Fig. 41.1) at a university medical center at 8 months of age. A tone burst auditory brainstem response evaluation conducted shortly after the VRA assessment confirmed the results of the behavioral evaluation. She was fitted with behind-the-ear (BTE) hearing aids when she was 8 months old. Real ear probe microphone assessment indicated an excellent match to the Desired Sensation Level (DSL) 5.0 targets for multiple speech input levels (e.g., 55, 65, and 75 dB Sound Pressure Level, SPL). Harper was enrolled into Auditory-Verbal therapy where she and her family received therapy from a Listening and Spoken Language Specialist (LSLS) on a weekly basis. Of note, Harper passed her newborn hearing screening for both ears. The cause of her hearing loss is unknown.

Harper's parents possessed a strong desire for her to develop optimally her auditory and spoken-language abilities. Both of her parents previously performed as actors in theatres on Broadway, and they both continued to work in the arts and music industry. Her father was the Chairperson of the Drama Department at a major university, and her mother held an executive position in a large civic arts center. Because of their occupational and recrea-tional interests, both parents placed a high value on Harper's music and oratory aptitude.

Harper's hearing loss progressively worsened throughout her early childhood years. By the time she was 3 years old, she had a severe to profound hearing loss, bilaterally (see ▶ Fig. 41.2). She was fitted with high-power BTE hearing aids to provide sufficient audibility in light of her shift in hearing sensitivity. Standardized speech and language evaluation conducted when she was 3 years old indicated that her speech, auditory, recep-tive, and expressive language were all within normal limits rel-ative to her normal-hearing peers of the same age (i.e., standard scores were at or near 100). Aided word recognition assessment indicated fair speech recognition at presentation levels consis-tent with average conversational-level speech and poor speech recognition for low-level (e.g., "softly spoken") speech (see ▶ Table 41.1). Additionally, the vast majority of Harper's errors on speech recognition assessment at an average conversational level occurred for high-frequency phonemes (e.g., /h/ and frica-tives). Her errors for low-level speech recognition assessment were widespread across phoneme class. Additionally, her par-ents reported that she seemed to struggle significantly with speech recognition in noisy environments. Although standar-dized speech and language evaluation indicated satisfactory progress (i.e., age-appropriate speech and language develop-ment), Harper's LSLS expressed concern that her hearing loss was impeding her progress. Recent testing indicated Harper's nonverbal IQ score to be almost 2 standard deviations above the mean for her age. Harper's LSLS suggested that given her exceptional cognitive aptitude, Harper's standardized speech and language scores should likely be higher, but are partially arrested by her impoverished auditory capacity.

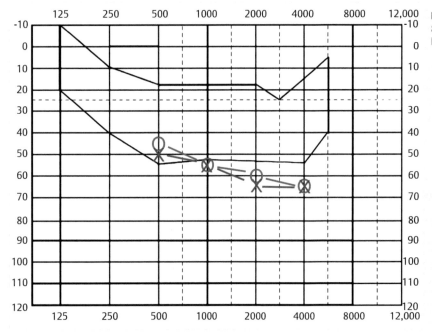

Fig. 41.1 Audiogram obtained when Harper was 8 months of age. O, right ear air conduction; X, left ear air conduction.

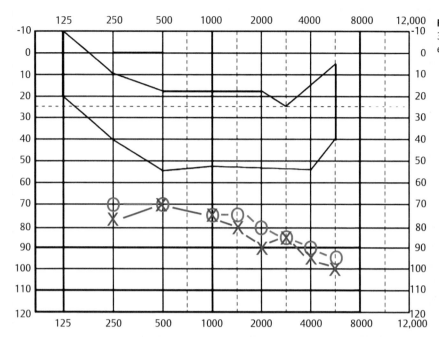

Fig. 41.2 Audiogram obtained when Harper was 3 years of age. O, right ear air conduction; X, left ear air conduction.

Table 41.1 Aided speech recognition results obtained when Harper was 3 years of age

Condition	LNT: 60 dBA	LNT: 50 dBA
Hearing aid: bilateral	75%	17%
Hearing aid: right	75%	17%
Hearing aid: left	67%	8%

LNT, Lexical neighborhood test

Table 41.2 Aided speech recognition results obtained when Harper was 4 years of age

Condition	PBK50: 60 dBA	PBK50: 50 dBA	BKB-SIN
Hearing aid	50%	8%	+16 dB SNR
Cochlear implant	88%	72%	+12 dB SNR
Bimodal	96%	84%	+4 dB SNR

PBK, phonetically balanced kindergarten; BKB-SIN, Bamford-Kowal-Bench-Speech in Noise Test

Given the aforementioned limitations in Harper's speech recognition abilities along with her family's and LSLS's concern regarding her functional hearing and spoken-language progress, the decision was made to pursue a cochlear implant for her left ear. At 3 years of age, Harper received a Cochlear Nucleus Freedom (24RE) implant with the Contour Advance electrode array, and almost immediately showed improvement in her auditory, speech, and language development. Audiologic assessment conducted when she was 4 years old indicated excellent word recognition scores for average conversational-level speech and good recognition for low-level speech (see ► Table 41.2). Although word recognition with the cochlear implant was significantly better than what she was able to obtain with the hearing aid, it was apparent that the hearing aid was making a substantial contribution to her ability to hear in the bimodal condition. Also, Harper's sentence recognition in noise was significantly better with bimodal use relative to her performance with the cochlear implant alone. Additionally, standardized speech and language assessment conducted when she was 4 years old indicated receptive and expressive language scores that were 2 standard deviations above the mean for children of her age with normal hearing. Furthermore, Harper's parents reported that she became more confident when interacting with others in public and that she was quite talented as a singer and actress on the theatrical stage. Specifically, they noted that Harper possessed "perfect vocal pitch." She transitioned out of Auditory-Verbal therapy but continued to be seen for annual comprehensive standardized speech and language assessment. Also, Harper was seen for quarterly audiologic appointments until she was 7 years old, at which time she began to be followed up for biannual audiologic assessments.

41.2 Assessment of Auditory and Spoken-Language Abilities

Harper continued to use bimodal hearing technology until she was 9 years old. At that time, she was seen at our clinic for audiologic assessment. As shown in ► Fig. 41.3, her hearing sensitivity of the nonimplanted ear continued to worsen. The results of speech recognition assessment are shown in ► Table 41.3. Her word recognition with the cochlear implant alone was excellent but almost nonexistent with use of the hearing aid alone. Of note, she did demonstrate good open-set speech recognition capacity with use of the hearing aid alone on a relatively simple test of sentence recognition in quiet, which is reflective of her high cognitive and spoken-language aptitudes, and of her associated ability to use contextual information in connected discourse in spite of her inability to readily recognize words in open-set. Also of note, her sentence recognition in noise with use of the cochlear implant and hearing aid together did not appear to be any better

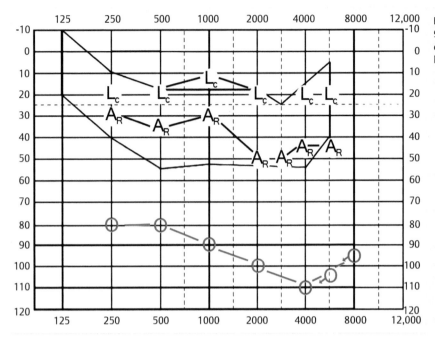

Fig. 41.3 Audiogram obtained when Harper was 9 years of age. O, right ear air conduction; L_C, left ear cochlear implant; A_R, right ear binaural hearing aid behind the ear; Arrows, no response.

Table 41.3 Aided speech recognition results obtained when Harper was 9 years of age

Condition	CNC: 60 dBA	HINTE-C quiet	BKB-SIN
Hearing aid	0%	92%	+ 20 dB SNR
Cochlear implant	96%	100%	+ 10 dB SNR
Bimodal	92%	100%	+ 8 dB SNR

CNC, consonant-nucleus-consonant; HINT, Hearing In Noise Test; BKB-SIN, Bamford-Kowal-Bench-Speech In Noise Test

than what she was able to achieve with the cochlear implant alone. Real ear probe microphone measures indicated that the hearing aid output was matched closely to the DSL 5.0 prescriptive targets for children. Aided warble tone thresholds indicated reduced access to low-level sounds with use of the hearing aid alone (see ▶ Fig. 41.3).

Her parents reported that Harper was doing well in school, but they expressed concern that she was beginning to struggle in noisy situations. Furthermore, they reported that Harper's classroom teacher reported that she frequently asked for repetitions in the classroom, and they noted that Harper seemed to be fatigued when she came home after a day in school. They also stated that she did not seem to be concerned when the battery of her hearing aid expired. More specifically, they reported that she was fine using the cochlear implant alone, but would panic anytime she had to rely solely on the hearing aid. Additionally, they noted that she seemed to have difficulty locating the source of sound. However, they did report that she continued to excel as a singer and actress. They expressed that they felt like she would likely hear speech better with the use of bilateral cochlear implants, but they expressed grave concern about giving up use of the hearing aid out of fear that her musical abilities would diminish. Standardized speech and language assessment indicated expressive and receptive language scores

that were approximately 2 standard deviations above the mean for children of the same age with normal hearing.

41.3 Questions for the Reader

1. Would you recommend a cochlear implant for the right ear?
2. What are the potential advantages and limitations of bilateral cochlear implantation relative to bimodal cochlear implantation for Harper?
3. What type of information should the clinician provide to the family to assist them in making the right decision for Harper?

41.4 Discussion of Questions

1. **Would you recommend a cochlear implant for the right ear?**

Yes, I did recommend a cochlear implant for Harper's right ear for a number of reasons. First, Harper's open-set word recognition with use of the hearing aid alone was very poor, and use of the hearing aid appeared to contribute little to nothing toward her ability to understand speech in noise. Also, audiologic assessment indicated that she had reduced access to low-level sounds with use of the hearing aid alone. More importantly, Harper's parents reported that she seemed to be struggling to communicate in noisy situations. It is well established that the vast majority of the school day is spent listening to speech in moderate- to high-level noise,[1] and it was also expected that she was likely subjected to moderate to high noise levels and unfavorable signal-to-noise ratios throughout her social and recreational activities.[2] Additionally, Harper's parents reported that she seemed to be very fatigued at the end of school day. This fatigue suggested that Harper was spending a great deal of energy concentrating on the tasks at hand in the classroom because she was having a difficult time communicating due to her hearing loss. Research has clearly shown that children struggling with communication secondary to hearing loss experience higher levels of fatigue and stress.[3,4,5] Further, Harper's listening and communication demands at school will likely increase as she transitions from the fourth to the fifth grade. In the fifth grade, lessons become more "lecture-based" and students are required to switch classrooms throughout the day to receive instruction from multiple teachers. Finally, Harper's parents reported that she was struggling to localize the source of sound. This difficulty is well established in bimodal hearing technology users.[6,7] The physiologic bases underlying this problem reside in the fact that the cochlear implant generally provides excellent audibility for sounds across the speech frequency range, while high-frequency audibility is often poor with use of the hearing aid. As a result, interaural level differences necessary to localize high-frequency sounds are not readily available. Likewise, the hearing aid provides a relatively good potential to preserve timing information that is important for localization of low-frequency sounds, while the auditory system does not readily process detailed timing information in response to electrical stimulation. As a result, interaural timing/phase cues required to localize low-frequency sounds are difficult to process.

2. **What are the potential advantages and limitations of bilateral cochlear implantation relative to bimodal cochlear implantation for Harper?**

Potential advantages of bilateral cochlear implantation relative to bimodal use:

- Improved access to low-level speech and environmental sounds.[8]
- Improvement in speech recognition in quiet and in noise is likely.[9,10]
- Improvement in localization is likely.[6,7]
- Improvements in the aforementioned areas will likely lead to better functional hearing performance in the classroom and to a reduction in stress and listening-related fatigue.

Potential disadvantages of bilateral cochlear implantation relative to bimodal use:

- Loss of fine temporal structure from use of a hearing aid for the right ear may diminish Harper's music aptitude and her appreciation of music.[11]
- Loss of access to an acoustical signal from use of a hearing aid for the right ear may diminish Harper's ability to identify the pitch of a talker or of her own voice.
- Harper may potentially reject the cochlear implant after 9 years of hearing aid use for the right ear.
- Residual acoustic hearing for the right ear may be lost during or after cochlear implantation.

3. **What type of information should the clinician provide to the family to assist them in making the right decision for Harper?**

To advocate for the benefits Harper may receive from bilateral cochlear implantation, the clinician should discuss the limitations associated with severe to profound degree of hearing loss in regard to the ability to understand speech in quiet and in noise. It is important to note that audibility for low-level speech and environmental sounds will almost definitely be improved for the right ear with use of a cochlear

implant. Also, the clinician should discuss the difficulties associated with localization for bimodal users and provide a basic explanation of the physiologic/acoustic bases underlying this difficulty. Additionally, the clinician should discuss Harper's current and future academic needs with a focus on the fact that academic and social/recreational demands will most likely escalate and become more sophisticated/complex and, as a result, will possibly exceed Harper's capabilities if she continues to use bimodal technology.

On the other hand, it is imperative for the clinician to adequately counsel Harper's family regarding the potential detriments of losing access to acoustical stimulation for the right ear. Particularly in light of Harper's and her family's affinity for music and the performance arts, the clinician is responsible for informing the family that Harper's music aptitude, her appreciation for music, and her ability to recognize pitch may suffer with the loss of her acoustic hearing in her right ear. Ideally, the family should be counseled to undergo a trial period in which Harper removes the hearing aid and plugs her right ear so that she is totally reliant only on the "electric hearing" she receives from her cochlear implant. This experience will allow the family to determine the value (or lack thereof) the acoustical hearing in the right ear has for music, performance theatre, and communication overall in social, recreational, and academic settings. Furthermore, the family should understand that there is a possibility that Harper may not immediately bond with or enjoy the cochlear implant for her right ear after using a hearing aid for 9 years for that ear. Finally, the family should be counseled regarding the likelihood of a loss of all residual acoustic hearing during or following cochlear implantation of the right ear.

41.5 Recommended Treatment

Harper received a Cochlear Nucleus CI422 implant for her right ear when she was 9 years old.

41.6 Outcome

Now at 10 years of age, Harper is a successful user of bilateral cochlear implants. She immediately accepted the cochlear implant for her right ear and showed steady progress in her ability to understand speech in quiet and in noise with that ear alone as well as in the bilateral cochlear implant condition. Her most recent results for aided audiologic assessment are provided in ▶ Table 41.4. As shown, open-set word recognition is excellent with use of each cochlear implant alone, and sentence recognition

Table 41.4 Aided speech recognition results obtained when Harper was 10 years of age

Condition	CNC: 60 dBA	CNC: 50 dBA	BKB-SIN
First CI	96%	84%	+ 11.5 dB SNR
Second CI	88%	82%	+ 14 dB SNR
Bilateral	96%	88%	+ 4 dB SNR

CNC, Consonant-Nucleus-Consonant; BKB-SIN, Bamford-Kowal-Bench-Speech In Noise Test

in noise is better in the bilateral condition relative to either unilateral condition. Further, sentence recognition in noise in the bilateral condition is significantly better than her previous performance with use of bimodal technology. Of note, Harper did lose all of her residual acoustic hearing in her right ear during the cochlear implant surgery process.

Most importantly, Harper and her parents reported that "listening is easier" in academic, social, and recreational settings. They reported that they have no regrets about pursuing bilateral cochlear implantation. They noted that Harper is typically not as fatigued at the end of the day in spite of the fact that the academic rigors at school have increased. Finally, they reported that Harper continues to excel in her development in the musical and theatrical arts. Specifically, they have reported that she continues to recognize the pitch of others' voices and of musical instruments with ease, and her own vocal pitch and quality are excellent. They also noted that her interest in performance arts has actually increased since receiving her second cochlear implant. Although this is in contrast to most reports that have typically indicated diminished music aptitude and pitch recognition with the loss of access to acoustic hearing,[11] it is consistent with the hypothesis that a period of access to acoustic hearing may serve to develop speech and auditory skills.[12] More research is needed in this area to further elucidate the roles of acoustic and electric hearing in auditory, spoken language, music, and academic/literacy development of children with hearing loss.

Currently, Harper is excelling in a typical fifth grade classroom placement. Her most recent standardized speech and language assessments showed that she continues to possess receptive and expressive language abilities that are almost 2 standard deviations above the mean for normal hearing children of the same age. It is important to remember that Harper's progress is a product of not only the hearing technology she has used throughout her lifetime but also, more importantly, the time, effort, and energy her family has invested in ensuring that she received the pediatric audiology and Auditory-Verbal therapy needed throughout her childhood. Also, her parents were diligent about implementing full-time hearing technology use as well as following the recommendations of her LSLS during all of Harper's waking hours.

References

[1] Cruckley J, Scollie S, Parsa V. An exploration of non. -. quiet listening at school. J Educ Audiol. 2011; 17:23–35

[2] Pearsons K, Bennett R, Fidell S. Speech Levels in Various Noise Environments (Report No. EPA-600/1-77-025). Washington, DC: U.S. Environmental Protection Agency; 1977

[3] Bess FH, Gustafson SJ, Corbett BA, Lambert EW, Camarata SM, Hornsby BW. Salivary cortisol profiles of children with hearing loss. Ear Hear. 2015

[4] Bess FH, Hornsby BW. Commentary: listening can be exhausting—fatigue in children and adults with hearing loss. Ear Hear. 2014; 35(6):592–599

[5] Werfel KL, Hendricks AE. The relation between child versus parent report of chronic fatigue and language/literacy skills in school-age children with cochlear implants. Ear Hear. 2016; 37(2):216–224

[6] Ching TY, Hill M, Brew J, et al. The effect of auditory experience on speech perception, localization, and functional performance of children who use a cochlear implant and a hearing aid in opposite ears. Int J Audiol. 2005; 44(12):677–690

[7] Gifford RH, Grantham DW, Sheffield SW, Davis TJ, Dwyer R, Dorman MF. Localization and interaural time difference (ITD) thresholds for cochlear implant recipients with preserved acoustic hearing in the implanted ear. Hear Res. 2014; 312:28–37

[8] Firszt JB, Holden LK, Skinner MW, et al. Recognition of speech presented at soft to loud levels by adult cochlear implant recipients of three cochlear implant systems. Ear Hear. 2004; 25(4):375–387

[9] Ching TY, Dillon H. Major findings of the LOCHI study on children at 3 years of age and implications for audiological management. Int J Audiol. 2013; 52(2) Suppl 2:S65–S68

[10] Gifford RH, Shallop JK, Peterson AM. Speech recognition materials and ceiling effects: considerations for cochlear implant programs. Audiol Neurootol. 2008; 13(3):193–205

[11] Gifford RH, Dorman MF, Brown CA. Psychophysical properties of low-frequency hearing: implications for perceiving speech and music via electric and acoustic stimulation. Adv Otorhinolaryngol 2010;67:51–60

[12] Nittrouer S, Caldwell A, Lowenstein JH, Tarr E, Holloman C. Emergent literacy in kindergartners with cochlear implants. Ear Hear. 2012; 33(6):683–697

42 Considerations for Hearing Technology Intervention for Precipitously Sloping Hearing Loss in Children

Jace Wolfe

42.1 Clinical History and Description

The patient, Jayden, now 11 years old, was seen at a pediatric audiology clinic at 10 years of age for audiologic evaluation to determine the optimal hearing technology required to best meet his diverse needs.

Jayden was adopted from China when he was 8 years old. Nothing was known of his birth history at the time of his adoption. He spoke Mandarin Chinese upon his arrival in the United States, and his adoptive parents began to teach him English once he began living in their home. His mother became concerned with Jayden's inability to readily learn English. The family also adopted a girl of the same age from China, and she became proficient with spoken English relatively quickly. Jayden's mother noted that her concern for his hearing and language development wavered because he always responded when someone spoke to him. However, she reported that he seemed to struggle to comprehend conversation and that he was adamant about directly facing the talker during conversational exchange. Furthermore, she noted that many of the English words he was developing were approximations of the actual words. Her concern was heightened when she purchased an alarm clock for him so that he could awaken on his own in the morning. She noted that he would not awaken to the alarm clock, which emitted a high-frequency alerting beep, and when she would enter his room to hit snooze on the alarm, he would not turn it off after it sounded again, even when he was awake.

Conditioned play audiometry using insert earphones was completed when Jayden was 9 years old and indicated a slight low-frequency sensory hearing loss that precipitously sloped to the severe range in the high frequencies for both ears (see ▶ Fig. 42.1). Distortion product otoacoustic emissions were absent, bilaterally. Tympanometry was normal for both ears, and ipsilateral acoustic reflexes were present within normal limits at 500 Hz and present at elevated presentation levels at 1,000 and 2,000 Hz, bilaterally. Monosyllabic word recognition was poor (e.g., less than 20% correct) when conducted under insert earphones at a high presentation level (e.g., 90 dB HL). Of note, it was difficult to determine whether Jayden's incorrect responses were attributed to his inability to recognize the target stimuli, to his own speech articulation errors, to his language delay due to the fact that Jayden had only been learning English for 8 months, or to all three factors.

A subsequent otologic evaluation was unremarkable. Magnetic resonance imaging revealed no abnormalities in the peripheral auditory system or in the auditory nervous system. The etiology of the hearing loss was not identified.

Jayden was fitted with behind-the-ear (BTE) hearing aids within 1 week of the diagnosis of his hearing loss. Real ear probe microphone assessment indicated an excellent match to the Desired Sensation Level (DSL) 5.0 targets for multiple speech input levels (e.g., 55, 65, 75 dB Sound Pressure Level, SPL). His hearing aids were equipped with nonlinear frequency compression, which was enabled in an effort to improve his access to high-frequency speech and environmental sounds. Jayden was simultaneously enrolled into Auditory-Verbal therapy where he and his family received therapy from a Listening and Spoken Language Specialist (LSLS) on a weekly basis.

Jayden's family expressed a desire for him to develop proficient English and Mandarin Chinese–spoken language. They

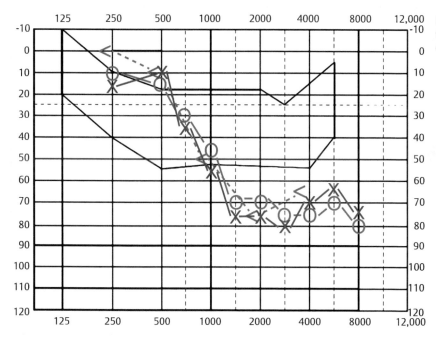

Fig. 42.1 Audiogram obtained when Jayden was 9 years of age. O, right ear air conduction; X, left ear air conduction; <, right ear bone conduction.

also noted that Jaden enjoys playing musical instruments and that he had developed a specific interest in the violin. They were eager to assist him in growing this musical interest. Additionally, they stated that Jaden participates in gymnastic practice several times a week, and he is involved in Boy Scouts of America. His parents want him to be able to communicate effectively in those activities.

42.2 Assessment of Auditory and Spoken-Language Abilities

Jayden was seen quarterly for audiologic assessment, hearing aid checks, and evaluation of aided hearing performance. Data logging indicated that he used his hearing aids during all waking hours. He also frequently used a remote microphone system, particularly in the classroom and in noisy situations. Despite his and his family's diligence with full-time hearing technology use and attendance to all audiology and Auditory-Verbal therapy sessions, his LSLS expressed concern that Jayden's speech and language progress was not occurring at a rate necessary for him to develop a level of competency required to succeed academically and to develop relationships with his peers. She also noted that he continued to only produce approximations of many English words and that he often omitted consonants in the initial and/or final word position, particularly fricatives. Standardized speech and language assessment conducted near his 10th birthday revealed significant delays in speech and language development (see ▶ Table 42.1).

Throughout his first year of audiologic monitoring, his low-frequency hearing sensitivity remained unchanged, but he experienced slight progression of his hearing loss (see ▶ Fig. 42.2). Of note, real ear probe microphone measures were conducted in an attempt to match the output of his hearing aids to the DSL 5.0 prescriptive target for children. Audiologic assessment conducted near his 10th birthday was consistent with a slight low-frequency

hearing loss sloping to a severe mid- to high-frequency hearing loss. Aided speech recognition assessment found poor word recognition in quiet and poor sentence recognition in noise (see ▶ Table 42.2). Also, aided sound-field warble tone thresholds indicated insufficient audibility throughout the mid- to high-frequency speech range. Of note, nonverbal IQ assessment was conducted and revealed that Jayden is an exceptionally bright child with no cognitive delays.

Table 42.1 Standardized speech and language scores obtained when Jayden was 10 years of age

Standardized tests	Prehybrid (standard score)
CELF-4: core language	44
CELF-4: receptive language	50
CELF-4: expressive language	51
PPVT-4: receptive vocabulary	50
EVT-2: expressive vocabulary	59

CELF-4, Clinical Evaluation of Language Fundamentals - Fourth Edition; PPVT-4, Peabody Picture Vocabulary - Fourth Edition; EVT-2, Expressive Vocabulary Test - Second Edition

In light of the unfavorable results obtained on his most recent standardized speech and language assessment and aided audiologic evaluation, Jayden's family, his LSLS, and pediatric audiologist met to discuss whether a cochlear implant should be considered as an option to optimize his progress.

42.3 Questions for the Reader

1. Would you recommend a cochlear implant for Jayden?
2. Are there any special considerations that should be taken into account in the selection of the most appropriate cochlear implant for Jayden?
3. What are the potential advantages and limitations of the specific cochlear implant recommendation indicated for Jayden?
4. What type of information should the clinician provide to the family to assist them in making the right decision for Jayden?

42.4 Discussion of Questions

1. **Would you recommend a cochlear implant for the right ear?**
   Yes, a cochlear implant was recommended for Jayden's right ear for a number of reasons. First, at the time of his most recent evaluation, Jayden had been living in the United States for almost 2 years and had used contemporary hearing technology during all waking hours for 1 year. Unfortunately, he had made very limited progress in his attempt to develop functional spoken English language. This was in spite of the fact that his family had been very diligent in adhering to every recommendation to facilitate language development made by Jayden's LSLS. Also, Jayden's open-set word recognition with use of the well-fitted hearing aids was very poor. Furthermore, an analysis of his responses for monosyllabic word recognition assessment indicated that the vast majority of his errors were omissions of or substitutions for high-frequency weighted phonemes. Despite the use of hearing aids with frequency-lowering technology, Jayden was unable to adequately recognize mid- to high-frequency phonemes on a consistent basis, a deficit that will most assuredly arrest his speech and language development. These findings are not particularly surprising given the unfavorable results of his aided threshold assessment (see ▶ Fig. 42.2), which indicated insufficient access to low-level sounds. In short, his auditory capacity with hearing aids was insufficient to develop adequate listening and spoken-language abilities.

   Additionally, Jayden's ability to understand speech in noise was very poor. It is well established that the vast majority of time of the school day is spent listening to speech in moderate- to high-level noise,[1] and it was also expected that Jayden will need to communicate adequately in moderate to high noise levels and unfavorable signal-to-noise ratios throughout his recreational (e.g., gymnastics and Boy Scouts) and social activities.[2] It is well known that children struggling with communication secondary to hearing loss experience higher levels of fatigue and stress, particularly when communicating in noisy situations.[3,4,5]

   Finally, in order for Jayden to excel in American classrooms, it is imperative that his hearing performance is

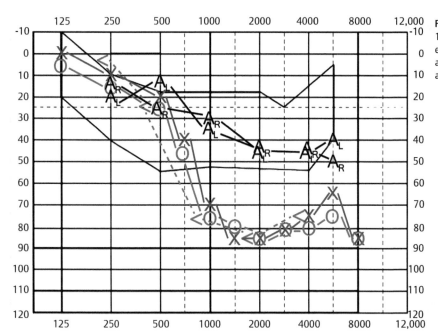

Fig. 42.2 Audiogram obtained when Jayden was 10 years of age. O, right ear air conduction; X, left ear air conduction; A_R, right ear binaural hearing aid behind the ear; A_L, left ear binaural hearing aid behind the ear; <, right ear bone conduction.

Table 42.2 Aided speech recognition results obtained when Jayden was 10 years of age

Condition	PBK words (60 dBA)	BKB-SIN (60 dBA)
Right hearing aid	20%	14.5 dB
Left hearing aid	20%	DNT
Bilateral hearing aids	36%	13 dB

PBK, phonetically balanced kindergarten; BKB-SIN, Bamford-Kowal-Bench-Speech In Noise Test

optimized, especially considering the fact that his listening and academic demands in the classroom will likely increase as he transitions from the third to the fourth grade, where lessons become more "lecture-based" and the curriculum becomes more challenging. Also, he will be required to switch classrooms throughout the day to receive instruction from multiple teachers. It is imperative that his hearing performance is optimized in order to be able to meet these academic demands and expectations.

2. **Are there any special considerations that should be taken into account in the selection of the most appropriate cochlear implant for Jayden?**

There are several factors unique to Jayden's case that should be considered when selecting the most appropriate hearing technology to meet his diverse hearing needs. First, Jayden is bilingual. Although sufficient access to high-frequency speech information (e.g., 2,000–9,000 Hz) is critical for understanding English speech,[6] Mandarin Chinese is a tonal language that possesses a greater dependence upon access to low- and mid-frequency speech information (e.g., below 2,000 Hz) for adequate intelligibility, particularly in noise.[7] As a result, it is imperative to select hearing technology that will provide Jayden with excellent access to low-level, high-frequency speech information to promote intelligibility of English speech, while also providing excellent access to the

spectral and temporal cues available in the low-frequency range of speech information to optimize his ability to understand a tonal language.

In addition, Jayden loves to play the violin. It is well established that musical proficiency is enhanced when listeners have access to fine temporal structure acoustical cues. The auditory system is better able to process fine temporal structure in response to acoustical stimulation relative to electrical stimulation.[8]

Additionally, Jayden frequently communicates in noisy situations. Research has shown that cochlear implant recipients' speech recognition in noise is better when listeners have sufficient access to binaural low-frequency information.[9] The binaural squelch effect and binaural summation are two phenomena supported by complex processing in the auditory nervous system, and likely require access to interaural timing cues that are aptly provided via acoustic stimulation, but are not provided via electrical stimulation.

Finally, in order to be able to localize sound, Jayden must be able to compare interaural timing differences in the low frequencies, and intermural level differences in the high frequencies. Research has shown that interaural timing cues are not processed and preserved effectively via electrical stimulation.[10] As a result, if he were to lose his residual acoustic hearing from cochlear implantation and be forced to rely on accessing low-frequency cues via electrical stimulation for the implanted ear, he would not have sufficient access to interaural timing differences critical for localization. Likewise, because of his suboptimal access to high-frequency sounds with hearing aid use, he would most likely struggle to make use of high-frequency, interaural level differences with use of bimodal hearing technology (e.g., use of a cochlear implant for the implanted ear and a hearing aid for the nonimplanted ear).

Given the aforementioned considerations, electric-acoustic stimulation (EAS) was suggested as an attractive option for Jayden. EAS technology involves the use of electrical stimulation via a cochlear implant to provide sufficient high-frequency stimulation and the use of amplification to optimize access to low-frequency sounds. Although many EAS options exist, one of the most viable is to insert the cochlear implant electrode array at a more shallow depth relative to a conventional cochlear implant electrode array insertion. For example, the Cochlear Nucleus Hybrid implant electrode array is inserted along the lateral wall of the cochlea to a depth of approximately 17 mm, which typically corresponds to an angular insertion depth of approximately 240 degrees (▶ Fig. 42.3 a). In contrast, the Nucleus CI422 electrode array is typically inserted along the lateral wall of the cochlea to a depth of 25 mm, which corresponds to an angular insertion depth of approximately 45 degrees (▶ Fig. 42.3 b). The shallower insertion depth of the Nucleus Hybrid electrode array avoids the apical regions of the cochlea and subsequently enhances the likelihood of low-frequency hearing preservation.[11,12] When low-frequency hearing is preserved, the recipient typically uses what is referred to as a hybrid/EAS sound processor (see ▶ Fig. 42.4), which delivers high-frequency sounds to the cochlear implant for electrical stimulation and low-frequency sounds to a receiver worn in the ear canal for acoustic amplification.

3. **What are the potential advantages and limitations of the specific cochlear implant recommendation indicated for Jayden?**
Potential advantages of EAS/hybrid cochlear implantation:
- With low-frequency hearing preservation, speech recognition in quiet and in noise for both English and Mandarin Chinese will likely be individually optimized relative to other technologies.[8,11,13] With low-frequency hearing preservation, music abilities will likely be individually optimized relative to other technologies.[8,13]
- With low-frequency hearing preservation, localization abilities will likely be individually optimized relative to other technologies because of the availability of interaural, low-frequency timing differences.[10]
- Improvements in the aforementioned areas will likely lead to better functional hearing performance in the classroom and social/recreational situations with a subsequent reduction in stress and listening-related fatigue.
- Potential disadvantages of EAS/hybrid cochlear implantation:

- Loss of low-frequency residual hearing in the implanted ear will most likely impair localization abilities.
- Loss of low-frequency residual hearing in the implanted ear may result in a reduction in speech recognition in quiet and in noise relative to the performance he would achieve with a cochlear implant with a full insertion of a conventional electrode array and use of a hearing aid for the opposite ear. Research is mixed in describing the results obtained for recipients who lose their residual hearing postimplant and have a cochlear implant with a shallow electrode array insertion depth.[14] However, hearing performance in the "electric-stimulation-only condition" is likely better with a full insertion relative to a shallow insertion.
- Loss of low-frequency residual hearing in the implanted ear will prevent him from having sound awareness for that ear when he is not using his cochlear implant.
- If Jayden loses his hearing and performs poorly with a cochlear implant with a shallow insertion depth, he may need to undergo a second surgery to receive a cochlear implant with a conventional insertion depth.

4. **What type of information should the clinician provide to the family to assist them in making the right decision for Jayden?**
The aforementioned relative advantages and limitations of EAS stimulation versus bimodal technology (e.g., conventional cochlear implant for one ear and a hearing aid for the opposite ear) should be discussed with the family. Most importantly, the family should be counseled regarding the risk that Jayden will lose his residual hearing during or after cochlear implantation. Although this risk is much higher with conventional cochlear implantation, the risk also exists with hybrid cochlear implantation.[11,14] Of note, preliminary research suggests that hearing preservation may be more likely with younger hybrid cochlear implant recipients.[15] The detriments associated with the loss of low-frequency acoustical hearing should be clearly defined for the family. Also, the clinician must be certain to counsel the family that Jayden's performance with a hybrid cochlear implant will likely be poorer than what he would achieve with a conventional cochlear implant if he were to lose his residual low-frequency hearing as a result of implantation or as a result of the natural progression of his hearing loss over time. It

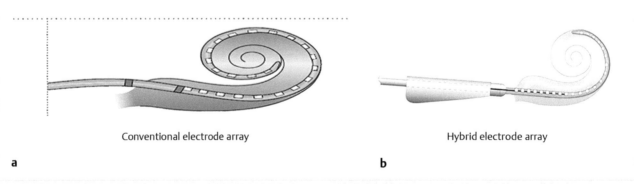

Conventional electrode array

Hybrid electrode array

a

b

Fig. 42.3 Illustration of a (**a**) Cochlear Nucleus Hybrid implant electrode array and (**b**) Cochlear Nucleus CI422 implant electrode array.

should be acknowledged that Jayden's low-frequency hearing sensitivity seemed to remain in the slight hearing loss range across time, so EAS is a viable consideration. However, it should also be noted that it is quite possible that his low-frequency hearing may progressively worsen over time, either as a result of cochlear implantation or of natural causes, even without cochlear implantation. Additionally, the family should be informed that Jayden may need to undergo another surgery to receive a conventional cochlear implant if his performance is poor with the shallow-inserted hybrid device.

42.5 Recommended Treatment

Jayden received a Cochlear Nucleus Hybrid implant for his right ear when he was 10 years old.

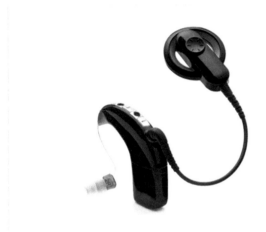

Fig. 42.4 Cochlear Nucleus 6 (CP910) electric-acoustic sound processor.

42.6 Outcome

Jayden's hybrid cochlear implant surgery was uneventful, and his low-frequency hearing sensitivity was preserved in entirety (see ▶ Fig. 42.5). ▶ Fig. 42.6 illustrates the fact that low-frequency acoustic stimulation was provided through approximately 1,000 Hz, and electrical stimulation from the cochlear implant was provided from approximately 1,000 to 8,000 Hz. Jaden immediately accepted EAS and showed steady progress in his ability to understand speech in quiet and in noise with the hybrid sound processor. His results for aided audiologic assessment conducted through the first 3 months of hybrid use are provided in ▶ Table 42.3. As shown, open-set word recognition and sentence recognition in noise have substantially improved with his use of the hybrid cochlear implant. Also, as shown, use of the hearing aid on the opposite ear seemed to provide little to no improvement in sentence recognition in noise. Further, Jayden showed rapid progress in his speech and language development following activation of his hybrid cochlear implant.

Most importantly, Jayden and his parents reported that they noticed immediate improvement in his ability to understand speech in most communication situations. Jaden also noted that he felt it was "easier to play" his violin after receiving the hybrid cochlear implant. They reported that they had no regrets about pursuing the hybrid cochlear implant. In fact, Jayden began to express reluctance to use the hearing aid for the left ear, and he requested a hybrid cochlear implant for that ear as well. Shortly before his 11th birthday, he underwent surgery to receive a Nucleus Hybrid cochlear implant for his left ear. His postsurgery audiogram is shown in ▶ Fig. 42.7. Also, the results of his most recent audiologic evaluation are provided in ▶ Table 42.4. Finally, his most recent standardized speech and language assessment indicated age-appropriate receptive and expressive spoken-language abilities.

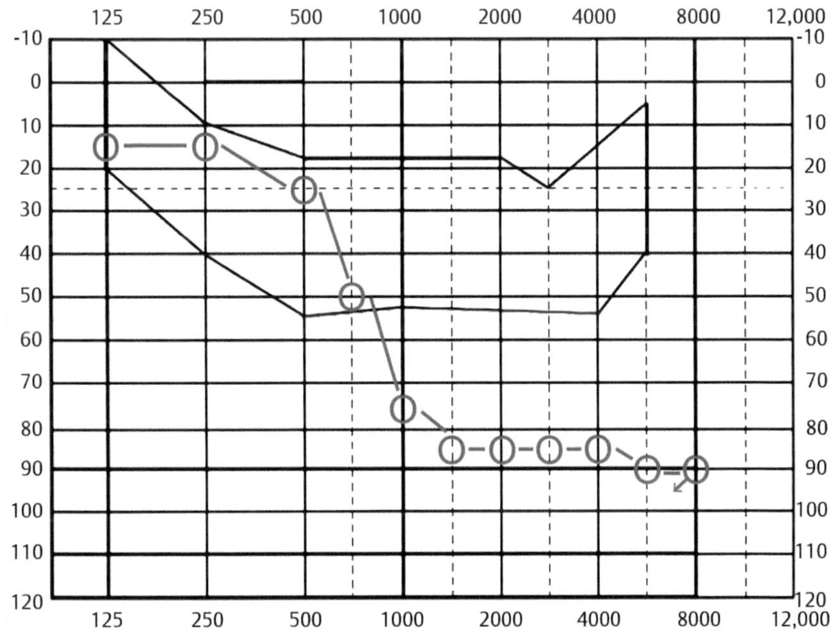

Fig. 42.5 Audiogram obtained after Jayden received a Cochlear Nucleus Hybrid implant for his right ear. O, right ear air conduction; Arrows, no response.

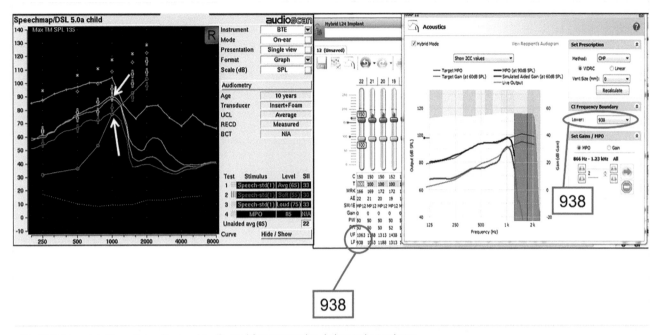

Fig. 42.6 Example of how the audio signal is allocated for acoustical and electrical stimulation.

Table 42.3 Aided speech recognition results obtained after Jayden had used his Cochlear Nucleus hybrid implant for 3 months

Tests	Prehybrid: right HA	Prehybrid: bilateral HAs	1 mo posthybrid: hybrid only	1 mo posthybrid: hybrid + left HA	3 mo posthybrid: hybrid only	3 mo posthybrid: hybrid + left HA
PBK-50 (60 dBA)	20%	36%	60%	64%	80%	76%
BKB-SIN (60 dBA)	14.5 dB	13 dB	7.5 dB	9 dB	5 dB	4 dB
CNC words (60 dBA)					92%	88%
AzBio sentences (60 dBA)					68%	77%

HA, hearing aid; CNC, consonant-nucleus-consonant

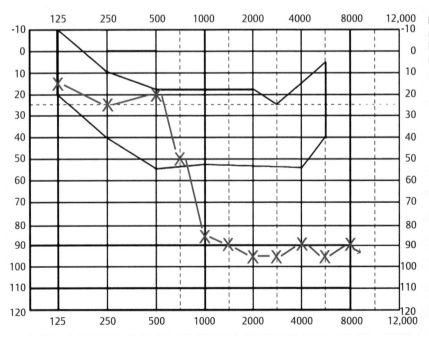

Fig. 42.7 Audiogram obtained after Jayden received a Cochlear Nucleus Hybrid implant for his left ear. X, left ear air conduction; Arrows, no response.

Table 42.4 Aided speech recognition results obtained when Jayden was 11 years of age (after receiving bilateral Cochlear Nucleus Hybrid implants)

Condition	CNC Words (60 dBA)	BKB-SIN (60 dBA)
Right hybrid	92%	4.5 dB
Left hybrid	88%	6.5 dB
Bilateral hybrid	96%	0.5 dB

CNC, consonant-nucleus-consonant; BKB-SIN, Bamford-Kowal-Bench-Speech In Noise Test

Currently, Jayden is excelling in a typical fifth grade classroom placement. He continues to be seen for quarterly audiology sessions to evaluate his aided hearing performance and to evaluate and program his hybrid cochlear implant sound processors. He is also seen for weekly Auditory-Verbal therapy, where he receives assistance with the continual optimization of his functional auditory and spoken-language abilities.

References

[1] Cruckley J, Scollie S, Parsa V. An exploration of non. -. quiet listening at school. J Educ Audiol. 2011; 17:23–35

[2] Pearsons K, Bennett R, Fidell S. Speech Levels in Various Noise Environments (Report No. EPA-600/1-77-025). Washington, DC: U.S. Environmental Protection Agency; 1977

[3] Bess FH, Gustafson SJ, Corbett BA, Lambert EW, Camarata SM, Hornsby BW. Salivary cortisol profiles of children with hearing loss. Ear Hear. 2015

[4] Bess FH, Hornsby BW. Commentary: listening can be exhausting—fatigue in children and adults with hearing loss. Ear Hear. 2014; 35(6):592–599

[5] Werfel KL, Hendricks AE. The relation between child versus parent report of chronic fatigue and language/literacy skills in school-age children with cochlear implants. Ear Hear. 2016; 37(2):216–224

[6] ANSI. ANSI S3.5-1997. American National Standard Methods for the Calculation of the Speech Intelligibility Index. New York, NY: ANSI; 1997

[7] Luo X, Fu QJ. Contribution of low-frequency acoustic information to Chinese speech recognition in cochlear implant simulations. J Acoust Soc Am. 2006; 120(4):2260–2266

[8] Gifford RH, Dorman MF, Brown CA. Psychophysical properties of low-frequency hearing: implications for perceiving speech and music via electric and acoustic stimulation. Adv Otorhinolaryngol 2010;67:51–60

[9] Gifford RH, Driscoll CL, Davis TJ, Fiebig P, Micco A, Dorman MF. A within-subject comparison of bimodal hearing, bilateral cochlear implantation, and bilateral cochlear implantation with bilateral hearing preservation: high-performing patients. Otol Neurotol. 2015; 36(8):1331–1337

[10] Gifford RH, Grantham DW, Sheffield SW, Davis TJ, Dwyer R, Dorman MF. Localization and interaural time difference (ITD) thresholds for cochlear implant recipients with preserved acoustic hearing in the implanted ear. Hear Res. 2014; 312:28–37

[11] Lenarz T, Stöver T, Buechner A, Lesinski-Schiedat A, Patrick J, Pesch J. Hearing conservation surgery using the Hybrid-L electrode. Results from the first clinical trial at the Medical University of Hannover. Audiol Neurootol. 2009; 14 Suppl 1:22–31

[12] Skarzyński H, Lorens A, Piotrowska A, Podskarbi-Fayette R. Results of partial deafness cochlear implantation using various electrode designs. Audiol Neurootol. 2009; 14 Suppl 1:39–45

[13] Incerti PV, Ching TY, Cowan R. A systematic review of electric-acoustic stimulation: device fitting ranges, outcomes, and clinical fitting practices. Trends Amplif. 2013; 17(1):3–26

[14] Miranda PC, Sampaio AL, Lopes RA, Ramos Venosa A, de Oliveira CA. Hearing preservation in. cochlear implant surgery. Int J Otolaryngol. 2014; 2014:468515

[15] Anagiotos A, Hamdan N, Lang-Roth R, et al. Young age is a positive prognostic factor for residual hearing preservation in conventional cochlear implantation. Otol Neurotol. 2015; 36(1):28–33

43 Teenager Rejecting Hearing Aids

Jane R. Madell

43.1 Clinical History and Description

Jake failed newborn hearing screening and was referred for a diagnostic audiological evaluation. Both auditory brainstem response (ABR) and behavioral observation audiometry (BOA) testing utilizing sucking responses were performed, and Jake was identified with a mild, rising to slight hearing loss, by both ABR and BOA (▶ Table 43.1). He accepted the hearing aids without difficulty. The family enrolled in an auditory-verbal therapy program, and Jake did well. He received a frequency modulation (FM) system when he began preschool and he did well through elementary school. In middle school, Jake refused the use of the FM system, and his grades started to fall. His parents continued to bring Jake for audiologic evaluations where he was tested with and without hearing aids. Jake's hearing loss was stable, and he continued to perform well with his hearing aids. Neither Jake nor his parents were completely forthcoming about the fact that Jake was not using hearing aids most of the time.

When Jake reached 10th grade, his grades became more of a concern. His grades consisted of an "A" in History, a "B" in Biology, and "C's" in Math, English, and Spanish. Jake recognized that his grades were not good, and the family sought assistance.

43.2 Questions for the Reader

1. Why might Jake be refusing hearing aids?
2. Should the audiologist have recognized sooner that there was a problem?
3. What should the audiologist do to deal with Jake's refusal to use hearing aids?

43.3 Discussion of Questions

1. **Why might Jake be refusing hearing aids?**
   There are many reasons why children reject hearing aids. The first thing to determine is how well they are hearing with the hearing aids. If a child is not hearing well with the hearing aids, there is no reason to use them. Real-ear measures for verification of the hearing aid fitting, and aided sound field testing for validation of the fitting (including aided thresholds and speech perception testing in different noise conditions), will provide more information about how well a child is actually receiving auditory information with the hearing aids. In Jake's case, the hearing aids were set appropriately, and he was hearing well with them.

Table 43.1 Audiologic test results at 3 weeks

	500 Hz	1,000 Hz	2,000 Hz	4,000 Hz
Right	30 dB HL	35 dB HL	35 dB HL	15 dB HL
Left	30 dB HL	40 dB HL	40 dB HL	15 dB HL

Teenage years are difficult for all children. They want to be like their peers, and having to use hearing aids can be distressing. In addition, teasing and bullying can be a problem in teenage years, which may contribute to rejection of technology. Although Jake denied that he was being bullied, the audiologist was not certain that he was not.

In Jake's case, he has sufficient hearing so that he is receiving some speech information, even when he is not wearing technology. Therefore, Jake may not realize how much academic and social information he actually is missing.

2. **Should the audiologist have recognized sooner that there was a problem?**
   During the annual evaluations, the audiologist should routinely discuss hearing aid use. By asking in a friendly manner how often the hearing aids are worn and in what conditions they are used, and gently probing to find out how the child feels about the hearing aids, the audiologist might have learned about the hearing aid rejection earlier. Data logging can also provide very useful information to assist in knowing how many hours/day hearing aids are being worn.

   Counseling can also be useful. Showing the child his or her audiogram, with aided and unaided test results, can provide a good counseling opportunity. Discussing what the child hears at normal and soft conversational levels, with and without hearing aids in sound field, provides useful counseling information.

3. **What should the audiologist do to deal with Jake's refusal to use hearing aids? What questions can she ask?**
   The first thing for the audiologist to do is to try to find out why Jake is refusing hearing aids. If the audiologist has had a relationship with him over the years, he is more likely to be willing to discuss the issue. Possible questions to ask include
   - Do you hear well with your hearing aids?
   - Are kids teasing you or bullying you about your hearing loss or the need to use hearing aids?
   - Why are you refusing to wear hearing aids? Do you not like the way the hearing aids look? If you had a different hearing aid (like a completely in-the-ear-hearing aid), would you wear that?
   - Would you consider using your hearing aids in classes where you have poor grades?
   - What do you think your future life choices will be if you continue to get poor grades? If you heard more of what happens in the classroom, do you think you would do better?
   - Are you aware that your parents report that you listen to TV at a very loud level?

43.4 Further Counseling

The audiologist showed Jake his (unaided) audiogram that was drawn on the speech banana with phonemes displayed (▶ Fig. 43.1). The audiologist was able to show Jake that with his hearing loss of around 40 dB HL, he was missing a great deal of speech information at normal conversational levels, and was not even hearing speech at soft conversational levels of 30 to

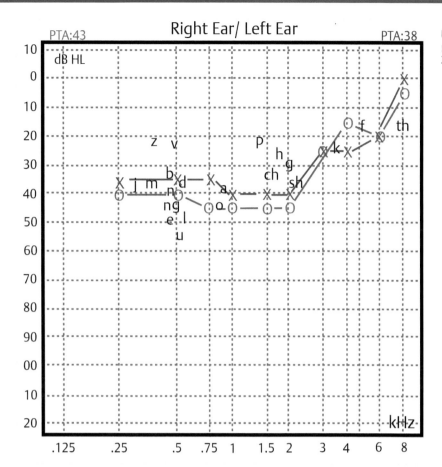

Fig. 43.1 Unaided thresholds on audiogram with phonemes displayed. O, right ear air conduction; X, left ear air conduction.

35 dB HL. He was stunned to see a visual description of what he was missing (▶ Table 43.2, ▶ Table 43.3). The speech perception testing was reviewed. Seeing clearly how much speech he was able to hear with no hearing aids, and in the same test conditions with hearing aids, was also valuable for counseling. Aided thresholds at 15 to 20 dB HL throughout the frequency range provided additional support to indicate what Jake could and could not hear.

The audiologist and Jake discussed the following reasons to wear hearing aids:
- The effect of not hearing well on academics and on social conversations, including missing social cues.
- The effect of not hearing well on his level of fatigue as the day progresses, and how fatigue affects his ability to learn in school and to engage in social conversations.
- The need to stimulate his brain (auditory cortex) to keep it functioning maximally.
- The necessity of continued acquisition of knowledge.
- For younger children, not wearing hearing aids has a significant effect on language learning and literacy. Jake already has language, so language development is less of an issue. However, there is still the critical issue of learning new language and new information.

Table 43.2 Audiologic test results at 15 years

	250 Hz	500 Hz	1,000 Hz	2,000 Hz	3,000 Hz	4,000 Hz	6,000 Hz	8,000 Hz
Right	35	30	35	35	25	15	10	10
Left	40	35	40	40	25	15	10	10
Right aid		20	20	20	20	15		
Left aid		20	15	20	25	15		

Table 43.3 Speech perception using CNC words

	Right	Left	Soundfield	Right aid	Left aid	Binaural
75 dB	96%	94%				
50 dB HL			28%	86%	82%	92%
35 dB HL			CNT	76%	72%	72%
50 dB HL + 5 SNR			CNT			68%

Abbreviation: SNR, signal-to-noise ratio.

Jake put his hearing aids back on. He was encouraged to pay attention to what bothered him about the hearing aids, so he could explain it to the audiologist who could offer adjustments. Jake and the audiologist talked about the fact that it is not fair that he has a hearing loss, but that we just have to deal with the situations we have. Jake received empathy from the audiologist, and he appreciated acknowledgement of his feelings.

At 1-month follow-up, Jake reported that he was hearing well with the hearing aids. He began the month by wearing the hearing aids only in the classes in which he was getting a "C" grade. He is now wearing his hearing aids full time in school, except for gym and lunch. He is not wearing them at home yet, so the TV continues to be a problem for the rest of the family.

44 Facilitating Full-Time Hearing Aid Use in Children

Darcy Stowe, Lindsay Hanna, Elizabeth Musgrave, and Tessa Hixon

44.1 Clinical History and Description

Mandy, a 4-year-old girl, participated in an intervention initiative to increase hearing aid wear-time and ultimately speech and language outcomes. Mandy reportedly referred on her newborn hearing screening, bilaterally, and was referred to the clinic for diagnostic auditory brainstem response (ABR) testing. Personal medical history was unremarkable, and there was no family history of hearing loss at the time of diagnosis. Mandy was diagnosed with a moderate sensorineural hearing loss bilaterally and was fitted with clinic loaner hearing aids in March 2011, at 1 month of age, and with her own personal hearing aids in June 2011. She began auditory-verbal therapy (AVT) services immediately following the hearing aid fitting but had inconsistent attendance for both audiology and AVT appointments. The family was referred to the state's early intervention program as an additional support, but the family was unable to commit to the program at that time. The family discontinued services in December 2011.

Approximately 1.5 years later, at 2 years old and under the care of her grandparents, Mandy returned to the clinic for an audiologic evaluation and to resume AVT services. She was fitted with new hearing aids in May 2013 and began attending therapy on a weekly basis. Again, attendance was inconsistent until she began attending a language-rich, reverse mainstream preschool class for children with hearing loss in September 2014; the classroom utilized children with normal hearing sensitivity as peer models.

44.2 Audiologic Testing

Early identification via ABR testing and intervention via appropriately fitted hearing aids for both ears would suggest that Mandy had the opportunity to meet developmental milestones in a typical manner. As seen in ▶ Fig. 44.1, electroacoustic measures revealed excellent access to soft, average, and loud speech bilaterally at the time of the initial hearing aid fitting. As noted in ▶ Fig. 44.2, behavioral testing at 2.5 years old revealed good access to auditory information in the 250- to 6,000-Hz frequency range in the binaural condition; testing could not be reliably

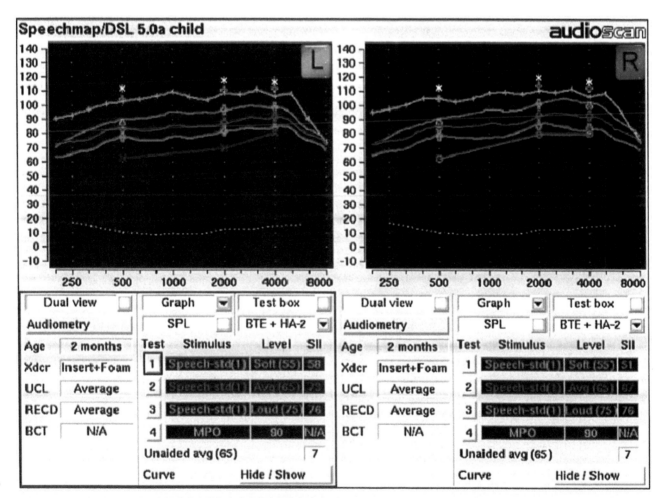

Fig. 44.1 Electroacoustic measures at Mandy's initial hearing aid fitting.

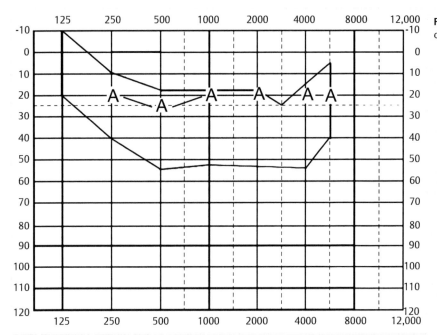

Fig. 44.2 Aided behavioral testing at 2.5 years old. A, binaural hearing aids behind the ear.

Table 44.1 Speech and language evaluation results at 3.10 years

Testing date: January 13, 2015 Child's chronological age: 3.10 years				
Standardized test		Standard score (85–115 WNL)	Percentile	Age equivalent
Preschool Language Scale, 5th ed.[a]	Auditory comprehension	76	5	2.7
	Expressive communication	82	12	2.9
	Total language score	78	7	2.8
Expressive Vocabulary Test, 2nd ed.[b]		81	19	2.10
Peabody Picture Vocabulary Test, 4th ed.[c]		70	2	2.4
Goldman-Fristoe Test of Articulation, 2nd ed.[d]		71	8	< 2.0

WNL, within normal limits.
[a]Zimmerman IL, Steiner VG, Pond E. Preschool Language Scales—5th ed. (PLS-5). San Antonio, TX: Pearson; 2011.
[b]Williams KT. Expressive Vocabulary Test. 2nd ed. Minneapolis, MN: NCS Pearson; 2007.
[c]Dunn M, Dunn LM. Peabody Picture Vocabulary Test. 4th ed. Circle Pines, MN: AGS; 2007.
[d]Goldman R, Fristoe M. Goldman-Fristoe Test of Articulation 2. 2nd ed. Circle Pines, MN: American Guidance Services; 2000.

completed with each hearing aid alone at that time because of patient fatigue. Data logging revealed consistent, limited use of the hearing aids, with an average of 3.8 hours of use per day.

As seen in ▶ Table 44.1, speech, language, and articulation scores were all below what was expected for Mandy's chronological and/or hearing age at the time of testing.

44.3 Questions for the Reader

1. Review the history provided later. For this family, what were some contributing factors to less-than-optimal hearing aid wear-time?
2. What is the ethical responsibility of an audiologist or speech-language pathologist (SLP) in the ongoing management for a child with hearing loss?

44.4 Discussion of Questions

1. **Review the history provided later. For this family, what were some contributing factors to less-than-optimal hearing aid wear-time (see later)?**

Mandy demonstrated inconsistent attendance for both audiology and AVT appointments from the time she was initially fitted with loaner hearing aids until they discontinued services in December 2011. At the time of diagnosis, Mandy's father had recently been incarcerated, and her mother was having difficulty with Mandy's diagnosis of hearing loss in addition to the daily responsibilities of raising three children as a single mom. Mandy's grandmother provided some support during that time but was still inconsistent in bringing Mandy to scheduled appointments. Mandy initially exhibited less-than-optimal hearing aid wear, reportedly due to poor-fitting earmolds and excessive feedback from the devices. Once Mandy was fitted with her personal hearing aids, she continued to exhibit poor follow-up with appointments and less-than-optimal hearing aid wear-time.

When Mandy and her family returned to the clinic in April 2013, she was living with her grandparents who were concerned about device use and delayed speech and language skills. Data logging consistently indicated less than 2 hours of daily hearing aid use due to the transition of Mandy moving in with her grandparents (i.e., establishing a routine, setting limits, etc.). The urgency of normalizing Mandy's life took precedence over management of the hearing technology.

2. **What is the ethical responsibility of an audiologist or SLP in the ongoing management for a child with hearing loss?**
Due to the critical nature and timing of conversations with families of children with hearing loss, providers must be equipped with tools to have difficult conversations. Providers are tasked with sharing critical information about hearing loss, brain development, and necessary steps to achieve listening and spoken language outcomes if that is what the family desires. First, audiologists and SLPs must be willing to join in difficult conversations or even initiate the difficult conversations for the sake of the child's development. If parents or family members are made aware of the critical nature of time in relation to the child's brain development, they are likely to move forward with purposeful urgency toward their desired outcomes. It should be noted that failure to provide a child with the necessary support required to facilitate the basic need of language development can be considered as neglect. Consideration may be given to reporting such cases to the appropriate child welfare agency.

Second, audiologists and SLPs must be thorough in documenting, in the patient's visit note, all aspects of counseling with families, in addition to other evaluative data. The provider must reflect when and what information was conveyed to the family in order to have that conversation on record, and thus be able to access it at a later date as needed. Finally, providers should be in continual dialogue with other team members in order to convey consistent information and assist the family of a child with hearing loss in achieving optimal outcomes. Teaming between an audiologist and SLP provides critical and timely information in moving forward. An audiologist can provide necessary information regarding thresholds, data logging, and troubleshooting to the SLP. The SLP can also discuss that information with the family during weekly sessions to provide support to facilitate full-time hearing technology use. Likewise, SLPs can give the audiologist feedback regarding auditory skill development in order to assist the audiologist in how to best serve the child with hearing loss. It takes a team effort to maximize the listening and spoken language outcomes of children with hearing loss.

44.5 Intervention Initiative

Facilitating Audition in the Home (FAITH) is an intervention initiative developed by clinicians at Hearts for Hearing. FAITH is a platform for difficult conversations with the goals of family education and achievement of optimal hearing aid wear-time. Mandy and her family were enrolled in the FAITH initiative in January 2015, when Mandy was 3.10 years old.

The FAITH program consists of the following components for clinic use and carryover into the home:

44.5.1 Data logging

Because it was measureable, data logging of hearing aid wear-time was obtained as the primary component to evaluate the success of the FAITH intervention initiative. Measurements were obtained preintervention, 2 months postintervention, 3 months postintervention, and 12 months postintervention.

Currently, there is no standard for optimal hearing aid wear-time; what may be acceptable to one clinician may not be acceptable to another. The FAITH initiative committee researched typical sleep patterns in infants and toddlers and developed minimum recommended technology wear-times per age (▶ Table 44.2).

44.5.2 Family and Educational Support

The FAITH initiative provided a central resource for the family. This resource, housed in a binder, included many documents: contact information for team members, audiograms, speech-language evaluations, minimum recommended technology wear-time chart, daily wear-time logs, parent/family questionnaires, equipment troubleshooting resources, speech, language, and auditory skill development milestones, and a glossary of terms.

Table 44.2 Minimum recommended technology wear-time by age

Age of child	Average sleep-time (day naps and night-time)	Minimum recommended wear-time
0–3 mo	16–17 h	6 h
3–6 mo	14–15 h	8 h
6–12 mo	13–14 h	9 h
1–3 y	12–14 h	10 h
3–4 y	11–14 h	11 h
>4 y	8–12 h	12 h

44.5.3 Family Questionnaires

The FAITH initiative committee developed a Daily Life Questionnaire, adapted from the Boys Town National Research Hospital Amplification in Daily Life Questionnaire, to evaluate the family's perceived use of hearing technology in various daily situations. The questionnaire also encouraged the family to estimate their child's average daily wear-time.

Additionally, the family was asked to complete a questionnaire, either the LittlEars or Parents' Evaluation of Aural/oral performance in Children (PEACH), depending on the child's age, to evaluate auditory skills relative to peers with normal hearing sensitivity.

44.5.4 Aural Rehabilitation

As initially recommended, Mandy and her grandmother continued to attend weekly AVT sessions. Through the FAITH resource binder, the family was educated regarding various topics including auditory brain development, speech and language milestones, and current research regarding auditory and spoken language outcomes in relation to hearing technology practices.

44.6 Additional Testing

44.6.1 Audiological

Mandy was seen by her audiologist for routine monitoring every 3 months. Data logging at 2 months postintervention revealed an average of 9.4 hours of device use per day. Data logging at 3 months postintervention revealed an average of 12.3 hours of device use per day. Follow-up behavioral testing, as seen in ▶ Fig. 44.3, revealed no major change in hearing sensitivity and good access to the 250- to 6,000-Hz frequency range in the binaural condition; ear-specific aided testing was attempted, but reliable responses could not be obtained at that time due to patient fatigue.

44.6.2 Family Questionnaires

The Daily Life Questionnaire revealed family-estimated technology wear-times of 9 to 11 hours per day at 2 months postintervention and 12 hours per day at 3 months postintervention.

44.7 Additional Questions to the Reader

1. What types of programs or strategies could be employed in the intervention to achieve optimal wear-time?
2. What was the minimum recommended wear-time for Mandy at the time the intervention initiative was implemented?
3. What follow-up conversations with the family would be useful to ensure continued success?

44.8 Discussion of Additional Questions

1. **What types of programs or strategies could be employed in the intervention to achieve optimal wear-time?**
   In order for Mandy to utilize her hearing aids during all waking hours and achieve optimal wear-time, her caregivers must be invested and involved in the process. The clinic involved the caregivers in regular data logging by making sure they knew weekly what Mandy's average hearing aid wear-time was and how that compared to the goal. Caregivers were also asked to estimate wear-time and have the child be engaged in that process.

   With the FAITH binder, the caregivers were given specific information regarding goals for optimal wear-time based on the child's age and sleeping patterns. It also included a parent questionnaire rating their comfort level with the hearing technology and its maintenance.

   The importance of attendance to all audiology appointments, AVT sessions, and twice-weekly classroom experiences was stressed as a priority for the family. Keeping them engaged in these appointments also gave regular times for feedback and checking in to make sure optimal wear-time was being achieved and was consistent.

2. **What was the minimum recommended wear-time for Mandy at the time the intervention initiative was implemented?**
   As seen in ▶ Table 44.2, the minimum recommended wear-time for a 3.10-year-old, Mandy's age at the onset of the intervention initiative, is 11 hours per day.

3. **What follow-up conversations with the family would be useful to ensure continued success?**
   The providers working with Mandy identified three key areas that would likely facilitate meaningful conversations regarding hearing aid wear-time over time. First, using the FAITH central resource on a consistent basis at audiology and AVT appointments was key. This binder will continue to be filled with new information from audiograms and data logging resources which will serve as a platform for continued conversations—whether those be to encourage the family in doing well with utilizing hearing technology during all waking hours or to encourage the family of the need to work toward goals of optimal wear-time again.
   Second, the audiologist will continue with regular data logging at each routine audiology appointment and share this information with the family. Just because a family has achieved optimal wear-time for their child with hearing loss does not mean that the data logging needs to cease or stop being reported to the family. Continue investing the family in the process of goal-setting.
   Finally, the SLP will maintain an annual speech-language evaluation protocol to assess progress toward goals and to provide timely recommendations for future treatment. This session with recommendations will easily lead to conversations regarding maximizing Mandy's speech, language, and listening outcomes.

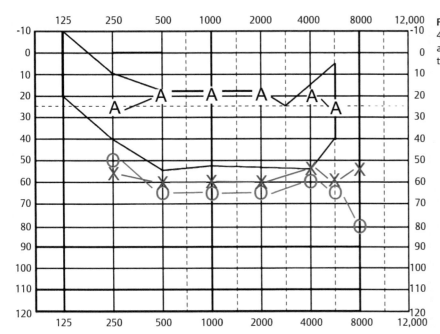

Fig. 44.3 Unaided and aided behavioral testing at 4 years old. O, right ear air conduction; X, left ear air conduction; A, binaural hearing aids behind the ear.

44.9 Outcomes

In January 2014, Mandy began attending preschool. Mandy's participation in the class provided additional assistance to the family by supporting the clinicians in recommendations for optimal hearing aid wear-time, exposing Mandy to other children wearing hearing technology, and increasing the expectations for speech and language development. Additionally, Mandy's auditory, speech, and language progress allowed her to be able to communicate the need and benefit of her hearing aids to her grandparents which ultimately increased hearing aid wear-time in conjunction with the implementation of the FAITH intervention initiative. Over time, Mandy's grandparents recognized the importance and benefit of optimal hearing aid wear-time and introduced an incentive program for Mandy's use of the hearing aids to encourage optimal wear-time as part of the implementation of the FAITH initiative. Mandy and her family no longer have a need to incentivize the program because Mandy wears her hearing aids all waking hours.

The PEACH questionnaire, completed 6 months postintervention, revealed auditory skills within the expected range in quiet and slightly below the expected range in noise (▶ Fig. 44.4). At that time, Mandy was also fitted with an ear-level remote microphone system, and behavioral testing revealed significant improvement in performance.

As of August 2015, Mandy attends a mainstream prekindergarten class in her neighborhood public school, attends AVT sessions on a weekly basis with her grandmother, and wears her hearing aids consistently.

44.9.1 Audiologic

Data logging at 12 months postintervention revealed an average of 13.7 hours of device use per day. As part of the FAITH initiative, Mandy participated in an activity to depict her hearing aid wear-time relative to her goal at the given data logging intervals (▶ Fig. 44.5).

44.9.2 Speech and Language

Current speech, language, and articulation scores are provided in ▶ Table 44.3. As shown, improvement has been achieved in most areas. Mandy's family and her service providers are working together diligently in an effort to facilitate continued progress. Continuation of full-time use of hearing technology and consistent attendance to audiology and AVT sessions will be necessary to optimize outcomes.

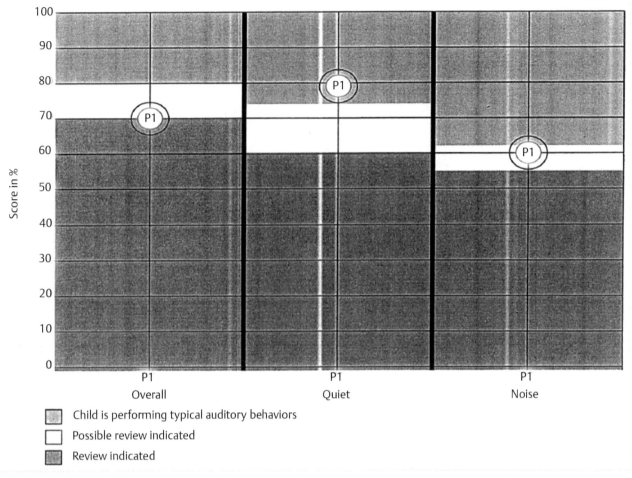

Fig. 44.4 PEACH outcomes 6 months postintervention.

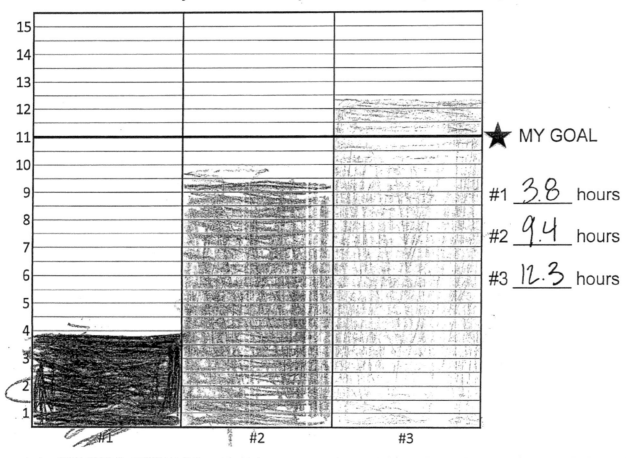

Fig. 44.5 Mandy's hearing aid wear-time log.

Table 44.3 Speech and language evaluation results at 5.1 years

Testing date: March 25, 2016 Child's chronological age: 5.1 years		Standard score (85–115 WNL)	Percentile	Age equivalent
Standardized test				
Preschool Language Scale, 5th ed.[a]	Auditory comprehension	90	25	4.8
	Expressive communication	76	5	3.9
	Total language score	82	12	4.2
Expressive Vocabulary Test, 2nd ed.[b]		101	53	5.3
Peabody Picture Vocabulary Test, 4th ed.[c]		96	39	4.9
Goldman-Fristoe Test of Articulation, 2nd ed.[d]		71	5	2.7

WNL, within normal limits.

[a]Zimmerman IL, Steiner VG, Pond E. Preschool Language Scales. 5th ed. (PLS-5). San Antonio, TX: Pearson; 2011.
[b]Williams KT. Expressive Vocabulary Test. 2nd ed. Minneapolis, MN: NCS Pearson; 2007.
[c]Dunn M, Dunn LM. Peabody Picture Vocabulary Test. 4th ed. Circle Pines, MN: AGS; 2007.
[d]Goldman R, Fristoe M Goldman-Fristoe Test of Articulation 2. 2nd ed. Circle Pines, MN: American Guidance Services; 2000.

Suggested Readings

[1] Byrd S, Shuman AG, Kileny S, Kileny PR. The right not to hear: the ethics of parental refusal of hearing rehabilitation. Laryngoscope. 2011; 121(8):1800–1804

[2] Ching TY, Dillon H, Marnane V, et al. Outcomes of early- and late-identified children at 3 years of age: findings from a prospective population-based study. Ear Hear. 2013; 34(5):535–552

[3] Fielding D, Duff A. Compliance with treatment protocols: interventions for children with chronic illness. Arch Dis Child. 1999; 80(2):196–200

[4] Moeller MP, Hoover B, Peterson B, Stelmachowicz P. Consistency of hearing aid use in infants with early-identified hearing loss. Am J Audiol. 2009; 18(1):14–23

[5] Muñoz K, Nelson L, Blaiser K, Price T, Twohig M. Improving support for parents of children with hearing loss: provider training on use of targeted communication strategies. J Am Acad Audiol. 2015; 26(2):116–127

[6] Muñoz K, Preston E, Hicken S. Pediatric hearing aid use: how can audiologists support parents to increase consistency? J Am Acad Audiol. 2014; 25 (4):380–387

[7] Muñoz K, Preston E, Hicken S. Pediatric hearing aid use: how can audiologists support parents to increase consistency? J Am Acad Audiol. 2014; 25 (4):380–387

[8] Sjoblad S, Harrison M, Roush J, McWilliam RA. Parents' reactions and recommendations after diagnosis and hearing aid fitting. Am J Audiol. 2001; 10 (1):24–31

[9] Tsiakpini L, Weichbold V, Kuehn-Inacker H, Coninx F, D'Haese P, Almadin S. LittlEARS Auditory Questionnaire. Innsbruck, Austria: MED-EL; 2004

[10] Walker EA, Spratford M, Moeller MP, et al. Predictors of hearing aid use time in children with mild-to-severe hearing loss. Lang Speech Hear Serv Sch. 2013; 44(1):73–88

45 Progressive Hearing Loss

Rollen Cooper and Dawn Violetto

45.1 Clinical History and Description

Amelia was brought to the audiology clinic at the age of 23 months after her family moved to the area from another state. Her mother stated that Amelia was born after an unremarkable pregnancy and delivery, but failed her newborn hearing screening and a rescreening prior to discharge from the birthing hospital. Records indicate that when she was 17 days old, visual reinforcement audiometry (VRA) and behavioral observation audiometry (BOA) were attempted, and a speech startle response was obtained at 80 dB. A week later, automated auditory brainstem response (AABR) and otoacoustic emissions (OAEs) testing were performed, and Amelia did not pass either test.

Amelia was aided, bilaterally, at the age of 2 months with Phonak Extra 311 BTE hearing aids potentially using the VRA/BOA in combination with the AABR results, and began receiving early intervention services. Due to chronic middle ear infections, pressure equalization (PE) tubes were placed when Amelia was 10 months old. While under sedation, only click ABR testing was performed and revealed thresholds at 80 dB in the left ear and 75 dB in the right ear, "indicating a severe hearing loss, bilaterally, in the mid to high frequencies." When she was approximately 14 months old, binaural sound field testing utilizing narrowband noise and warbled pure tones testing showed unaided responses at 70 dB HL across 500, 1,000, 2,000, and 4,000 Hz, with aided responses at 30 dB HL at 500 and 1,000 Hz and 35 dB at 2,000 and 4,000 Hz.

Standardized speech and language testing was performed through the state's early intervention program when Amelia was 19 months old. Two tests were administered, giving slightly differing results: the Rossetti Infant-Toddler Language Scale (RITLS) showed an age equivalent score of 6 to 9 months, but the SKI-HI Language Development Scale showed an age equivalent score of 9 months.

Amelia's mom reported that Amelia continuously pulls out her hearing aids and the devices are only worn for a few hours per day. She also stated that Amelia communicates using only jargon and nonsense words, and she feels that Amelia's speech and language development are poor.

45.2 Audiologic Testing

Testing at 23 months was conducted over two sessions (▶ Fig. 45.1). A four-frequency audiogram and speech awareness thresholds were obtained for each ear using VRA through inserts. Word recognition testing was not obtained due to Amelia's limited vocabulary and language. Results indicated a severe rising to moderate symmetrical hearing loss. Real-ear-to-coupler difference (RECD) measures were completed, and, then, predicted real-ear measures proceeded in the 2cc coupler due to lack of patient cooperation. Data logging indicated an average use of 3 hours in the left hearing aid and 4 hours in the right hearing aid. Results indicated that, at their current settings, Amelia's hearing aids were meeting DSL V targets for loud sounds only and were significantly under target for low to mid frequencies for soft (55 dB SPL) and medium sounds (65 dB SPL). Adjustments were made to Amelia's Phonak Extra 311 devices to best fit DSL V targets. However, the hearing aids were set to maximum available gain settings in the higher frequencies, and were still not meeting prescribed targets. It was, therefore, recommended that Amelia be fitted with Phonak Naida V SP BTE hearing aids, and they were ordered. Upon arrival, in situ real-ear measures were completed

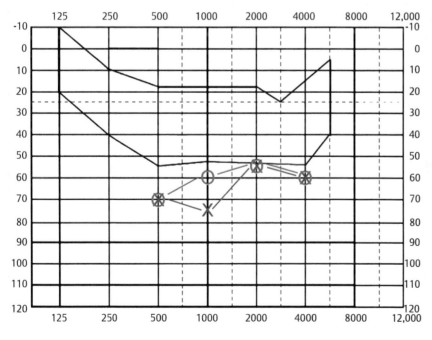

Fig. 45.1 Audiogram obtained at 23 months. O, right ear air conduction; X, left ear air conduction.

with the new Naida SP BTEs and showed that the hearing aids were meeting all targets for all inputs. Given that Amelia's new hearing aids were appropriate for her hearing loss and programmed via real ear measures (REMs), her access to auditory information was improved, so she became a consistent hearing aid user. Data logging at a subsequent appointment indicated an average of 9 hours use per day. Approximately 6 months later when Amelia was 25 months old, the Rossetti was administered again and results showed an age equivalency of 22 months.

45.3 Questions for the Reader

1. What is the appropriate testing for diagnosing a hearing loss in newborn infants? Was the testing done at 17 days developmentally appropriate?
2. What does the standardized testing show about Amelia's communication skills? What does the discrepancy between the two tests signify?
3. What kind of testing can be performed to demonstrate how Amelia's listening skills are developing?

45.4 Discussion of Questions

1. **What is the appropriate testing for diagnosing a hearing loss in infants?**
   According to the AAA and ASHA pediatric protocols, for infants under 6 months, use of behavioral observation is appropriate. VRA is not appropriate for a 17-day-old infant, because the baby cannot yet sit alone nor have the developed head/motor control to perform the conditioned response of turning the head to the sound. VRA is intended to be used in infants approximately 5 to 36 months of developmental age to gain an estimation of hearing thresholds based on minimum response levels that are closely tied to perceptual thresholds. At 17 days of age, Amelia could not have developmentally performed the VRA task.

   It should also be noted that a startle response may be observed from 60 to 90 dB HL even when peripheral hearing is normal, and the startle reflex is highly influenced by physiologic conditions (i.e., hunger and fatigue). Amelia's testing at 17 days of age consisted of VRA and startle response which was noted at 80 dB HL, neither of which could diagnose the configuration or extent of the hearing loss across the speech frequency range. However, hearing aids were fitted based on these questionable results.

   After failing the AABR and OAEs, a nonsedated or sedated ABR should have been performed at that time. However, an ABR was not performed until 10 months of age. When the ABR was performed, testing used only a click stimulus, even though the child was sufficiently sedated in the OR after PE tube placement to complete a full tone pip/burst audiogram. A click stimulus may elicit a response from the auditory system at the best-hearing frequency across a range from approximately 750 to 4,000 Hz and does not provide sufficient, frequency-specific information for setting hearing aids appropriately. Although the audiology clinic complied with JCIH 1, 3, and 6 recommendations, their methodology and accuracy were compromised, resulting in poorly underfit hearing aids and speech and language delays manifesting at the time of first evaluations at the new center.

   A complete audiologic test battery consisting of a health and history interview, parent interview, otoscopic examination, 1,000-Hz tympanograms, acoustic reflex threshold assessment, DPOAEs, tone burst/pip air conduction, and bone conduction ABR assessment, performed at a minimum of 500 and 4,000 Hz, would be preferable for diagnosing a hearing loss and for estimating the slope/configuration of the hearing loss—all necessary for the accurate fitting of hearing aids.

2. **What does the standardized testing show about Amelia's communication skills? What does the discrepancy between the two tests signify?**
   The RITLS is a criterion-referenced test that evaluates the preverbal and verbal communication skills for children from birth to the age of 3 years, 11 months regardless of hearing status. The SKI-HI Language Development Scale was designed to assess the communication skills of children with hearing loss from birth to the age of 5. The expressive language score for the SKI-HI allows for credit to be given for gestures, signs, and spoken communication, whereas the expressive language score for the Rossetti does not. Children with hearing loss can be evaluated with both of these measurements; however, it is common to see a discrepancy in the expressive language score as was seen with Amelia. If the clinician is looking at the development of a child's spoken language skills and wants to analyze them in comparison to their typically hearing peers, the Rossetti will give a more accurate representation than the SKI-HI.

3. **What kind of testing can be performed to demonstrate how listening skills are developing?**
   A clinician must be measuring a child's functional listening skills to determine what kind of progress the child is making. There are two excellent tests that measure the listening skills for children younger than 3 years: the LittlEARS and the Infant Toddler Meaningful Auditory Integration Scale. Both of these measurements have been standardized on children with typical hearing. They give the clinician valuable information on the progress (or lack thereof) that a baby is making in terms of their functional listening skills with or without devices. This information is important to consider when making decisions about types of hearing devices and how to program them. For children who have mastered the skills measured in these tests (score of 27 or higher on the LittlEARS) or for a child older than 2 years, the Parents' Evaluation of Aural/Oral Performance of Children can be administered to measure listening skills in both quiet and noisy environments.

45.5 Additional Testing

About the time that Amelia turned 3 years old, her mother noted that Amelia seemed to be declining even with her hearing aids. Audiological testing demonstrated that the hearing loss in Amelia's left ear had deteriorated to the severe-profound level

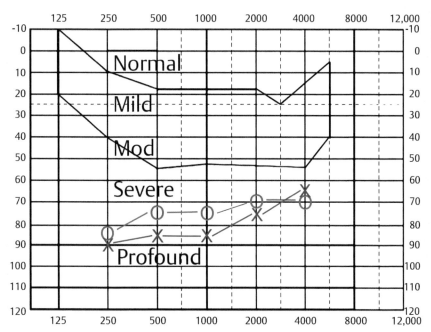

Fig. 45.2 Audiogram prior to left cochlear implantation. O, right ear air conduction; X, left ear air conduction.

(▶ Fig. 45.2). Formal speech perception testing was performed using the Northwestern University Children's Perception of Speech (NU-CHIPS), revealing a score of 60% on the left side and 88% on the right side. Amelia was fitted with a new loaner device, a Phonak Naida V UP using REM, based on the new audiogram on the left side. Amelia was closely monitored by her classroom teacher, speech-language pathologist, and audiologist. Speech perception testing was repeated using the NU-CHIPS 2 months later, and the results showed a decrease to 40%. Amelia and her family were referred to a cochlear implant center, and within 4 months Amelia had received a cochlear implant for her left ear.

Because of her history, Amelia continued to be closely monitored by our clinic for progression of hearing loss in the right ear. Approximately a year after the progression in her left ear, a sharp decrease in speech perception skills was noted in the right ear (▶ Fig. 45.3). Amelia stated that she did not want to wear her right hearing aid anymore and asked when she could get another cochlear implant. Six months later, her cochlear implant on the right side was activated.

45.6 Additional Questions for the Reader

1. If you suspect a progressive hearing loss, how often would you test a child?
2. Which members of a child's educational team would you consult regarding a child with a progressive hearing loss? What information would you want from them?
3. If a child still has good access to auditory information with one ear, is it necessary to look for alternatives to improving access to sound in the other ear?

45.7 Discussion of Additional Questions

1. **If you suspect a progressive hearing loss, how often would you test a child?**
   Given that a progression of the hearing loss was noted in the left ear, we tested Amelia every 3 months. However, after consultation with the classroom teachers, speech-language pathologist, and parents, Amelia was tested any time a change was noted in her functional performance at home or in the classroom, especially as she had a history of chronic middle ear disorder. Temporary fluctuations of hearing thresholds were noted with severe retraction of the tympanic membranes or the presence of middle ear fluid, along with the eventual progression of hearing loss and decrease of speech perception skills in each ear. Prior to cochlear implantation, a magnetic resonance imaging and computer tomography scan were performed and no abnormalities were noted on either study.

2. **Which members of a child's educational team would you consult regarding a child with a progressive hearing loss? What information would you want from them?**
   For any child with hearing loss, and especially with progressive hearing loss, it is imperative to have good communication with all members of the child's educational team. A professional who works with the child regularly, such as a speech-language pathologist, a teacher of the deaf, or a listening and spoken language specialist, would be able to note a lack of progress or a regression in skills.

   The audiologist would need to obtain ear-specific information on responses to pure tones across the speech spectrum and collect information on the child's speech perception skills and his or her ability to demonstrate comprehension

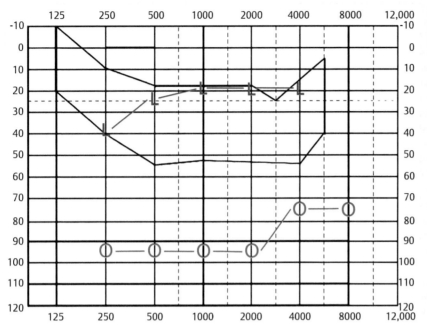

Fig. 45.3 Audiogram obtained prior to right cochlear implantation. O, right ear air conduction; L, left ear hearing aid.

of monosyllabic words and connected speech from both a close and far distance and with and without background noise.

Also, if the child is no longer able to detect all Ling sounds in the ear with progressive hearing loss, then he or she will no longer have the needed brain access to sound/auditory information for auditory neural development for the development of listening and spoken language skills.

It is equally important to communicate with the child's parents or caregivers to see what differences they note in the child's home environment. If a child is experiencing a progressive hearing loss on one side, the parent may observe that the child experiences difficulty understanding speech from the poorer side as well as demonstrates increased difficulty localizing sound and understanding speech in the presence of background noise.

3. **If a child still has good access to auditory information with one ear, is it necessary to look for alternatives to improving access to sound in the other ear?**
   For children with hearing loss, audiology services must be aggressive; children with hearing loss need to have optimal access to auditory information in both ears so they can develop listening and spoken language skills commensurate with their typically hearing peers. Children who do not have good access to sound in one ear are at great risk for developing significant delays in speech and language, and for experiencing academic failure.

45.8 Treatment

After the activation of her first left cochlear implant, Amelia received additional, individual aural habilitation sessions with the new device. Within 4 months, her listening skills with the cochlear implant reached the same level as her listening skills while wearing both her implant on her left ear and the hearing

Table 45.1 Standardized testing results upon graduation from a listening and spoken language program

Standardized test	Standard score (85–115 is the average range)
Peabody Picture Vocabulary Test, 4th ed., Form A	104
Expressive Vocabulary Test, 2nd ed., Form A	118
The Clinical Evaluation of Language Fundamentals, 4th ed. (Receptive Language)	101
The Clinical Evaluation of Language Fundamentals, 4th ed. (Expressive Language)	118
Goldman Fristoe Test of Articulation, 2nd ed.	113

aid on her right side. Amelia followed a similar protocol when her right cochlear implant was activated (▶ Fig. 45.4). At the time of writing this case, Amelia was 6 weeks postactivation and was able to identify monosyllabic words differing only in vowels and to correctly sequence three critical elements in a message.

45.9 Outcome

During her preschool years, Amelia was placed in a listening and spoken language preschool program for children with hearing loss. There, she was able to receive individualized therapy, small group instruction, and proactive audiological management. By the time she was 5 years old, all standardized speech and language testing scores were within the average range, with expressive vocabulary and expressive language scores being above average (▶ Table 45.1). Amelia was then successfully mainstreamed into a first grade classroom in her neighborhood school with minimal hearing itinerant services and the use of a personal remote microphone system.

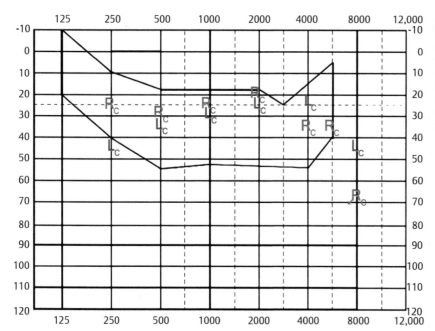

Fig. 45.4 Most recent audiogram with both cochlear implantations activated. Slight adjustments were made to both maps after this audiogram was completed for better detection of soft sounds and to balance the maps obtained using FRESH noise and warbled pure tones. RC, right ear cochlear implant; LC, left ear cochlear implant; Arrows, no response.

Suggested Readings

[1] American Speech-Language-Hearing Association. Executive Summary for JCIH Year 2007 Position Statement: Principles and Guidelines for Early Hearing Detection and Intervention Programs. 2007. Available at: www.asha.org

[2] American Speech-Language-Hearing Association. Guidelines for the Audiologic Assessment of Children from Birth to 5 Years of Age [Guidelines]. 2004. Available at: www.asha.org/policy

[3] Audiologic Guidelines for the Assessment of Hearing in Infants and Young Children. 2012. Available at: http://audiology-web.s3.amazonaws.com/migrated/201208_AudGuideAssessHear_youth.pdf_5399751b249593.36017703.pdf

[4] Ching T, Hill M. Parents' Evaluation of Aural/Oral Performance of Children. Australian Hearing; 2005

[5] Cole E, Flexer C. Children with hearing loss: developing listening and talking: birth to six. San Diego, CA: Plural Publishing; 2007

[6] Kühn-Inacker H, Weichbold V, Tsiakpini L, Coninx S, D'Haese P. Little Ears: Auditory Questionnaire. Innsbruck: MED-EL; 2003

[7] SKI-HI Language Development Scale. 2004. Available at: https://hopepubl.com/proddetail.php?prod=401

[8] The Rossetti Infant-Toddler Language Scale. 2006. Available at: https://www.linguisystems.com/products/product/display?itemid=10041

[9] Bagatto M, Moodie S, Malandrino A, Richert F, Clench D, Scollie S. The University of Western Ontario Pediatric Audiological Monitoring Protocol. The LittleEARS Auditory Skill Questionnaire; 2011

[10] Zimmerman-Phillips S, Osberger MJ, Robbins AM. Infant-Toddler Meaningful Auditory Integration Scale. Sylmar, CA: Advanced Bionics Corp; 1997

46 Fitting Frequency-Lowering Technology to Children

Danielle Glista, Marianne Hawkins, and Susan Scollie

46.1 Clinical History and Description

Bentley is a 12-year-old girl with a mild sloping to profound hearing loss in the right ear and a moderately severe sloping to profound loss in the left ear (▶ Fig. 46.1). Air- and bone-conduction thresholds measured at octave and interoctave frequencies are consistent with asymmetrical, sensorineural hearing loss (SNHL). Acoustic immittance measures were unremarkable. Results from the Threshold Equalizing Noise (TEN) test (version ER-3A) suggest the presence of cochlear dead regions at 4,000 Hz on the right side and at 2,000, 3,000, and 4,000 kHz on the left side; this test only assesses for the presence of dead regions from 500 to 4,000 Hz.

Bentley's mother reports that Bentley was born with a hearing loss, but did not receive amplification until the age of 4 years and after the family relocated to Canada. Since then, Bentley has consistently worn high-power digital behind-the-ear (BTE) hearing aids coupled to occluded personal earmolds. At the age of 9 years, Bentley was enrolled at a public school offering a Hearing Support program for hearing-impaired children. This program included intervention from a speech-language pathologist (SLP) and auditory-verbal therapist and the use of remote microphone hearing assistance technology in the classroom. This support has carried through to current day and incorporates training around the audibility/production of high-frequency sounds.

Bentley is currently wearing high-power BTE hearing aids. Hearing levels and wideband real-ear-to-coupler difference values were assessed using insert phones coupled to personal earmolds. Hearing aid verification was completed using the Audioscan Verifit2 test box. For the purposes of this case study, coupler-based measures are displayed to illustrate the fitting steps that were taken. On-ear verification would be the preferred method for a child of this age. The shape and gain of the conventional hearing aid fitting were verified according to Desired Sensation Level (DSL) v5.0 child targets; these were met up to 4 kHz in the right ear and 2 kHz in the left for soft (±5 dB), average (±3 dB), and loud sounds (±5 dB) and for the maximum power output (MPO) to a 90-dB sound pressure level (SPL) swept pure tone (±5 dB). Electroacoustic measures suggest that the hearing aid response rolls off in the high frequencies, limiting audibility achieved above 4 kHz in the better ear and above 2 kHz in the poorer ear. Bentley's SLP reports indicated that Bentley was having difficulty with her production of high-frequency consonants. Further parent report suggests Bentley has difficulty participating in social activities outside of the structured classroom environment, particularly in the home, which she shares with her five younger siblings.

46.2 Additional Audiologic Testing and Electroacoustic Measurement with Conventional Amplification

Aided speech recognition assessments were completed in the sound booth using an average presentation level (65 dB SPL) and with Bentley wearing both hearing aids. Bentley scored 58% correct on the consonant-nucleus-consonant (CNC) word recognition test from the new Minimum Speech Test Battery (MSTB). Three additional tests were performed to further probe Bentley's ability to hear and discriminate different speech sounds. First, performance on the University of Western Ontario (UWO) Plurals Test was measured at 58% correct, indicating

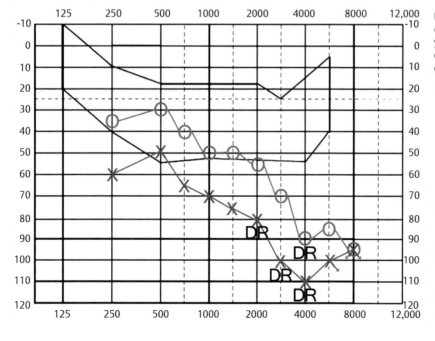

Fig. 46.1 Unaided air-conduction thresholds obtained with conventional audiometry at 12 years of age. O, right ear air conduction; X, left ear air conduction; Arrows, no response; DR, dead region.

difficulty detecting word-final fricatives. Vowel recognition testing was scored at 86% correct, with performance for normal-hearing listeners generally falling above 95% correct. Last, Bentley's ability to discriminate between /s/ and /ʃ/ sounds was assessed to be at 75% correct, indicating some difficulty discriminating between high-frequency phonemes. Although the initial fitting appointment did not permit aided speech sound detection testing, this will be included in the follow-up appointment (e.g., the Ling 6(HL) Test of speech sound detection). Overall, Bentley's performance with conventional amplification was poor to satisfactory.

This prompted the use of further hearing aid verification measures to assess candidacy for frequency-lowering (FL) technology. Recall, Bentley's conventional fitting is below DSL targets above 2 and 4 kHz on the left and right side, respectively. Real-ear measures using high-frequency speech sounds were completed to further assess high-frequency audibility with conventional amplification. All advanced hearing aid features (e.g., digital noise reduction) were disabled for these measures. High-frequency phonemes, /s/ and /ʃ/, were presented at an average level (▶ Fig. 46.2). Refer to Glista et al[1] and Scollie et al[2] for details on the development and validation of the /s/ and /ʃ/ verification signals referred to in this case study. Electroacoustic results suggested that Bentley could not hear an aided female /s/ on the left side, but that she has partial audibility of the /ʃ/ sound. On the right side, partial audibility of the /s/ sound could be achieved, along with full audibility of the /ʃ/ sound.

46.3 Questions for the Reader

1. Does Bentley have access to the entire speech spectrum to allow for optimal speech recognition?
2. What factors should be considered when assessing candidacy for FL hearing aids?
3. What type of verification procedures should be used when fitting FL hearing aids?

46.4 Discussion of Questions

1. **Does Bentley have access to the entire speech spectrum to allow for optimal speech recognition?**

Taking into consideration the asymmetrical nature of Bentley's hearing loss, ability to provide amplification across a broad bandwidth of speech has been judged per ear using hearing aid verification. Even with high-power digital hearing aids, the aided response for both the right and left fitting rolls off in the high frequencies; this effectively has limited audibility achieved above 4 kHz when you consider the better ear and above 2 kHz when you consider the poorer ear. For the worse ear (left), phoneme-based verification results suggest that high-frequency sounds such as /s/ will be inaudible, with partial access to other high-frequency phonemes. For the better ear, we observed partial audibility of high-frequency phonemes. We know from the literature that the peak energy of a female or child /s/ can lie beyond 8,000 Hz.[3] Validation measure results suggest that Bentley's abilities to recognize words and detect word-final plurality markers, in quiet and when fitted binaurally, are below satisfactory. Therefore, Bentley may experience difficulty understanding the high-frequency tokens of female and child speech with her conventional hearing aid fitting; speech perception will likely be worse for the left ear when compared to the right.

2. **What factors should be considered when assessing candidacy for FL hearing aids?**

After fine-tuning multilevel output curves and MPO, for the conventional fitting, the next step in determining candidacy for FL includes the use of modified verification measures to assess high-frequency audibility (▶ Fig. 46.2). Specifically, if the /s/ sound cannot be made audible with the conventional fitting, FL fitting may provide some benefit. Additional factors that were considered when evaluating Bentley's candidacy for FL included the following:

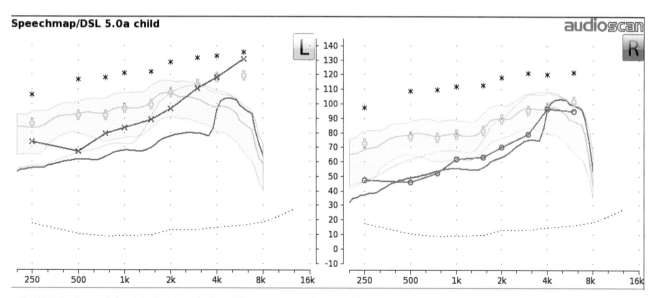

Fig. 46.2 Real ear aided output for a standard speech passage, /ʃ/ and /s/, measured with conventional amplification. All screen shots shown in this case are from the Audioscan Verifit2 test box, with measurements completed at a presentation level of 65 dB SPL.

- *The configuration and degree of her hearing loss*: Bentley presents with a profound loss in the high frequencies for both ears. The literature suggests that children with this type of loss may be more likely to benefit from FL such as frequency compression.[4]
- *Hearing instrument/electroacoustic factors*: Has the gain response been maximized for the conventional fitting and has an appropriate device been chosen based on the audiogram? Does the conventional fitting fail to meet DSL targets across all frequencies? Does the hearing aid provide FL capabilities? In Bentley's case, all these statements would be considered true, further indicating that she may be a candidate for FL.
- *Other factors related to parental/professional report*: Validation measure results suggest that Bentley may not have access to the full speech spectrum. These findings were consistent with parental report, indicating some difficulty participating in conversation at school, and likely relate to SLP report of difficulty with the production of high-frequency phonemes. Literature in this area suggests that fricative/affricate development can be more challenging for pediatric listeners presenting with a hearing deficit in the high frequencies coupled with hearing aid bandwidth and gain limitations associated with this frequency region.[5]

3. **What type of verification procedures should be used when fitting FL hearing aids?**

It is important to verify that an appropriate amount of FL has been provided, so fine-tuning of the settings is often needed. For Bentley's fitting, FL settings were determined separately per ear based on the large asymmetry.[6] In the case of symmetrical SNHL, FL settings can often be determined based on the better ear. Protocols for fitting FL exist in the literature and can be useful to clinicians when verifying and fine-tuning FL (refer to the suggested readings for further details). As discussed earlier, the first step includes verification of the shape and gain of the conventional hearing aids. From this, the fitter can determine the frequency at which the output of the hearing aid falls below audibility for a given audiogram, referred to as the MAOF: maximum audible output frequency.[7] This helps determine a "range" in which to position the frequency-lowered signal. This range allows for the fitter to use the weakest possible setting, while still maximizing audibility of high frequencies based on the hearing aid(s) response, audiogram, and chosen FL settings. ▶ Fig. 46.3 displays the MAOF range that was established for Bentley's fitting.

The next step was to determine if audibility of high-frequency phonemes could be improved with FL; this was accomplished by verifying the response for /s/ without FL and evaluating whether the full spectrum of /s/ was audible. As seen in ▶ Fig. 46.2, real-ear measures suggest that the /s/ could not be made audible on the left side and that Bentley was likely receiving partial audibility of the /s/ spectrum on the right side. Lastly, FL was enabled and fine-tuned for Bentley's fitting (this fine-tuning process is displayed for the left ear in ▶ Fig. 46.4). Here, the strength of the FL setting was adjusted until the upper shoulder of the /s/ was audible and fell within the MAOF range for both the right and left ear. This fitting did not incorporate information related to cochlear dead regions. Further research is needed to determine if FL settings should be chosen to accommodate for the presence of cochlear dead regions. For the purpose of this case, the information from the TEN test was not incorporated into the fitting.

46.5 Diagnosis and Recommended Treatment

Based on the audiological history, in combination with results from the verification and validation measures reported for the

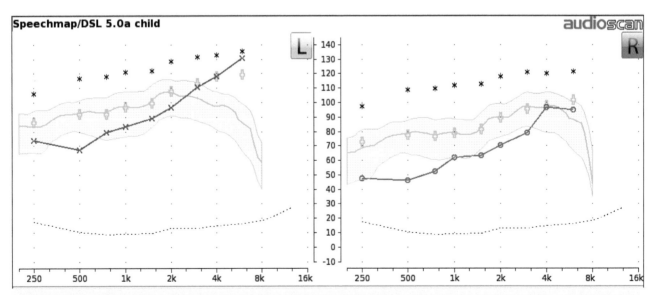

Fig. 46.3 Binaural real-ear aided output for a standard speech passage with the conventional fitting, displaying the long-term average speech spectrum (LTASS) with peak and valley measurements for a presentation level of 65 dB SPL. The MAOF range spans from the point at which the LTASS crosses the hearing threshold line to the point at which the peaks of speech cross the threshold line. For the right ear, the MAOF has been marked at an extrapolated point extending from the hearing threshold line.

conventional fitting, FL was activated in Bentley's fitting. The type of FL available in the hearing aids that Bentley was wearing used adaptive nonlinear frequency compression signal processing. Real ear measurement results suggest improved audibility for /s/ for both the left and right side, when compared to measures made with the conventional fitting (▶ Fig. 46.5).

46.6 Outcomes

The hearing aid fitting validation measures were completed again, with FL enabled, to evaluate any performance differences. Overall, Bentley received substantial benefit from activating FL in her hearing aids. Performance change between conventional and FL fittings was assessed using 95% confidence intervals; all reported changes were judged to be significant. Bentley's CNC word recognition scores increased to 72% correct; her UWO Plurals scores went up to 73% correct; and a 12% improvement in vowel recognition was measured. Improvements noted across speech recognition/detection measures are likely related to high-frequency audibility provided via FL technology. Reported vowel recognition scores are within the normal range with FL enabled.

An 11% decrement in scores associated with /s-ʃ/ discrimination was also measured. It is worth noting that these improvements were measured at the time of initial activation of FL. Literature suggests that children may need a period of time to acclimatize to FL technology to achieve maximum speech recognition ability.[8,9] It is possible that with time Bentley may learn to better discriminate between novel sounds made audible with FL. Counselling around this topic was provided to Bentley and her family. Bentley continues to see an SLP offering therapy sessions that include practice of the production of /s/ and /ʃ/ sounds in relation to new audibility provided with the FL fitting. Based on the degree/asymmetrical nature of the hearing loss presented in this case and the age of the participant, follow-up appointments should include monitoring of hearing loss progression and assessment of cochlear implantation (CI) candidacy. Current literature suggests that some listeners may benefit from the inclusion of FL signal processing in bimodal device fittings.[10] Given that candidacy guidelines for CI vary greatly depending on the child's country of residence, a formal assessment would need to be completed for this case to establish candidacy.

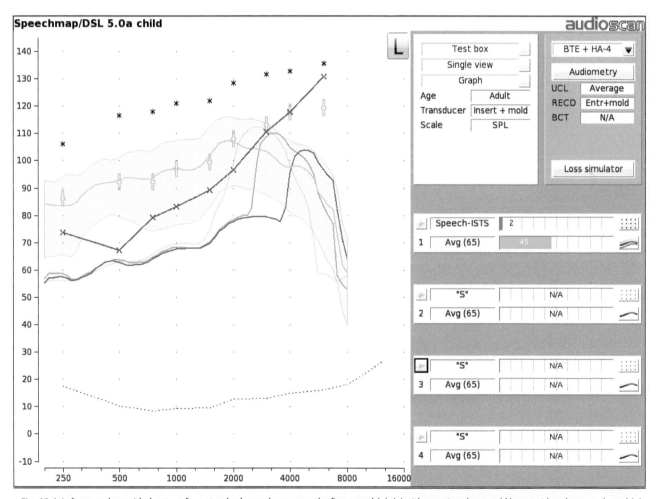

Fig. 46.4 Left ear real-ear aided output for a standard speech passage, the fine-tuned /s/, /s/ with a setting that would be considered too weak, and /s/ with FL off (/s/ spectra reported from left to right). The upper shoulder of the /s/ can be seen within the MAOF range and has been made audible for the fine-tuned /s/. However, for the weak setting and with FL off, the /s/ is inaudible for the listener.

Speechmap/DSL 5.0a child

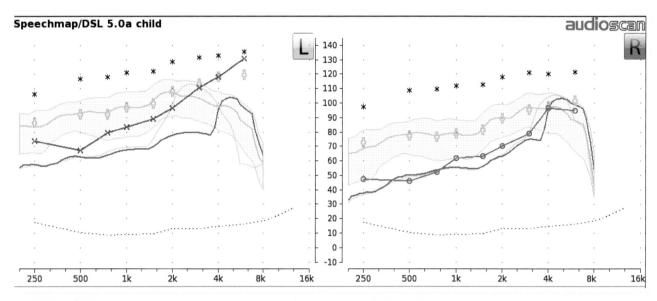

Fig. 46.5 Binaural real-ear aided output for a standard speech passage, /s/ for the fine-tuned FL setting and /s/ without FL, measured with the Audioscan Verifit2 test box at a presentation level of 65 dB SPL.

References

[1] Glista D, Hawkins M, Scollie S. An update on modified verification approaches for frequency lowering devices. AudiologyOnline Article 16932. Available at: www.audiologyonline.com

[2] Scollie S, Glista D, Seto J, et al. Fitting frequency-lowering signal processing applying the American academy of audiology pediatric amplification guideline: updates and protocols. J Am Acad Audiol. 2016; 27(3):219–236

[3] Stelmachowicz PG, Pittman AL, Hoover BM, Lewis DE. Aided perception of /s/ and /z/ by hearing-impaired children. Ear Hear. 2002; 23(4):316–324

[4] Glista D, Scollie S, Bagatto M, Seewald R, Parsa V, Johnson A. Evaluation of nonlinear frequency compression: clinical outcomes. Int J Audiol. 2009; 48 (9):632–644

[5] Moeller MP, Hoover B, Putman C, et al. Vocalizations of infants with hearing loss compared with infants with normal hearing: Part I–phonetic development. Ear Hear. 2007; 28(5):605–627

[6] John A, Wolfe J, Schafer E, et al. Original research: In asymmetric high-frequency hearing loss, NLFC helps. Hear J. 2013; 66(9):26–29

[7] McCreery RW, Brennan MA, Hoover B, Kopun J, Stelmachowicz PG. Maximizing audibility and speech recognition with nonlinear frequency compression by estimating audible bandwidth. Ear Hear. 2013; 34(2):e24–e27

[8] Wolfe J, John A, Schafer E, et al. Long-term effects of non-linear frequency compression for children with moderate hearing loss. Int J Audiol. 2011; 50 (6):396–404

[9] Glista D, Scollie S, Sulkers J. Perceptual acclimatization post nonlinear frequency compression hearing aid fitting in older children. J Speech Lang Hear Res. 2012; 55(6):1765–1787

[10] Davidson LS, Firszt JB, Brenner C, Cadieux JH. Evaluation of hearing aid frequency response fittings in pediatric and young adult bimodal recipients. J Am Acad Audiol. 2015; 26(4):393–407

47 Removing Reluctance in Remote Microphone Use

Linda Thibodeau and Brett Shonebarger

47.1 Clinical History and Description

JM is a 13-year-old 8th grade student in a large public school district. He is a bilateral cochlear implant (CI) user and successful oral communicator. JM had a normal birth with no family history of hearing loss. At 13 months, he contracted meningitis, resulting in a profound bilateral hearing loss. He received a Cochlear N24 CI in his right ear at 16 months; his left Cochlear Freedom CI was implanted at 3 years, with "significant ossification" noted by the surgeon. At age 9 years 9 months, he was upgraded to bilateral, Cochlear N5 speech processors.

From the time of diagnosis to 3 years old, he received Early Childhood Intervention (ECI), which included medical, audiological, and speech services. Per the Individuals with Disabilities Education Act (IDEA) Part C, an Individual Family Service Plan (IFSP) was developed to address JM's development and his family's concerns and goals, and included a plan for monitoring outcomes.

Postimplantation audiological history showed successful development of speech understanding in the right ear but significant difficulty in using the left speech processor. Most recent speech testing (age 9 years) by his speech-language pathologist indicated that his articulation ability was in the 50th percentile for his age, assessed via Arizona Articulation Proficiency Scale (AAPS-3). Speech goals at this time pertained to understanding critical elements in a phrase, retaining auditory information, following simple commands, understanding figurative language, recalling details from stories, and using new vocabulary. JM is currently managed by a CI audiologist, as well as an educational audiologist contracted with his school district.

47.2 Audiologic Testing

47.2.1 Clinic Testing

At age 9 years 9 months, testing was completed with the new Cochlear N5 speech processors. The Hearing in Noise Test for Children (HINT-C) was presented at 55 dB HL (70 dB SPL) in sound field while JM was wearing both Nucleus 5 speech processors. Conditions ranged from quiet to +0 dB signal-to-noise ratio (SNR). As shown in ▶ Table 47.1, JM achieved better scores as the SNR improved from 0 to +10 dB.

Table 47.1 Hearing in Noise Test for Children (HINT-C) scores while listening with both Nucleus 5 speech processors

Condition	Score (%)
Quiet	98
+10 dB SNR	86
+5 dB SNR	64
+0 dB SNR	16

During JM's most recent audiological evaluation at age 13 years 10 months, speech recognition was performed. This provides more useful information than measuring frequency-specific thresholds in the sound field. JM was able to accurately repeat the six Ling sounds, bilaterally. JM repeated consonant-nucleus-consonant (CNC) words that were presented at 55 dB HL (70 dB SPL) in quiet while listening with each implant. He achieved scores of 98 and 92% for phonemes and words, respectively, in the right ear, and 24 and 12% for phonemes and words, respectively, in the left ear. AzBio sentences were presented at 55 dB HL (70 dB SPL) at a +10 dB SNR while JM listened with both implants. He obtained a score of 61% words correct. Telemetry results were within normal limits bilaterally. Channels 22 and 13 in the left ear had previously been deactivated per the manufacturer's recommendation. At the session's conclusion, JM's audiologist recommended that he wear his speech processors during all waking hours. She noted that it was particularly important to consistently wear his left processor with the right processor in order to improve the benefit received from the devices to the extent possible.

47.2.2 Classroom Speech-in-Noise Testing

When JM entered 7th grade, the educational audiologist sought to demonstrate the benefits of frequency modulation (FM) remote microphone systems to him and his teachers. He had used a remote microphone system in his previous school with limited success. Attempts to provide an optimal arrangement included ear level FM receivers, which he refused because they weighted down his speech processors. JM preferred using an induction neckloop arrangement. However, he disliked using the system in general, mainly due to the perceived struggle of using the transmitter; he felt that the process of giving the transmitter to teachers often delayed the start of his classes. From his perspective, the system did not provide benefit worth the embarrassment and hassle of using it, and he considered discontinuing use of remote microphone systems altogether. JM wanted a transmitter that he could keep at his desk. At this time, his educational audiologist mentioned a remote microphone system "like a pen" (Phonak Roger Pen) and demonstrated the use of the "pen" system, along with other transmitter/receiver configurations. However, in order to justify making a change from the traditional transmitter in that school district (Phonak inspiro), speech recognition was evaluated with a trial remote microphone system that was similar to a Roger Pen. The trial included a Phonak EasyLink transmitter and a MyLink+ neckloop.

The speech-in-noise test setup used in the educational setting is shown in ▶ Fig. 47.1. The Bamford-Kowal-Bench Speech-in-Noise (BKB-SIN) test was converted into a movie file and sentence prompts in text format were added to align with the progressive increases in noise level. The audiologist sat 4 feet in front of JM. Behind JM was a Bluetooth Jam speaker from which

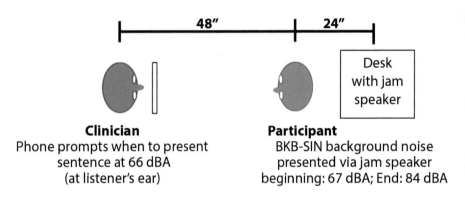

48"   24"

Desk
with jam
speaker

Clinician
Phone prompts when to present
sentence at 66 dBA
(at listener's ear)

Participant
BKB-SIN background noise
presented via jam speaker
beginning: 67 dBA; End: 84 dBA

Fig. 47.1 Speech recognition in noise setup for testing in educational setting.

the background noise was presented. This noise was played from a video via smartphone held by the clinician, and the sentences were presented with monitored live voice to allow microphone position effects to be realized during the testing. The audiologist held a small sound level meter to monitor voice intensity while watching the video on the smartphone, which provided cues to the correct timing for the each sentence presentation.

The scores obtained for several equipment arrangements are shown in ▶ Table 47.2. Because he benefited from the EasyLink arrangement, JM and the audiologist decided to pursue a trial using this transmitter and a MyLink receiver. The agreement was made that if he consistently used this trial remote microphone system with success, a recommendation would be made for the school district to purchase the Roger Pen digital transmitter.

During this trial period, JM sent an email to his educational audiologist describing his excitement about the remote microphone system. "I was wondering when you planned to come see me again. I'm very excited about the new FM system and have been researching and telling my parents and teachers about it. I like the one I'm using and it is working O.K., but I would really love to use the newer model. I can't wait to see you!!" It should be noted that this is not the typical greeting an educational audiologist receives from students.

After a month of successful and responsible use of the Easy-Link FM system, JM was fit with a Roger Pen and Roger MyLink neckloop. The arrangements that can be used with implants and hearing aids can be determined through consulting the Roger Configurator as shown in ▶ Fig. 47.2. At this time, the audiologist counseled JM on using the system for the best possible benefit. She informed him and his teacher that the remote microphone system will help the most when worn by the teacher, either clipped on or in a shirt pocket, or using a lanyard to put the transmitter in close proximity to the teacher's mouth. JM and the teacher worked together later that day to read the instruction manual and practice using the Pen.

JM and teachers reported success during the first year of using the Roger Pen—but not without challenges. At one point, JM lost the Pen in the school's parking lot; it was later found in pieces, crushed by an unaware driver. The device was covered under the manufacturer's warranty and was quickly replaced.

After a year of successful device use and regular check-ups (with no other incidences of loss), the audiologist returned to

Table 47.2 Bamford-Kowal-Bench Speech-in-Noise (BKB-SIN) with multiple FM and digital transmitter/receiver configurations

Condition	Score (%)
CI only	19
CI + MyLink + Inspiro	100
CI + MyLink + EasyLink worn by talker	95
CI + MyLink + EasyLink held by JM	42
CI + Roger X + Roger Pen worn by talker	100

Abbreviation: CI, bilateral cochlear implant.

reevaluate JM's use and benefit with the remote microphone system. He reported doing well in school, even excelling in advanced placement (AP) classes. During lectures, he kept the Roger Pen at his desk, pointed toward the teacher. When classes required more hands-on group work, he was able to point the Pen toward talkers in his group, improving his ability to participate in activities with peers. Also, he was able to easily connect to his computer using the Pen.

Testing was completed with the BKB-SIN materials and the Jam speaker using the setup as shown in ▶ Fig. 47.1. The results obtained in four equipment arrangements are shown in ▶ Table 47.3. During the Roger Pen condition, the signal from the Roger Pen was delivered to both JM's CI speech processors via a Roger MyLink and the t-coil program.

JM was counseled on appropriately using the Roger Pen based on his BKB-SIN scores. His best speech understanding in noise was achieved with the microphone close to the talker—that is, when the teacher was wearing the microphone. Although keeping the Pen at his desk during lectures has the potential for better speech understanding in noise than the CI-only condition, increasing distance between the talker and microphone can eliminate benefit entirely. In this case, preferential seating is still a critical component of classroom hearing success. Alternative options for use may include keeping the Roger Pen on the teacher's desk depending on the teacher's mobility during lectures, or having the teacher wear the Pen during lecture, and then JM holding the Pen for group work.

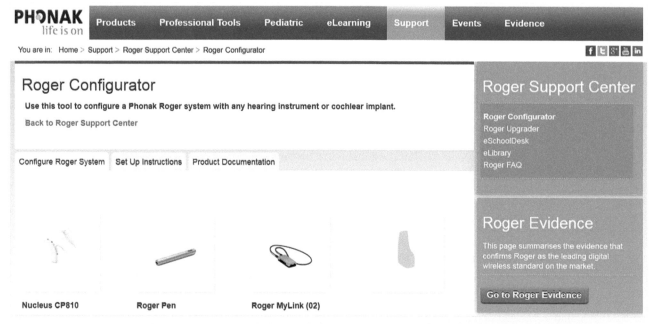

Fig. 47.2 Phonak/Roger Configurator. Hearing aid and speech processor make/model can be selected to explore available remote microphone options.

Table 47.3 BKB-SIN test results with Roger Pen transmitter and Roger MyLink receiver

Condition	Score (%)	Score (dB SNR loss)
CI only (4 ft)	64	7.5
CI + Roger Mylink + Roger Pen on talker (4 ft)	96	–0.5
CI + Roger Mylink + Roger Pen on desk (4 ft)	78	4.0
CI + Roger Mylink + Roger Pen on desk (8 ft)	58	9.0

Abbreviations: CI, bilateral cochlear implant; 4 ft, talker 4 feet away from JM; 8 ft, talker 8 feet away from JM.

47.3 Questions for the Reader

1. What are the pros/cons of using a remote microphone system like the Roger Pen versus a traditional transmitter?
2. Why not use a Phonak Clip-on microphone?
3. How might a student demonstrate responsibility to use the Roger Pen?

47.4 Discussion of Questions

1. **What are the pros/cons of using a remote microphone system like the Roger Pen versus a traditional transmitter?**
   - Pros:
     - Better speech recognition in noise with digital modulation system.[1,2]
     - Greater acceptance by the student.
     - Ability to manage the microphone settings by the student.
     - Can easily use in both lecture and group discussion settings, with automatic transitions between the two settings.
     - Less conspicuous.
   - Cons:
     - Easier to lose or break.
     - Need additional counseling for the student on managing the microphone and how to achieve best benefit.

2. **Why not use a Phonak Clip-on microphone?**
   The Clip-on microphone does not result in as much benefit as the Roger Pen.[3]

3. **How might a student demonstrate responsibility to use the Roger Pen?**
   - Be motivated by a trial with a less optimal remote microphone system (MyLink + I = inspiro).
   - Connect with a designated teacher daily about use of the remote microphone system.

47.5 Additional Testing

The following additional testing and information could provide a more comprehensive picture of JM's auditory and educational function:
- Ear-specific BKB-SIN testing.
- Speech processor telecoil mixing ratio.
- Screening Instrument for Targeting Educational Risk (SIFTER).
- Listening Inventories for Education (LIFE).

47.6 Final Diagnosis and Recommended Treatment

Educational audiologists have three goals when working with their students with hearing loss. First, they counsel school administrative staff, teachers, and parents on the needs of these students within educational contexts. In addition, they reduce effects of noise, distance, and reverberation experienced by the students in the classroom by providing recommendations as well as fitting, verification, and troubleshooting of assistive technology. Finally, they work to instill good communication health habits, such as self-advocacy, in the students and their families. However, if the student is reluctant to use the wireless technology or refuses it completely, these goals cannot be achieved. Therefore, all options must be considered to find a suitable arrangement that will be accepted by the older student. Ultimately, accomplishment of these goals should result in students who can function as independent and successful communicators in their future college and career endeavors. JM was pleased with the Roger Pen and MyLink arrangement and excited to use it daily. Speech recognition testing confirmed the benefit and limitations of various microphone placement options.

47.7 Outcome

Throughout the process of managing JM, the audiologist counseled school staff and JM's parents on hearing loss, JM's CIs, and remote microphone technology. They were all highly involved and provided valuable input throughout the process. Overall, JM has been very successful with the Phonak Roger Pen. Thorough fitting and verification ensured that the technology was providing the greatest possible benefit. Using the nontraditional remote microphone system seems to have shifted his perception of assistive technology use. Rather than dreading "delaying the class" as he gives the teacher his traditional transmitter, he is excited about the system, researches it in his spare time, and openly uses it for both lecture and group discussions.

Future management should include discussion of transition to college/career settings. During one of his appointments, JM indicated that he wants to attend college and eventually be a "businessman." In both college and the business world, effective communication is critical to success—meaning self-advocacy and assistive technology will continue to be an important part of JM's daily function. Phonak's Guide to Access Planning is one resource designed to address this transitional period.[4] It provides self-assessments and educational resources for students and parents on self-advocacy skills (writing accommodations letters, explaining hearing loss and needs, knowledge of legislature related to disability), assistive technology, and other resources for individuals who are Deaf or Hard of Hearing. GAP and other materials can be used as a springboard for discussions that guide the student in developing knowledge and skills necessary for successful transition into adulthood.

References

[1] Thibodeau L. Comparison of speech recognition with adaptive digital and FM remote microphone hearing assistance technology by listeners who use hearing aids. Am J Audiol. 2014; 23(2):201–210

[2] Wolfe J, Morais M, Schafer E, et al. Evaluation of speech recognition of cochlear implant recipients using a personal digital adaptive radio frequency system. J Am Acad Audiol. 2013; 24(8):714–724

[3] Wolfe J, Duke MM, Schafer E, et al. Evaluation of performance with an adaptive digital remote microphone system and a digital remote microphone audio-streaming accessory system. Am J Audiol. 2015; 24(3):440–450

[4] Guide to Access Planning (GAP). Available at: https://www.phonak.com/com/en/support/children-and-parents/guide-to-access-planning.html. Accessed May 26, 2016

Suggested Readings

[1] American National Standards Institute (ANSI). American National Standard Specification of Performance Measurement of Hearing Assistance Devices/Systems. ANSI S3.47–2009. New York, NY: ANSI

[2] American Academy of Audiology. Clinical Practice Guidelines: Remote Microphone Hearing Assistance Technologies for Children and Youth from Birth to 21 Years. 2008. Available at: www.audiology.org/resources

[3] Thibodeau LM, Johnson C. Wireless technology to improve communication in noise. Semin Hear. 2014; 35(03):157

48 Poor Performance with a Cochlear Implant: A Case of Overinsertions

Casey Stach and Teresa Zwolan

48.1 Clinical History and Description

JD is a 13-year-old girl who transferred care to our cochlear implant clinic following a move from out of state. She was diagnosed with a profound hearing loss of unknown etiology following a failed newborn screening at birth. At 12 months of age, her right ear was implanted with an Advanced Bionics device. She experienced significant facial nerve stimulation when using the device and failed to make progress despite regular participation in auditory verbal therapy (AVT). When she was 29 months of age, the device was explanted and replaced with a Nucleus CI24RCS device, but she continued to demonstrate poorer than expected results. At 36 months of age, her left ear was implanted with a Nucleus CI24RE device. JD preferred the sound quality of her left ear, and she continued to report inconsistent sound quality in the right ear despite participation in regular mapping appointments. She continued to receive weekly AVT services.

48.2 Audiologic Testing

Upon transfer to our facility, we performed speech processor mapping, assessment of sound-field detection thresholds, speech perception testing, speech and language testing, and a transorbital plain film to evaluate placement of the electrode arrays. JD's evaluation revealed normal mapping parameters for the left ear, and a wider than typical pulse width of 37 μs/phase and a narrow electrical dynamic range for the right ear. Several electrodes had been deactivated in each ear for an unknown reason. Sound-field detection thresholds fell within the expected range for the left ear but were slightly elevated for the right ear. Speech perception scores are displayed in ▶ Table 48.1 and indicate poor performance for each ear. Speech and language scores are displayed in ▶ Table 48.2 and ▶ Table 48.3 and revealed profound speech/language delays on auditory-only tasks as well as voice quality, reflective of severe-to-profound hearing loss.

A transorbital plain film revealed overinsertion of both the right and left electrode arrays (▶ Fig. 48.1). A computed tomography (CT) scan was performed and confirmed overinsertion of each electrode array. The device manufacturer was contacted,

and integrity testing of the internal devices was performed. This testing revealed no obvious problem with either electrode array.

48.3 Questions for the Reader

1. Do you agree that JD's electrode arrays appear to be overinserted? Do you believe that overinsertion of the electrode arrays could be the cause of JD's poor outcome with her cochlear implants despite early implantation and good intervention?
2. What type of intervention, if any, would you recommend for JD?
3. Were transorbital plain film X-rays helpful in this case? Why or why not?

Table 48.1 Word and sentence recognition for the right, left, and bimodal conditions when recorded stimuli were presented at a level of 60 dB SPL at time of transfer

	Ped AzBio sentences	HINT sentences	LNT monosyllabic words
Right CI	0%	4%	0%
Left CI	0%	20%	0%
Bilateral CIs	0%	30%	36%

Abbreviations: AzBio, pediatric AzBio sentences (Spahr et al[1]); CI, cochlear implant; HINT, Hearing-in-Noise Test (HINT) sentences (Nilsson et al[2]); LT, Lexical Neighborhood Test (Kirk et al[3]).

Table 48.2 Speech and language evaluation results on the Peabody Picture vocabulary (PPVT) Test 4 (Dunn and Dunn[4]) and the Oral and Written Language Scales II (OWLS II) (Carrow-Woolfolk[5]) at time of transfer

	PPVT-4 receptive vocabulary	OWLS II listening comprehension	OWLS II oral expression
Raw score	165	80	76
Standard score	92	69	84
Age equivalent	11 y, 8 mo	8 y, 11 mo	10 y, 11 mo
Description	Low average	Severe	Average

Table 48.3 Speech and language evaluation results on the Woodcock Johnson IV (Semrud-Clikeman and Teeter Ellison[6]) tests of oral language (subtests 2 and 6), listening comprehension (combined subtests of 2 and 6), oral language (subtest 5), and passage comprehension (subtest 4) at time of transfer

	WJ IV #2	WJ IV #6	WJ IV 2&6	WJ IV #5	WJ IV #4
Raw score	10	6	–	5	37
Standard score	48	16	21	27	–
Age equivalent	6 y	2 y, 10 mo	4 y, 6 mo	3 y, 2 mo	11 y, 7 mo
Description	Profound	Profound	Profound	Profound	Average

48.4 Discussion of Questions

1. **Do you agree that JD's electrode arrays appear to be overinserted? Do you believe that overinsertion of the electrode arrays could be the cause of JD's poor outcome with her cochlear implants despite early implantation and good intervention?**

   When evaluating performance with a cochlear implant, several factors need to be considered. When one considers that several of JD's historical factors would facilitate a good outcome with cochlear implants (early bilateral implantation; normal cognition and development; early, intensive and consistent participation in AVT with strong parental involvement; and the absence of any cochlear anomalies), other factors should be investigated that may negatively impact performance. In this case, our team agreed that poor performance could be due to surgical placement of the electrode array, which was confirmed with X-rays and CT scans.

2. **What type of intervention, if any, would you recommend for JD?**

   One of the risks associated with explant/reimplant of an electrode array is reduced performance with the second device. This was particularly concerning with JD since she had already received two devices in her right ear. Although she demonstrated good detection skills in the right ear, she did not demonstrate any of the expected open-set speech recognition skills.

3. **Were transorbital plain film X-rays helpful in this case? Why or why not?**

   Without the transorbital plain film X-rays, we would have assumed proper placement of the electrode arrays. JD would have continued on the path of detecting sound with her cochlear implants, but not understanding speech.

48.5 Final Diagnosis and Recommended Treatment

Following a review of her test results, explant/reimplant of each ear was recommended. This procedure was performed sequentially, so JD would not be without sound. The right ear was explanted first, followed by the left ear 1 month later. JD was reimplanted with two CI24RE (CA) devices.

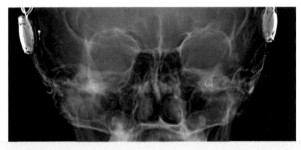

Fig. 48.1 Transorbital plain film showing placement of the electrode arrays in the right and left ears.

48.6 Outcome

At this time, JD is approximately 6 months postexplant/reimplantation of both ears. ▶ Fig. 50.2 displays the postoperative explant transorbital plain films compared to the original films. Sound-field detection results are as expected for each ear, and fall in the 10 to 25 dB range from 250 to 4,000 Hz. JD's 6 month postexplant/reimplant speech perception scores are displayed in ▶ Table 48.4 and indicate significant improvement in open-set speech recognition, particularly when using both implants. Her speech and language scores are provided in ▶ Table 48.5 and ▶ Table 48.6, and although she continues to experience a significant delay, she made marked gains on several measures

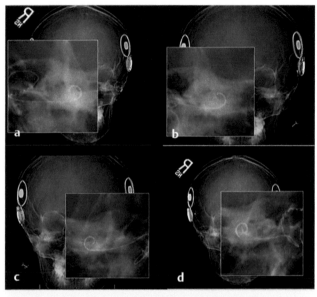

Fig. 50.2 Postoperative transorbital X-rays for the right and left cochlear implants compared to films prior to explant/reimplant.

Table 48.4 Pediatric AzBio sentences and CNC monosyllabic word (Peterson and Lehiste[7]) scores 6 months postexplant/reimplants

	Ped AzBio Sentences	CNC monosyllabic words
Right CI	23%	20%
Left CI	48%	28%
Bilateral CIs	81%	DNT

Table 48.5 Speech and language evaluation results on the Peabody Picture vocabulary (PPVT) Test 4 and the Oral and Written Language Scales II (OWLS II), scores 6 months post explant/reimplants

	PPVT-4 receptive vocabulary	OWLS II listening comprehension
Raw score	178	97
Standard score	96	85
Age Equivalent	13 y, 9 mo	10 y, 7 mo
Description	Average	Low average

Note: OWLS II oral expression could not be tested due to time constraints.

Table 48.6 Speech and language evaluation results on the Woodcock Johnson IV tests of oral language (subtests 2 and 6), listening comprehension (combined subtests of 2 and 6), oral language (subtest 5), and passage comprehension (subtest 4). Scores 6 months post explant/reimplants

	WJ IV #2	WJ IV #6	WJ IV 2&6	WJ IV #5	WJ IV #4
Raw score	7	29	–	7	37
Standard score	<40	58	40	40	–
Age equivalent	5 y	6 y, 4 mo	5 y, 6 mo	3 y, 7 mo	11 y, 7 mo
Description	Profound	Severe-profound	Profound	Profound	Average

during this brief period. Her understanding of oral directions (without lip-reading) improved 42 months across a 10-month time period (from previous speech and language evaluation). In addition, her vocal resonance was perceived to be improved. Receptive language indicated a gain of 2 years, in 10 months' time.

This case study demonstrates the importance of performing a comprehensive examination when patients experience a poorer than expected outcome with a cochlear implant. It is not acceptable to state that some children just do not do well. Before making a decision that this child "will not be a CI success," it is essential to examine every possibility. In this case, a simple transorbital X-ray revealed that device placement likely contributed to her lack of progress with the cochlear implants. The cost in 2016 of a transorbital plain film in the United States averages $86.00, without physician fees (www.healthcarebluebook.com, 2016). We recommend that all clinics consider performing transorbital X-rays on all patients postoperatively to ensure optimal placement of the array.

References

[1] Spahr AJ, Dorman MF, Litvak LM, et al. Development and validation of the pediatric AzBio sentence lists. Ear Hear. 2014; 35(4):418–422

[2] Nilsson M, Soli SD, Sullivan JA. Development of the Hearing in Noise Test for the measurement of speech reception thresholds in quiet and in noise. J Acoust Soc Am. 1994; 95(2):1085–1099

[3] Kirk KI, Pisoni DB, Osberger MJ. Lexical effects on spoken word recognition by pediatric cochlear implant users. Ear Hear. 1995; 16(5):470–481

[4] Dunn LM, Dunn DM. Peabody Picture Vocabulary Test. 4th ed. (PPVT-4). Upper Saddle River, NJ: Pearson Education; 2007

[5] Carrow-Woolfolk E. OWLS-II Oral and Written Language Scales. 2nd ed. Upper Saddle River, NJ: Pearson Education; 2011

[6] Semrud-Clikeman M, Teeter Ellison PA, eds. Child Neuropsychology: Assessment and Interventions for Neurodevelopmental Disorders. New York, NY: Springer; 2009:119

[7] Peterson GE, Lehiste I. Revised CNC lists for auditory tests. J Speech Hear Disord. 1962; 27:62–70

Suggested Readings

[1] Aschendorff A. Imaging in cochlear implant patients. GMS Curr Top Otorhinolaryngol Head Neck Surg. 2011; 10:Doc07

[2] Fishman AJ, Roland JT, Jr, Alexiades G, Mierzwinski J, Cohen NL. Fluoroscopically assisted cochlear implantation. Otol Neurotol. 2003; 24(6):882–886

[3] Jain R, Mukherji SK. Cochlear implant failure: imaging evaluation of the electrode course. Clin Radiol. 2003; 58(4):288–293

[4] Shpizner BA, Holliday RA, Roland JT, Cohen NL, Waltzman SB, Shapiro WH. Postoperative imaging of the multichannel cochlear implant. AJNR Am J Neuroradiol. 1995; 16(7):1517–1524

[5] Viccaro M, Covelli E, De Seta E, Balsamo G, Filipo R. The importance of intraoperative imaging during cochlear implant surgery. Cochlear Implants Int. 2009; 10(4):198–202

[6] Vogl TJ, Tawfik A, Emam A, et al. Pre-, intra- and post-operative imaging of cochlear implants. RoFo Fortschr Geb Rontgenstr Nuklearmed. 2015; 187(11):980–989

[7] www.heathcarebluebook.com. 2016. Available at: https://www.healthcarebluebook.com/page_ProcedureDetails.aspx?id=457&dataset=MD&g=X-Ray%3a+Skull

[8] Zwolan T, Stach CJ. Programming pediatric cochlear implant systems. In: Eisenberg L, ed. Clinical Management of Children with Cochlear Implants. San Diego, CA: Plural Publishing; 2009:113–131

[9] Zwolan T, Stach CJ. Diagnosis and management of cochlear implant malfunction. In: Young N, Kirk K, eds. Cochlear Implants in Children: Learning and the Brain. New York, NY: Springer Publishing; 2016

49 Personal Roger System Fitting

Amy Lynn Birath

49.1 Clinical History and Description

MK, a 5-year-old boy, was seen for fitting and evaluation of a personal Phonak Roger DM (digital modulation) system to use in conjunction with his Phonak Sky Q70 SP hearing aids.

MK was born full-term following an essentially healthy pregnancy via emergency cesarean section due to breech position. He weighed 7 pounds, 10 ounces at birth and had no breathing, sucking, or swallowing difficulties. There was some concern over loss of birth weight, but weight was regained following a few days of breastfeeding.

MK's hearing loss initially was suspected following a failed newborn hearing screening at each ear; however, his parents were not notified of these results until 7 weeks after discharge from the hospital. At 10 weeks of age, auditory brainstem response testing was completed and suggested mild sloping to moderately-severe hearing loss at each ear. MK and his family enrolled in the parent–infant program of a nonprofit center for children who have hearing loss. Through this program, MK and his family received parent support and coaching, direct child therapy targeting the development of audition, speech, and spoken language, and audiologic services. Behavioral hearing testing completed at this center confirmed MK's hearing loss and determined that it is sensorineural in nature. Continued testing has indicated that his hearing loss is stable. The cause of MK's hearing loss is unknown. He initially was fitted with loaner hearing aids at 3 months of age, then with personal hearing aids at 9 months of age, and finally with a personal Phonak Dynamic FM (frequency modulation) system to use in conjunction with his hearing aids at 2 years of age.

MK currently is 5 years old and is enrolled in kindergarten at his local elementary school. For his fifth birthday, MK received new Phonak Sky Q70 SP hearing aids and a personal Phonak Roger digitally modulated (DM) adaptive remote microphone (RM) system. His hearing aids were programmed and fitted using real-ear measurements based on recommendations from the *American Academy of Audiology Clinical Practice Guidelines: Pediatric Amplification* protocol.[1] Real-ear-to-coupler difference (RECD) values were obtained for each ear using MK's personal earmolds. Desired Sensation Level (DSL) real-ear targets for gain and maximum output were generated based on the measured RECD values and current behavioral hearing testing results. The hearing aids were adjusted via speech mapping to meet amplification targets within 2 dB in response to the Audioscan Verifit calibrated speech stimulus presented at 55, 65, and 75 dB SPL, levels that represent soft, average, and loud speech, respectively. MK was given two programs in his hearing aids. The first, for use at home and other listening environments when not using his Roger system, is an adaptive program utilizing Phonak's SoundFlow feature. The SoundFlow feature analyses the acoustic environment and makes changes, including employing directional microphones when needed, to provide the best listening situation for the child based on the environment. The second, for use at school or other situations where hearing the primary speaker is of utmost importance, and where distance, background noise, and/or reverberation may interfere with hearing the primary speaker. The first program is a nonadaptive program employing omnidirectional microphones and the input from the Roger system. When using this second program, scene analysis is deactivated, and equal input is provided to the hearing aids by the hearing aid microphones and the Roger transmitter microphone, with neither attenuated. Following programming and fitting of MK's hearing aids, his Roger system was fitted and evaluated.

49.2 Audiologic Testing

In order to verify appropriate function of the Roger system, quantify need, determine appropriate receiver gain settings, and demonstrate benefit with the Roger system, both electroacoustic and behavioral assessments were completed, as suggested by the *American Academy of Audiology Clinical Practice Guidelines: Remote Microphone Hearing Assistance Technologies for Children and Youth from Birth to 21 Years* protocol.[2]

Using the *Roger Phonak Offset Protocol* (Roger POP),[3] electroacoustic verification of MK's Phonak Sky Q70 SP hearing aids with Phonak Roger 11 integrated receivers and Phonak Roger inspiro transmitter was completed and transparency between the two was confirmed for each hearing instrument (▶ Fig. 49.1).

Following transparency confirmation, speech perception testing (in addition to that administered during MK's most recent hearing evaluation) was completed in quiet and in background noise without and with the Roger system with each hearing instrument individually and in the binaural condition. Words were presented at 0 degrees azimuth (from the front), and background noise was presented at 270 degrees azimuth (from the left).

The recorded version (REC) of the Phonetically Balanced Kindergarten Word Test (PBK) was administered in quiet (presented at 60 dB SPL) and in background noise (presented at 60 dB SPL with a + 5 signal-to-noise ratio [SNR], with recorded multitalker babble presented at 55 dB SPL) with the transmitter turned off.[4] Then, in the same + 5 SNR noise condition, the transmitter was turned on, connected to the receivers, and placed in front of a single cone speaker approximately 6 inches down from center, and the PBK test was administered once again. Following testing in background noise, the receiver gain settings for each receiver were adjusted, and testing in background noise was repeated, until MK's performance on the PBK in noise approximated his performance on the PBK in quiet, to ensure optimal benefit from the Roger system and to validate its fitting (▶ Fig. 49.2).

49.3 Questions for the Reader

1. Why would a child with hearing loss need a personal DM adaptive RM system?
2. Why does an audiologist need to fit and evaluate a personal DM adaptive RM system?

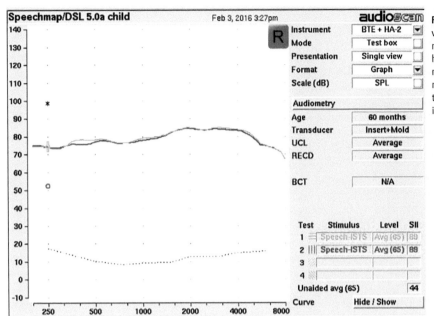

Fig. 49.1 Right hearing instrument transparency verification: Test 1: (Roger +)M65 is a measurement with 65 dB SPL ISTS speech input to the hearing instrument microphone with the Roger microphone muffled. Test 2: Roger (+M)65 is a measurement with a 65 dB SPL ISTS speech input to the Roger microphone with the hearing instrument microphone muffled.

TESTING/EVALUATION			
Speech Material: PBK-50 Word Lists	Source: 0° (Front-Facing Speaker)	Presentation Level/Mode: 60 dBA/REC	
Noise Material: Multi-Talker Babble	Source: 270° (Speaker facing left ear)	Presentation Level: *See Below*	
	RIGHT	**LEFT**	**BINAURAL**
Internal Device	N/A	N/A	
External Device	Phonak Sky Q70 SP	Phonak Sky Q70 SP	
External Device Settings	Junior Roger + Mic	Junior Roger + Mic	
FM/DM Receiver	Roger 11	Roger 11	
Receiver S/N	1429ALBJM	1429ALBJN	
FM/DM Transmitter (+S/N)	Roger Inspiro (1430MJBLA)		
Secondary Transmitter	N/A		
Speech in Quiet (no FM/DM)	23/25	22/25	24/25
Speech in Noise (no FM/DM)			
SNR = +5 dB	10/25	11/25	13/25
Speech in Noise (w/ FM/DM) @ +5 SNR			
Rcvr Gain = +0; Mix Ratio = 1:1	17/25	15/25	18/25
Rcvr Gain = +2; Mix Ratio = 1:1	22/25	17/25	22/25
Rcvr Gain = +4 Left only; Mix Ratio = 1:1	DNT	21/25	24/25

Fig. 49.2 Results of speech perception testing in quiet and background noise for Roger system fitting validation.

3. (A) Is MK benefitting from his personal Roger system? (B) If his school district had purchased and provided him with his Roger system without having it fitted and evaluated, would he be receiving optimal benefit from it?

49.4 Discussion of Questions

1. **Why would a child with hearing loss need a personal DM adaptive RM system?**

The negative impact of noise, distance, and reverberation on listening for children who have hearing loss is well documented.[5] For these children, hearing aids are provided which amplify acoustic information in order to improve access to that information. However, currently, hearing aids have limitations. As explained by Cole and Flexer, the biggest limitation of hearing aids is "their inability to make the details of spoken communication available under the following conditions: when there is competing noise, when the listener cannot be physically close to the speaker, or when both conditions exist together."[6] Use of remote microphone hearing assistance technology, such as a Roger system, is a way to improve the SNR for the listener and help combat the negative impact of noise and distance and the limitations of the hearing aids for children who have hearing loss.

In addition, it is important to know that not all remote microphone technology provides the same benefit. Thibodeau compared the speech perception performance of people using hearing aids in conjunction with fixed FM (e.g., traditional FM), adaptive FM (e.g., Dynamic FM), and DM adaptive (e.g., Roger) RM systems.[7] She found that the participants' performance in background noise was significantly better when using a DM adaptive RM system than when using fixed or adaptive FM systems, with the greatest benefits seen in the highest background noise levels.

Providing an improvement in the SNR for children using hearing aids and providing the greatest benefit from remote microphone technology for these children are two reasons a child with hearing loss would need a personal DM adaptive RM system.

2. **Why does an audiologist need to fit and evaluate a personal DM adaptive RM system?**

Much research has demonstrated the benefit of using remote microphone technology with children who have hearing loss. The use of this technology to improve speech understanding in background noise frequently is implemented in educational settings as part of a child's Individualized Educational Plan (IEP). Unfortunately, too often, these systems are purchased by the school district and provided to a child without appropriate fitting and evaluation of the system by an audiologist to ensure appropriate function and optimal benefit. There are three primary reasons these systems need to be fitted and evaluated.

First, these systems comprise complex electronic equipment, and even though the manufacturers intend for their products to meet certain specifications, sometimes the devices do not work properly, and on occasion, they do not work at all, even when new. If the system does not work at all, this likely will be obvious to the purchaser. On the other hand, if only a part of the system is malfunctioning, and the device powers on and appears to be working, the system will not be beneficial to the child, and potentially could be detrimental.

Second, if the system itself is working, it also has to function appropriately in conjunction with the child's hearing aids. This verification, described earlier, must be completed in a hearing aid test box. Without this transparency verification, it is impossible to know if the DM adaptive RM system is functioning appropriately in conjunction with the child's hearing aids.

Third, even if the system itself is working, and the system is functioning appropriately in conjunction with the child's hearing aids, performance validation assessment needs to be completed to ensure optimal benefit and performance when using the DM adaptive RM system. The goal of DM adaptive RM system use is to have essentially equivalent speech perception performance when using the system in poor listening conditions as when listening in quiet. The system's default receiver gain settings do not always allow for equivalent performance. As in this case, in order to approximate performance in quiet, both receivers needed a gain setting increase, and, in MK's case, each receiver needed a different gain setting. Without this speech perception validation, optimal benefit cannot be confirmed.

3. **(A) Is MK benefitting from his personal Roger system? (B) If his school district had purchased and provided him with his Roger system without having it fitted and evaluated, would he be receiving optimal benefit from it?**

(A) Yes, MK is benefitting from his personal Roger system. This is evident because his speech perception performance in background noise is approximating his performance in quiet with each device individually, and his performance is equivalent in quiet and in background noise in the binaural condition.

(B) No, if MK's school district had provided him with this Roger system without having it fitted and evaluated, he would not be receiving optimal benefit. The default receiver gain setting is 0. When MK was listening in background noise at receiver gain settings of 0, he received some benefit (72% correct in the binaural condition as compared to 52% correct in the binaural condition in noise without the Roger system), but not optimal benefit. In order for his performance in background noise to be equivalent to his performance in quiet (96% correct in the binaural condition), each of MK's receivers needed increased gain settings.

49.5 Final Diagnosis and Recommended Treatment

MK's personal Roger system was determined to be working appropriately, and it was fitted utilizing a +2 receiver gain for the right device and a +4 receiver gain for the left device. Orientation and training regarding appropriate use and troubleshooting of the Roger system were provided to MK's parents and teachers, including instructions for a daily listening check of the equipment and a daily functional listening check with MK using the Ling six sounds.[8] In addition, further validation is to be ongoing, to ensure that MK is benefitting from use of his personal Roger system in his educational environment, through completion of validation tools such as the *Listening Inventory for Education-Revised* (LIFE-R).[9]

49.6 Outcome

MK uses his personal Roger system throughout the school day, except during recess. For recess, his teacher changes his hearing aids to the first program (SoundFlow). Then, after recess, she changes back to the second program (Junior Roger + Mic) in his hearing aids and reconnects him to the Roger transmitter. MK also uses his Roger system in the car, in Sunday School at church, for Saturday Story Hour at the library, during soccer, when his family goes to the zoo, and on other similar outings.

References

[1] American Academy of Audiology Clinical Practice Guidelines. Pediatric amplification. June 2013. Available at: http://audiology-web.s3.amazonaws.com/migrated/PediatricAmplificationGuidelines.pdf_539975b3e7e9f1.74471798.pdf

[2] American Academy of Audiology Clinical Practice Guidelines. Remote microphone hearing assistance technologies for children and youth from birth to 21 years. April 2008 (updated April 2011). Available at: http://audiology-web.s3.amazonaws.com/migrated/HAT_Guidelines_Supplement_A.pdf_53996ef7758497.54419000.pdf

[3] Phonak AG. Roger Phonak Offset Protocol. June 2013. Available at: https://www.phonakpro.com/content/dam/phonakpro/gc_hq/en/products_solutions/wireless_accessories/roger_inspiro/documents/phonak_offset_protocol_roger_inspiro.pdf

[4] Haskins H. A Phonetically Balanced Test of Speech Discrimination for Children [unpublished Master's thesis]. Evanston, IL: Northwestern University; 1949

[5] Crandell CC, Smaldino JJ. Classroom acoustics for children with normal hearing and with hearing impairment. Lang Speech Hear Serv Sch. 2000; 31(4):362–370

[6] Cole EB, Flexer C. Children with Hearing Loss: Developing Listening and Talking. Birth to Six. 3rd ed. San Diego, CA: Plural Publishing; 2016

[7] Thibodeau L. Comparison of speech recognition with adaptive digital and FM remote microphone hearing assistance technology by listeners who use hearing aids. Am J Audiol. 2014; 23(2):201–210

[8] Ling D. Speech and the Hearing-impaired Child: Theory and Practice. Washington DC: Alexander Graham Bell Association for the Deaf; 1976

[9] Anderson KL, Smaldino JJ, Spangler C. Listening Inventory for Education – Revised (LIFE-R). 2011. Available at: http://www.successforkidswithhearingloss.com

50 Hypoplastic Cochlear Nerve

Kenneth Bodkin

50.1 Clinical History and Description

ES, a 9-month-old, was referred by her pediatrician because of parental concerns regarding her hearing. Pre-, peri-, and postnatal history was unremarkable. ES passed her newborn otoacoustic emissions hearing screening bilaterally. Two behavioral hearing tests by another audiologist revealed inconsistent responses to sound utilizing visual reinforcement audiometry (VRA), normal tympanic membrane motility, and present distortion-product otoacoustic emissions (DPOAEs).

50.2 Audiologic Testing

ES was re-evaluated at 13 months of age using bone conduction to condition to VRA (▶ Fig. 50.1). Test results revealed no

response at the limits of the audiometer in the sound field, and responses with bone conduction at vibrotactile levels. Robust DPOAEs were present bilaterally (▶ Fig. 50.2). An auditory brainstem response (ABR) under sedation was recommended.

ES had her sedated ABR at 14 months of age (▶ Fig. 50.3, ▶ Fig. 50.4, ▶ Fig. 50.5). The ABR was absent to tone bursts presented via air conduction (▶ Fig. 50.3) and bone conduction (▶ Fig. 50.4), but cochlear microphonics (▶ Fig. 50.5) were present for both ears.

ES was fitted with flexible behind-the-ear hearing aids so the gain/output could be adjusted during the trial period. The aids were initially set using simulated real ear, because ES would not allow the clinician to insert real-ear probe tubes in her ears. A moderate hearing loss was used to program the devices to DSL 5.0 (▶ Fig. 50.6). This was used as a relatively conservative starting point because a reliable behavioral audiogram could not be obtained. Behavioral

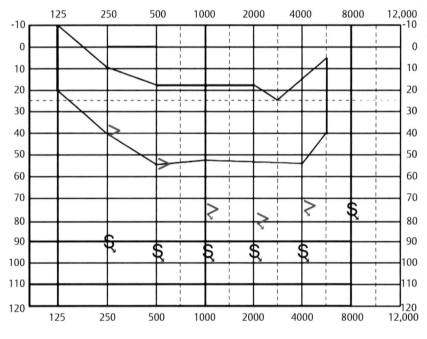

Fig. 50.1 Initial audiogram obtained using visual reinforcement audiometry conditioned with bone conduction at vibrotactile levels. >, left ear bone conduction; S, soundfield air conduction; Arrows, no repsonse.

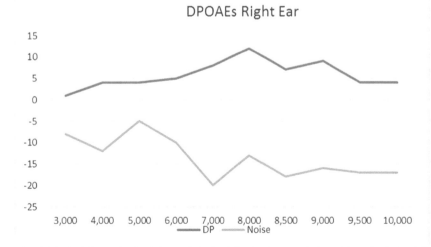

DPOAEs Right Ear

Fig. 50.2 Robust distortion-product otoacoustic emissions from the right and left ears.

Hackensack University Medical Center · Department of Audiology

30 Prospect Ave · Hackensack · NJ

Tel: 551-996-5327 · Fax: 551-996-0557

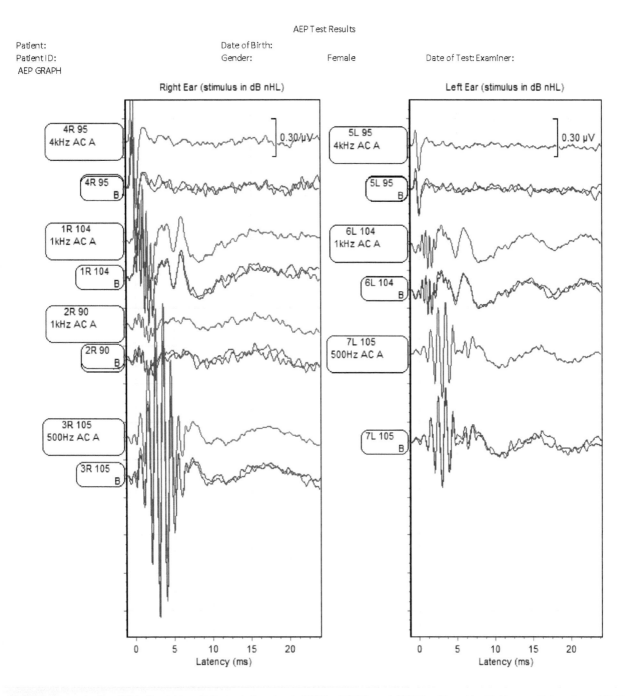

AEP Test Results

Patient: Date of Birth:

Patient ID: Gender: Female Date of Test: Examiner:

AEP GRAPH

Fig. 50.3 Air-conduction ABR in the right and left ears to tone bursts 500 Hz, 1000 Hz, and 4000 Hz with no identifiable wave V at equipment limits. (*continued*)

responses with the devices were monitored to determine if the devices were providing any benefit. The family was given the P.E.A.C.H. (parents' evaluation of aural/oral performance of children) to evaluate ES's behavior with the hearing aids. No significant change was noted on the P.E.A.C.H. as reported by ES's family over 2 weeks; therefore, the hearing aids were reprogrammed with significantly more gain/output using a profound hearing loss to determine the

hearing aid settings. Her behavior was monitored again over the next 2 weeks with no significant change in score on the P.E.A.C.H. (▶ Table 50.1). Aided cortical auditory evoked potentials (CAEP; ▶ Fig. 50.7, ▶ Fig. 50.8) were assessed at loud conversation levels (75 dB SPL). The results revealed no response in the right ear and a possible response for /t/ in the left ear. It was determined that ES should have a consultation with otolaryngology for a cochlear implant.

Right Ear (R)   Left Ear (L)

ABR WAVEFORM DATA

		Corr. Coef.	RN µV	Time (ms)											Amp (µV)		Ratio	SS	SE
				I	I'	II	III	IV	V	V'	I-III	III-V	I-V	I-I'	V-V'	(V-V')/(I-I')		
1	R 104		0.014															
2	R 90		0.019															
3	R 105		0.012															
4	R 95		0.020															
5	L 95		0.012															
6	L 104		0.011															
7	L 105		0.016															

TEST CONDITIONS

		Stimulus Level		Stimulus Type	Stimulus Rate (/sec)	Polarity	Electrodes +	Electrodes −	Mask Level (dB HL)	Notch Filter (Hz)	Algorithm	* Noise Adj. Sweeps	% Rej.	# of Stimuli
1	R 104	104 dB nHL	1000 Hz	ABR air-conducted 1000 Hz tone-burst 37.7	37.7 Alt.	Fz	A2			SOAP-Kalman	1488	0	2096
2	R 90	90 dB nHL	1000 Hz	ABR air-conducted 1000 Hz tone-burst 37.7	37.7 Alt.	Fz	A2			SOAP-Kalman	1176	0	1968
3	R 105	105 dB nHL	500 Hz	ABR air-conducted 500 Hz tone-burst 37.7	37.7 Alt.	Fz	A2			SOAP-Kalman	1564	0	2376
4	R 95	95 dB nHL	4000 Hz	ABR air-conducted 4000 Hz tone-burst 37.7	37.7 Alt.	Fz	A2			SOAP-Kalman	960	0	1264
5	L 95	95 dB nHL	4000 Hz	ABR air-conducted 4000 Hz tone-burst 37.7	37.7 Alt.	Fz	A1			SOAP-Kalman	1264	0	3072
6	L 104	104 dB nHL	1000 Hz	ABR air-conducted 1000 Hz tone-burst 37.7	37.7 Alt.	Fz	A1			SOAP-Kalman	1856	0	3264
7	L 105	105 dB nHL	500 Hz	ABR air-conducted 500 Hz tone-burst 37.7	37.7 Alt.	Fz	A1			SOAP-Kalman	1128	0	2256

Alt.=Alternating; Ipsi.=Ipsilateral % Rej.=Percent Rejected

Using the SOAP-Kalman Weighted algorithm, 2000 "noise adjusted sweeps" is comparable to 2000 "accepted sweeps" used in conventional averaging.

PROTOCOL DETAILS

Protocol	Stimulus Type	Stimulus Rate (/sec)	Window	Ramp # of Cycles	Filter Cutoff (Hz) High Pass	Filter Cutoff (Hz) Low Pass	Filter Rolloff (dB/Octave) High Pass	Filter Rolloff (dB/Octave) Low Pass	ART (µV)	Max. # of Stimuli
ABR air-conducted 1000 Hz tone-burst 37.7	1000 Hz	37.7 Black.		2-0-2	30	1500	12	24		33930
ABR air-conducted 500 Hz tone-burst 37.7		37.7 Black.		2-0-2	30	1500	12	24		33930
ABR air-conducted 4000 Hz tone-burst 37.7	4000 Hz	37.7 Black.		2-0-2	30	1500	12	24		33930

ART=Artifact Rejection Threshold; Rec.Win.= Recording Window; Trans. Type=Transducer Type; Win. = Windowing; Black.=Blackman

Fig. 50.3 (continued)

50.3 Diagnosis

ES was referred for a magnetic resonance imaging (MRI) with cochlear nerve protocol by her otolaryngologist because of her lack of responsiveness to sound and the presence of DPOAEs. The MRI revealed that both cochlear nerves were poorly visualized and were likely hypoplastic. The significant risks for using a cochlear implant in a child with questionable cochlear nerves were reviewed with the family. The cochlear implant team consulted with another facility regarding candidacy for an auditory brainstem implant. Because there appeared to be some auditory function on the CAEP, the consultant recommended the cochlear implant. The family eventually decided to pursue a cochlear implant for her right ear.

At 2 years of age, ES received her cochlear implant. She was activated 1 month later. During the initial activation, ES startled to sound. She was MAPped again 2 weeks later, and the family noted that she was responding to sound at home. ES was MAPped again in another month and tested in the booth. Results revealed that she was responding at mild/moderate hearing loss levels (▶ Fig. 50.9). ES was enrolled in the auditory-oral track at the Hearing Impaired Preschool Program.

50.4 Questions for the Reader

1. Is this child a good candidate for a cochlear implant?
2. How much benefit do you expect the patient to receive from the cochlear implant?
3. The family wants ES to communicate using spoken language. What can be done to facilitate spoken language? Should a manual mode of communication be included?

Hackensack University Medical Center · Department of Audiology
30 Prospect Ave · Hackensack · NJ
Tel: 551-996-5327 · Fax: 551-996-0557

AEP Test Results

Patient: Date of Birth:
Patient ID: Gender: Date of Test: Examiner:
AEP GRAPH

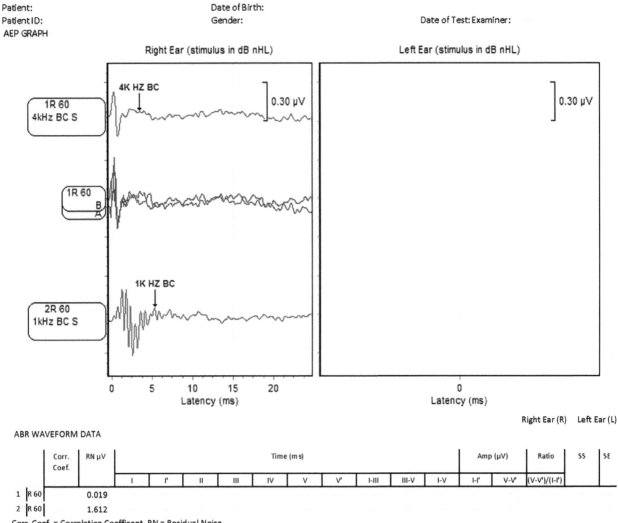

ABR WAVEFORM DATA

	Corr. Coef.	RN µV	Time (ms)													Amp (µV)		Ratio	SS	SE
			I	I'	II	III	IV	V	V'	I-III	III-V	I-V	I-I'	V-V'	(V-V')/(I-I')				
1	R 60	0.019																		
2	R 60	1.612																		

Corr. Coef. = Correlation Coefficent, RN = Residual Noise

TEST CONDITIONS

		Stimulus Level	Stimulus Type	Stimulus Rate (/sec)	Polarity	Electrodes +	Electrodes -	Mask Level (dB HL)	Notch Filter (Hz)	Algorithm	* Noise Adj. Sweeps	% Rej.	# of Stimuli
1	R 60	60 dB nHL	4000 Hz	37.7	Alt.Split	Fz	A1			SOAP-Kalman	1356	0	2216
		ABR bone conducted 4000 Hz tone-burst 37.7											
2	R 60	60 dB nHL	1000 Hz	37.7	Alt.Split	Fz	A1			SOAP-Kalman	1188	0	2152
		ABR bone conducted 1000 Hz tone-burst 37.7											

Alt.Split=Alternating Split; Contra.=Contralateral % Rej.=Percent Rejected
Using the SOAP-Kalman Weighted algorithm, 2000 "noise adjusted sweeps" is comparable to 2000 "accepted sweeps" used in conventional averaging.

PROTOCOL DETAILS

Protocol	Stimulus Type	Stimulus Rate (/sec)	Window	Ramp # of Cycles	Filter Cutoff (Hz) High Pass	Filter Cutoff (Hz) Low Pass	Filter Rolloff (dB/Octave) High Pass	Filter Rolloff (dB/Octave) Low Pass	ART (µV)	Max. # of Stimuli
ABR bone conducted 4000 Hz tone-burst 37.7	4000 Hz	37.7	Black.	2-0-2	30	1500	12	24		33930
ABR bone conducted 1000 Hz tone-burst 37.7	1000 Hz	37.7	Black.	2-0-2	30	1500	12	24		33930

ART=Artifact Rejection Threshold; Rec.Win.= Recording Window; Trans. Type=Transducer Type; Win. = Windowing; Black.=Blackman

Fig. 50.4 Unmasked bone-conduction auditory brainstem response on the right mastoid to tone bursts 1,000 and 4,000 Hz with no identifiable wave V at equipment limits.

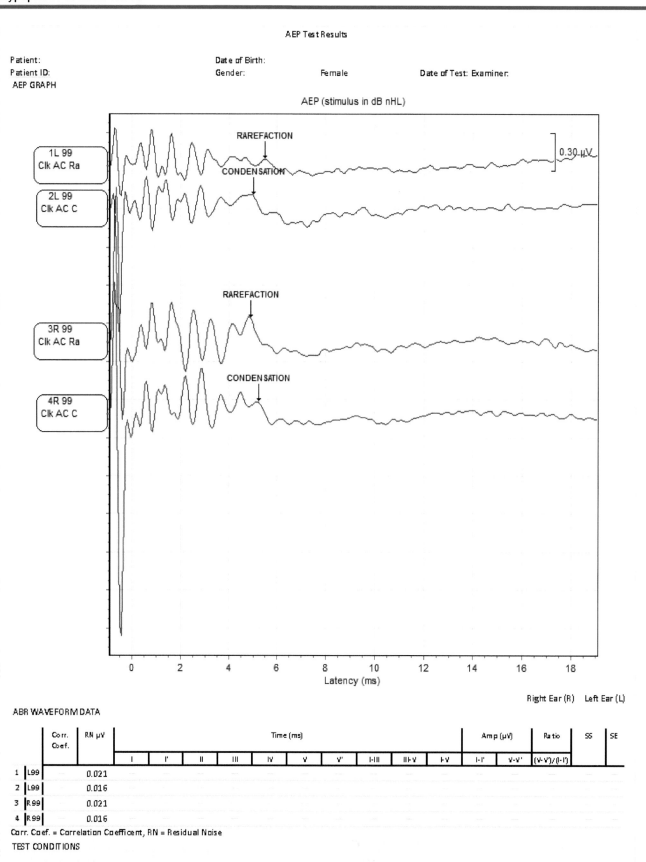

Fig. 50.5 Air-conduction click stimuli to rarefaction and condensation polarity revealed a cochlear microphonic with a latency that extends beyond 3 μs in both ears. (*continued*)

Patient: Date of Birth: Date of Test:

Patient ID: Gender: Female   Examiner:

TEST CONDITIONS

		Stimulus Level	Stimulus Type	Stimulus Rate (/sec)	Polarity	Electrodes +	-	Mask Level (dB HL)	Notch Filter (Hz)	Algorithm	* Noise Adj. Sweeps	% Rej.	# of Stimuli
1	L 99	99 dB nHL click Neuro ABR 19.1 cps		19.1 Rarefac.	Fz	A2				SOAP-Kalman	1572	0	1600
2	L 99	99 dB nHL click Neuro ABR 19.1 cps		19.1 Condens.	Fz	A2				SOAP-Kalman	1516	0	2136
3	R 99	99 dB nHL click Neuro ABR 19.1 cps		19.1 Rarefac.	Fz	A2				SOAP-Kalman	1300	0	1880
4	R 99	99 dB nHL click Neuro ABR 19.1 cps		19.1 Condens.	Fz	A2				SOAP-Kalman	1436	0	2544

Rarefac.=Rarefaction; Condens.=Condensation; Contra.=Contralateral; Ipsi.=Ipsilateral % Rej.=Percent Rejected

Using the SOAP-Kalman Weighted algorithm, 2000 "noise adjusted sweeps" is comparable to 2000 "accepted sweeps" used in conventional averaging.

PROTOCOL DETAILS

Protocol	Stimulus Type	Stimulus Rate (/sec)	Window	Ramp # of Cycles	Filter Cutoff (Hz) High Pass	Low Pass	Filter Rolloff (dB/Octave) High Pass	Low Pass	ART (µV)	Max. # of Stimuli
Neuro ABR 19.1 cps	click	19.1			30	2400	12	24		15930

ART=Artifact Rejection Threshold; Rec.Win.= Recording Window; Trans. Type=Transducer Type; Win. = Windowing

Fig. 50.5 (*continued*)

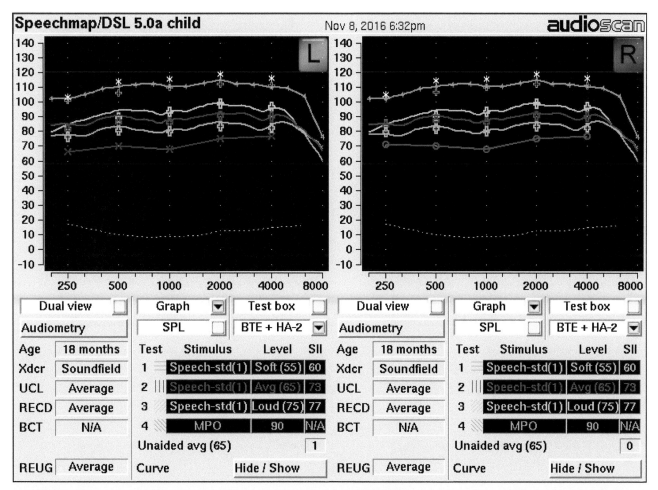

Fig. 50.6 Simulated real ear to DSL 5.0 targets using a conservative approach to amplification.

50.5 Discussion of Questions

1. **Is this child a good candidate for a cochlear implant?**
   The family and the surgeon felt the possible benefits of the cochlear implant, even with hypoplastic cochlear nerves, outweighed the surgical risks. The family understood that it was not possible to predict if ES's brain would receive sufficient auditory information with a cochlear implant. They also understood that ES might be a candidate for a brainstem implant if she did not perceive sound via the cochlear implant.

2. **How much benefit do you expect the patient to receive from the cochlear implant?**
   ES was responding to sound. She began to vocalize and approximate speech sounds. This favorable beginning suggested that she has the potential to continue to develop listening and speech skills with intensive spoken language intervention and family involvement. Her progress was continually monitored by her auditory-verbal therapist. Even with the cochlear implant and intensive speech therapy, ES was unable to make fundamental improvements in speech/language. Unfortunately, patients with hypoplastic cochlear nerves often have poorer outcomes than other causes of hearing loss.

3. **The family wants ES to communicate using spoken language. What can be done to facilitate spoken language? Should a manual mode of communication be included?**

ES was enrolled in a listening and spoken language program to facilitate the family's desire for her to communicate using spoken language. The cochlear implant team ensured that the family understood that a Total Communication option may need to be considered if it was determined that ES had limited success in learning to use audition for developing spoken language.

50.6 Outcome

At 2 years, 2 months of age, ES was MAPped and tested again. She was accompanied by her parents and teacher of the deaf (TOD), who is also a certified auditory-verbal therapist. The TOD noted significant improvements in ES's responsiveness to sound. She noted that ES was vocalizing and approximating speech sounds. The parents also noted continued improvements in her responsiveness to sound at home. The results of the P.E.A.C.H. (▶ Table 50.1) demonstrated improvement in functional performance with the cochlear implant in comparison to the hearing aids. However, ES's overall aural/oral performance remained limited. Attempts to obtain open-set speech recognition were made, but her scores did not exceed chance levels. She was enrolled in an auditory-oral program with supplemental speech therapy. Unfortunately, ES did not make significant strides in her speech/language development and has been transitioned to the preschool program that uses a Total Communication approach. ES's language skills using a manual mode of communication are reportedly at or above same-age peers.

Table 50.1 P.E.A.C.H. (parents' evaluation of aural/oral performance of children) results with unaided, initial hearing aid settings, increased gain/output, and cochlear implant conditions. Calculated differences between unaided, aided, and cochlear implant conditions

Name:

MR#:

P.E.A.C.H. items	1 unaided	2 aided	3 aided	CI 4	Δ 1–2	Δ 2–3	Δ 3–4
Responds to name in quiet	1	1	1	2	0	0	1
Follows verbal instructions in quiet	1	1	1	1	0	0	0
Responds to name in noise	0	0	1	2	0	1	1
Follows verbal instructions in noise	0	0	0	0	0	0	0
Follows story read aloud	0	0	0	0	0	0	0
Participates in conversation in quiet	0	0	0	0	0	0	0
Participates in conversation in noise	0	0	0	0	0	0	0
Participates in conversation in car	0	0	0	0	0	0	0
Recognizes familiar voices	0	0	1	2	0	1	1
Talks on phone	0	0	0	0	0	0	0
Recognizes environmental sounds	1	1	1	2	0	0	1
Quiet score	8.33	8.33	12.50	20.83	0.00	4.17	8.33
Noise score	5.00	5.00	10.00	20.00	0.00	5.00	10.00
Overall score	13.33	13.33	22.50	40.83	0.00	9.17	18.33

ACA ASSESSMENT REPORT

Client ID: Date of Test:

Name: Time:

Gender: Clinician:

DOB: Hearing Centre: Audiology Department

Test Conditions

Ear Assessed:Right   Aided: Yes

Stimuli Used:/m/, /t/, /g/   Intensity Levels (dB SPL):75   Stimuli Presentation:Free Field

Masking Used:None Masking Level (ref. to stimuli):N/A Masking Presentation:N/A **Averaged Cortical Responses**

Obtained

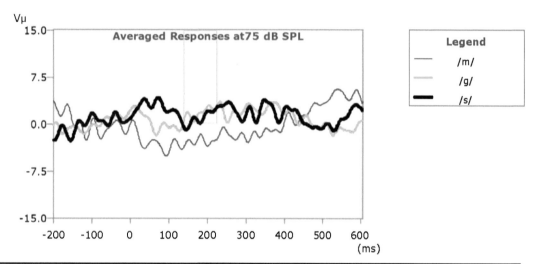

Results of Statistical Analysis

Detection

Were client's responses to the stimuli presented significantly
different from noise? (i.e. p <= 0.05)

	/m/	/t/	/g/	/s/
75 dB SPL	0.304		0.775	0.200

| **Latency Results** | **Additional Notes** |

Latencies for responses at75 dB SPL (ms)   No response to /m/, /g/, and /s/ at 75 dB SPL.

	/m/	/t/	/g/	/s/
P1				
N1				
P2				

Fig. 50.7 Aided cortical auditory evoked potential for the right ear.

ACA ASSESSMENT REPORT

Client ID: Date of Test:

Name: Time:

Gender: Clinician:

DOB: Hearing Centre: Audiology Department

Test Conditions

Ear Assessed:Left   Aided: Yes

Stimuli Used:/m/, /t/, /g/   Intensity Levels (dB SPL):75   Stimuli Presentation:Free Field

Masking Used:None Masking Level (ref. to stimuli):N/A Masking Presentation:N/A **Averaged Cortical Responses**

Obtained

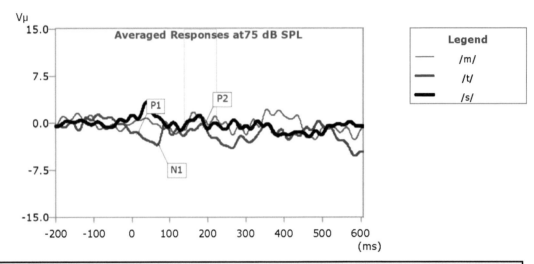

Results of Statistical Analysis

Detection

Were client's responses to the stimuli presented significantly different from noise? (i.e. p <= 0.05)

	/m/	/t/	/g/	/s/
75 dB SPL	0.509	**0.039**		0.956

Latency Results	Additional Notes

Latencies for responses at75 dB SPL (ms)

	/m/	/t/	/g/	/s/
P1		13		
N1		68		
P2		188		

No response to /m/ and /s/; questionable response to /t/.

Fig. 50.8 Aided cortical auditory evoked potential for the left ear.

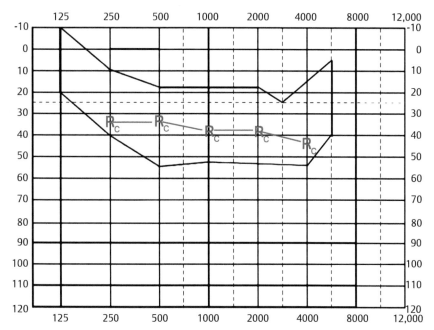

Fig. 50.9 Aided audiogram with the cochlear implant. RC, right ear cochlear implant.

Suggested Readings

[1] Feirn R, Sutton G, Parker G, Sirimanna T, Lightfoot G, Wood S. (2012). Guidelines for the Assessment and Management of Auditory Neuropathy Spectrum Disorder in Young Infants Version 2.1

[2] Guidelines for Identification and Management of Infants and Young Children with Auditory

[3] Neuropathy Spectrum Disorder, ed. Northern, 2008. Available from the Bill Daniels Center for Children's Hearing, The Children's Hospital, Aurora, CO

[4] Valero J, Blaser S, Papsin BC, James AL, Gordon KA. Electrophysiologic and behavioral outcomes of cochlear implantation in children with auditory nerve hypoplasia. Ear Hear. 2012; 33(1):3–18

51 Complicated Mapping

Rose Wright and Lisa S. Davidson

51.1 Clinical History and Description

RW's birth and family history are unremarkable for hearing loss. She passed her newborn hearing screening and was later diagnosed with a severe to profound hearing loss at 1 year, 4 months of age. She received her first cochlear implant (CI), a Cochlear Nucleus CI512, for her left ear at 2 years, 4 months. She enrolled in an auditory oral school for the children who are deaf and hard or hearing at age 5 and transferred her audiologic care to the school upon enrollment. At that time, she was using bimodal devices (CI and a hearing aid [HA] at the nonimplanted ear).

51.2 Audiologic Testing

Upon RW's enrollment and transfer of audiologic care, an unaided and aided assessment was completed. All testing was performed using frequency modulated warble tones and conditioned play audiometry (CPA), with good reliability. Unaided testing was performed via insert earphones, and aided testing was performed in the sound field. Unaided results indicated a bilateral, profound sensorineural hearing loss. Despite device optimization of the HA using desired sensation level (DSL) targets on the Audioscan Verifit with measured Real Ear to Coupler Differences (RECDs), audibility at her right, HA side was poor.[1] Aided speech perception testing conducted in the CI alone, HA alone, and bimodal conditions failed to show a bimodal benefit. RW subsequently received a Cochlear Nucleus CI422 at her right ear at 5 years, 11 months. Surgery and initial activation of the device occurred at her medical hospital. Subsequent programming was completed at the Listening and Spoken Language LSL School. ▶ Table 51.1 shows RW's implant thresholds at the left ear (first CI). ▶ Fig. 51.1 provides the map thresholds, and ▶ Table 51.2 provides the implant thresholds, at the right (second CI) at 4 weeks post initial activation.

Based on research literature suggesting that CI thresholds should approximate 20-dB HL for the optimal detection of speech ranging from soft to loud, RW's corresponding CI thresholds of 35- to 40-dB HL indicate fair.[2,3,4,5,6] RW's CI speech detection was much better (15-dB HL); however, we often note a mismatch between tones and speech for very young CI users adjusting to a new hearing experience. In these cases, we carefully monitor speech detection thresholds and frequency specific frequency-modulated (FM) tones to determine optimal audibility. Mapping procedures included measuring Thresholds (Ts) at first hearing across the array using a CPA task and set at first detection. Comfort levels (Cs) were set across the array using a five-point, loudness-scaling task, and set at "loud but ok." Further adjustments were made to RW's map to optimize thresholds. Changes included increasing Ts and Cs globally by 3 units, and an additional 2 units at 3,000 and 4,000 Hz. At 6 weeks post initial activation, RW's device was remapped based on high compliance levels and Ling confusion. Programming changes included increasing pulse width to 50 μs due to voltage compliance limitations, enabling electrodes 1 and 2, counted Ts, and loudness scaling of Cs (▶ Fig. 51.2).

Table 51.1 Cochlear implant (CI) thresholds in dB HL in the left ear

Condition	250 Hz	500 Hz	1,000 Hz	2,000 Hz	4,000 Hz	6,000 Hz
Left CI, aided	25 dB	30 dB	30 dB	30 dB	30 dB	30 dB

Table 51.2 Implant thresholds in dB HL 4 weeks post initial activation

Condition	250 Hz	500 Hz	1,000 Hz	2,000 Hz	4,000 Hz	6,000 Hz
Right CI thresholds	35 dB	35 dB	35 dB	40 dB	45 dB	40 dB

Table 51.3 Right implant thresholds in dB HL at 6 weeks post activation

Condition	250 Hz	500 Hz	1,000 Hz	2,000 Hz	4,000 Hz	6,000 Hz
Right cochlear implant thresholds	20 dB	20 dB	25 dB	25 dB	25 dB	25 dB

CI detection (▶ Table 51.3) indicates good audibility, which is in good agreement with speech detection at 15-dB HL. While detection indicates audibility, it does not indicate clarity. RW's speech language pathologist reported RW consistently misses /m/, and guesses for /i/ and /a/ at her right ear. These phoneme errors may be due to limited experience with the CI or to a pitch difference between ears. Auditory training did not help clear up errors, indicating the phoneme confusions may be due to the latter.

Zwolan et al[7] evaluated electrode discrimination in a group of 11 CI subjects. They investigated whether removal of electrodes that were indiscriminable in pitch from other adjacent electrodes in the array would result in an improved ability to understand speech. The authors identified electrodes that failed to elicit distinguishable pitch differences from adjacent electrodes by using a pitch ranking procedure. They found that the majority of participants showed significant improvement with the pitch-ranked map (some electrodes deactivated) compared to the full map. These findings indicate that a reduction of electrodes may improve perception of envelope cues. Based on this literature, pitch ranking was completed using a simplified same/different task. Electrical stimulation at Cs was presented at two different electrodes, and RW reported if the pitch was the same or different. At the left CI, all electrodes were distinguished as different in pitch. At the right CI, every third electrode was distinguished as different. An "experimental" map with only the electrodes that were distinguished as different was created at the right CI (▶ Fig. 51.3). The rationale for this map was to help envelope cues become more salient and reduce possible current spread, as suggested by Zwolan et al.[7]

Upon activation of the experimental map, immediate improvements were noted. RW was able to identify 100% of the Ling sounds at her right CI alone. Further adjustments were attempted to enable more electrodes; however, Ling sound confusion returned as soon as any changes were made. A 2-week

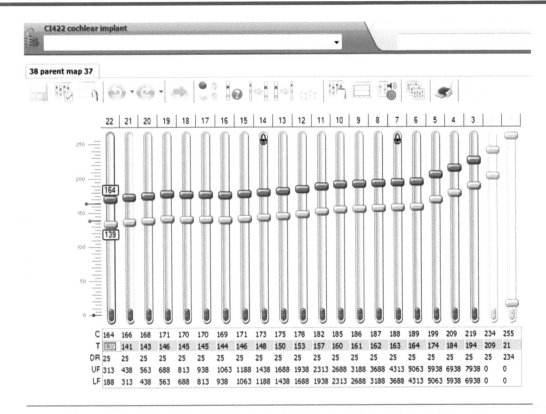

Fig. 51.1 Map programming characteristics for the right cochlear implant ear. Map T and C levels for active electrodes 3 to 22 are shown in green and red, respectively, and noted in table below map. The upper and lower frequency boundary assignments are listed in the table for electrodes 3 to 22. C, comfort level; T, threshold level; DR, dynamic range; UF, upper frequency; LF, lower frequency.

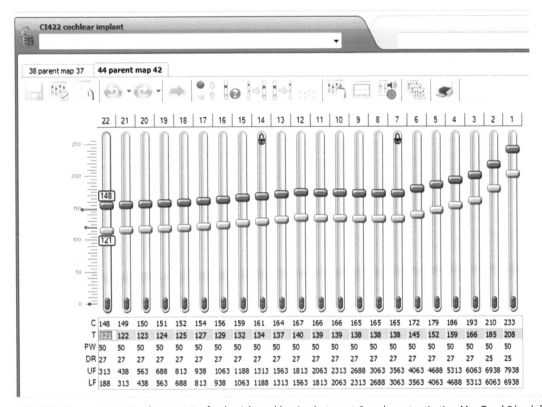

Fig. 51.2 Map programming characteristics for the right cochlear implant ear at 6 weeks post activation. Map T and C levels for active electrodes 1 to 22 are shown in green and red, respectively, and noted in table below map. The upper and lower frequency boundary assignments are listed in the table for electrodes 1 to 22. C, comfort level; T, threshold level; DR, dynamic range; UF, upper frequency; LF, lower frequency.

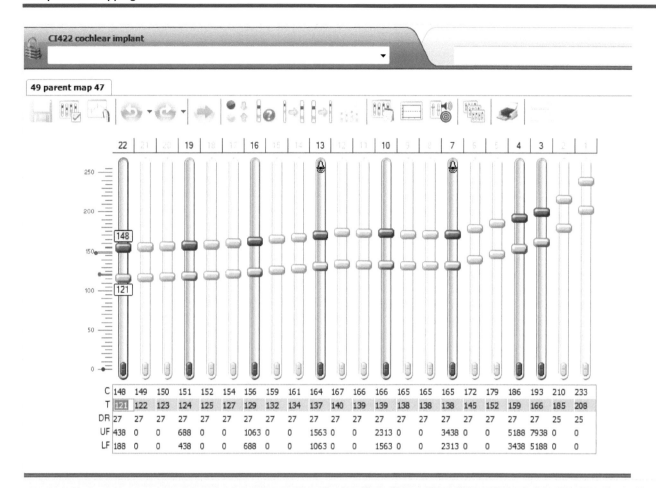

Fig. 51.3 Map programming characteristics for the experimental map for the right cochlear implant. Map T and C levels for active electrodes 3, 4, 7, 10, 13, 16, 19, and 22 are shown in green and red, respectively, and noted in table below map. The upper and lower frequency boundary assignments are listed in the table for active electrodes. C, comfort level; T, threshold level; DR, dynamic range; UF, upper frequency; LF, lower frequency.

trial ensued with the experimental map at the right CI. At the end of the 2-week trial, speech perception testing was assessed using the Consonant-Nucleus-Consonant (CNC) and Lexical Neighborhood Test (LNT) word lists, presented at 60-dB SPL (▸ Table 51.4).

No significant difference in speech perception was noted between the different conditions following the 2-week trial with the experimental map at the right CI. A 2-week trial with the full map ensued. When the full map was loaded, RW was able to identify 100% Ling sounds with both the experimental and full map. This was not the case previously. After a 2-week trial with the full map, speech perception was retested.

Results indicate a doubling of score on the LNT at the right CI alone with the full map post 2-week trial (▸ Table 51.5).

51.3 Questions for the Reader

1. Why was RW remapped at 6 weeks post initial activation? Explain rationale.
2. What other programming changes could have been made to influence compliance levels?
3. Why is speech perception testing essential for this case?

Table 51.4 Speech perception, post 2-week trial with experimental map at right cochlear implant (CI)

Condition	CNC words	CNC phonemes	LNT words	LNT phonemes
Left CI alone	48%	77%		
Both CIs (Right = experimental map)	48%	75%		
Both CIs (Right = full map)	44%	73%		
Right CI, experimental map			14%	35%
Right CI, full map			16%	45%

Abbreviations: CNC, consonant-nucleus-consonant; LNT, lexical neighborhood test.

51.4 Discussion of Questions

1. **Why was RW remapped at 6 weeks post initial activation? Explain rationale.**

   A mapping adjustment was needed for two reasons. First, Ling sound confusion suggests the need for a mapping

Table 51.5 Speech perception, post–2-week trial with full map at right cochlear implant (CI)

Condition	CNC words	CNC phonemes	LNT words	LNT phonemes
Both CIs (Right = full map)	50%	79%		
Right CI, full map			34%	53%

Abbreviations: CNC, consonant nucleus consonant; LNT, lexical neighborhood test.

adjustment. Second, remapping was warranted because C levels closely approached voltage compliance limitations. Approaching or exceeding voltage compliance levels can create a distorted signal because increases in current may not be able to be delivered by the implant at some electrodes, and channel interaction is also more likely.

2. **What other programming changes could have been made to influence compliance levels?**
In this case, pulse width was widened. Another change that may affect voltage compliance limitations is the use of alternative battery options (e.g., rechargeable batteries may provide more voltage capacity than disposable zinc-air batteries).

3. **Why is speech perception testing essential for this case?**
While important, aided detection only indicates audibility. Speech perception helps us understand the clarity of RW's signal. Several layers of speech perception were used throughout the case from detection of Ling sounds to recorded CNCs. Speech perception was also used as the outcome measure to compare the experimental and full map.

51.5 Final Diagnosis and Recommended Treatment

Based on improved speech perception scores, a full map was recommended. It is possible less information was necessary initially, but given time, introducing more information no longer compromised the signal or clarity. It is also possible that RW needed more time to acclimate to the new program containing a stimulus with a longer pulse width. Implant detection was verified with good audibility using the full map at the right CI (▶ Table 51.6).

Table 51.6 Implant thresholds, post 2-week trial with full map at right cochlear implant (CI)

Condition	250 Hz	500 Hz	1,000 Hz	2,000 Hz	4,000 Hz	6,000 Hz
Right CI thresholds	25 dB	25 dB	25 dB	30 dB	30 dB	25 dB

Table 51.7 Speech perception, 10 months post initial activation

Condition	CNC words (%)	CNC phonemes (%)
Both CIs	80	90
Right CI	72	89
Left CI	68	88

Abbreviations: CI, cochlear implant; CNC, consonant nucleus consonant.

51.6 Outcome

RW has since used a full map at her right CI. Speech perception completed 10 months post initial activation at the right CI indicates continued improvement (▶ Table 51.7).

References

[1] Scollie SD. Prescriptive procedures for infants and children. In Seewald RC, Bamford JM, eds. Proceedings of the third international conference. A Sound Foundation through Early Amplification. Stäfa, Switzerland: Phonak AG; 2004:91–104)

[2] Davidson LS, Geers AE, Nicholas JG. The effects of audibility and novel word learning ability on vocabulary level in children with cochlear implants. Cochlear Implants Int. 2014; 15(4):211–221

[3] Davidson LS, Skinner MW, Holstad BA, et al. The effect of instantaneous input dynamic range setting on the speech perception of children with the nucleus 24 implant. Ear Hear. 2009; 30(3):340–349

[4] Firszt JB, Holden LK, Skinner MW, et al. Recognition of speech presented at soft to loud levels by adult cochlear implant recipients of three cochlear implant systems. Ear Hear. 2004; 25(4):375–387

[5] Holden LK, Finley CC, Firszt JB, et al. Factors affecting open-set word recognition in adults with cochlear implants. Ear Hear. 2013; 34(3):342–360

[6] Skinner MW. Optimizing cochlear implant speech performance. Ann Otol Rhinol Laryngol Suppl. 2003; 191:4–13

[7] Zwolan TA, Collins LM, Wakefield GH. Electrode discrimination and speech recognition in postlingually deafened adult cochlear implant subjects. J Acoust Soc Am. 1997; 102(6):3673–3685

52 A Case of Pediatric Hyperacusis

Jenne Tunnell

52.1 Clinical History and Description

DR was a 5-year-old boy referred to audiology by his psychologist to evaluate and treat for hyperacusis. At his initial visit, his mother rated his perception of hyperacusis as 4/10 on a severity scale (10 being the most severe) (▶ Fig. 52.1). He had no medical, neurological, or traumatic history that would predispose him to hyperacusis. His sleep patterns were age-appropriate, and his mother denied a predisposition to anxiety or depression. He wore hearing protection (plugs/muffs) when exposed to dangerously loud noise levels, but not otherwise. His reactions to moderate- to high-level sounds varied; he might withdraw from the situation, refuse to participate, cover his ears, and sometimes he would cry. It would take him 5 to 60 minutes to recover from adverse sound exposure.

The following is a list of sounds or types of sounds that were bothersome to DR (in order of severity, starting with the most severe): fire trucks, fire alarms, motorcycles, gunshots, monster trucks, semi-trucks, and loud voices. DR's mother reported that she stayed at home so DR did not have to attend daycare. She reported that the home was quiet and that the TV volume is low. DR reportedly did not tolerate noisy children or adults with loud voices.

DR's mother also reported that he had none of the following characteristics or traits: high-risk indicators for hearing loss, history of otitis media or any chronic ear or upper respiratory disease, predisposing medical or neurologic history, or exposure to loud noise or ototoxic agents.

52.2 Initial Evaluation

At the first assessment, conditioned play audiometry was performed under insert earphones. Results were repeatable and reliable and showed hearing within normal limits bilaterally (▶ Fig. 52.2). There was a slight asymmetry in the high frequencies as the right ear responses were as low as –10 dB at 6,000 Hz. Speech reception thresholds were 5 dB for each ear. DR's most comfortable listening level for speech was 35 dB HL for each ear. Acoustic immittance measures showed normal type A tympanograms, suggesting intact and appropriately mobile tympanic membranes. DR's mother denied any significant history of recurring otitis media.

Frequency-specific loudness discomfort levels (LDLs) were measured using Jastreboff's recommended measurement protocol,[1] which calls for the clinician to present a tone at the child's hearing threshold and increase the presentation level in 5-dB increments. This procedure is completed with pure tones at octave frequencies from 250 to 8,000 Hz. Jastreboff recommends measuring each frequency twice, and taking the second measurement, as this is likely the more accurate of the two. He stresses the importance of ensuring that the children understand that they have the control to stop the testing at any moment. The clinician established trust with DR prior to testing, and they practiced "stop" behaviors so that DR understood

that he was in control of how loud the sounds would ultimately become. DR's responses are shown in ▶ Table 52.1.

52.3 Interpretation and Counseling

DR exhibited abnormal sensitivity to sound. Normal comfort levels for speech should occur at 60 to 70 dB SPL. Typically, children allow 90 dB HL or louder for frequency-specific LDLs. The test results were explained to DR's mother, and she was given a copy of the findings. She was counseled about hyperacusis and sound therapy as well as habituation exercises that should be done in tandem with behavioral health visits. She was provided with information about web sites with links to downloadable sound therapy MP3 s. An appointment was made for follow-up for further evaluation and to establish a plan of care.

52.4 Treatment

52.4.1 What's Been Done Before?

Stiegler and Davis[2] recommended that, when treating children with hyperacusis, simultaneous supports should be provided by caregivers to show that the sounds and environment are safe for the child. Koegel et al[3] successfully treated children with autism with a similar "successive approximation" approach, exposing children first to sounds in the distance and gradually bringing them closer.

52.4.2 Treatment Plan

▶ Fig. 52.3 outlines the treatment plan for DR, which was given to his mother at the first session.

52.5 Additional Testing

52.5.1 Session #2: Outcomes and Further Assessment

During the second session, the treatment plan was reviewed with DR's mother, and she reported that she had not had a chance to give the sound aversion diary to his teacher yet. She also reported that she did not feel it was necessary to follow up with the psychologist at present. She reported that all providers now had a good understanding of hyperacusis. She did keep a journal of aversion behaviors for a typical week and reported that the only noticeable aversion behavior, other than loud voices, was a church program where the preschool children at the church were putting on a very noisy Christmas show (sample journal entry provided in ▶ Fig. 52.4). At that point, DR wanted to leave the church; she reacted by comforting him, reminding him why they were there, and telling him that he had to stay. DR had been listening to pink noise one to two times a day for 15 minutes at a comfortable listening level using the iPad with headphones. He

Pediatric Hyperacusis Questionnaire

1. How long has your child had hyperacusis? _____

2. Has your child had multiple ear infections? _____yes ____ no

3. Has your child had a head injury? _____yes ____ no

4. Does your child have a hearing loss/hearing difficulty? _____yes ____ no

5. Has your child seen an Ear Nose and Throat doctor? _____ yes _____ no

    a.   If so, has your child had surgery on his/her ears? ____yes ____no

6. Do you associate the onset of hyperacusis with a specific event? _____ yes _____ no

7. In which ear is the sensitivity to sound a problem for your child?

    ___ Right ear only ____ Left ear only ____ Both ears

8. Does your child's hyperacusis vary? ____ yes ____no

9. Does your child complain of tinnitus (ringing/buzzing or other sounds in the ears)?

    ____No _____ Right ear _____ Left ear ____ Both ears

10. Does your child have trouble falling asleep? _____yes ____ no

11. Does your child have episodes of dizziness? _____yes ____ no

12. Does your child get frequent headaches? _____yes ____ no

13. How many hours of sleep does your child get in a night? _____

14. Does your child have anxiety or depression? _____yes ____ no

15. Does your child have a learning disability? _____yes ____ no

16. Does your child have an IEP or 504 plan at school? _____yes ____ no

17. Does your child have autism or a behavioral disorder? _____yes ____ no

18. Has your child been seen by a behavioral health professional ? _____yes ____ no

19. Is your child sensitive to other sensory stimuli (eg. Light, touch, etc.) _____yes ____ no

20. Has the hyperacusis affected your child's relationship with others? _____yes ____ no

21. Has the hyperacusis affected your child's social activities? _____yes ____ no

22. Does your child use ear protection? _____yes ____ no

    a.   If yes, what type of ear protection? _____

    b.   If yes, how often does your child use ear protection? _____

    _____

23. List the reactions experienced or expressed when your child is suffering from hyperacusis (e.g. self harm, flight, verbal or bodily expressions of anger, frustration, rage sorrow, confusion, or others):

    _____

    _____

    _____

24. How long does it take to recover from the reactions? _____

25. What are the activities or actions that can positively affect the reaction, either in the intensity or duration of the reaction? _____

    _____

    _____

Fig. 52.1 Pediatric hyperacusis questionnaire. (*continued*)

26. Please list your child's current medications (including over the counter):

_____

_____

_____

27. What, if any, treatments have you tried for the hyperacusis?

_____

_____

_____

28. Please list a typical week day's routines/activities for your child (eg. 7 a.m. wake up, get dressed, breakfast, daycare etc.)

Morning: _____

_____

_____

_____

_____

Lunchtime: _____

_____

_____

Evening : _____

_____

_____

Bedtime: _____

_____

_____

29. What daily living activities are affected by the hyperacusis? How does this impact the others in the household? _____

_____

_____

_____

_____

_____

_____

_____

_____

_____

_____

_____

_____

Fig. 52.1 (continued)

30. Please list the sounds or types of sounds that are bothersome to your child:

a. _____

b. _____

c. _____

d. _____

e. _____

f. _____

g. _____

h. _____

i. _____

j. _____

31. In the list above, please rank them from 1-10, with number 1 being the most bothersome sound, and 10 the least bothersome sound.

32. Please rate the severity of your child's hyperacusis on a scale of 1-10 (1=minimal>10= severe)

_____

33. Is there any other information you think would be helpful for us to know? _____

_____

Fig. 52.1 (*continued*)

was able to tolerate the pink noise as long as he was distracted by playing on the iPad. He plateaued at approximately a quarter of the volume scale for the first 10 days. By the 11th and 12th day, he was able to jump up to 60% of the dynamic range on the player and has been able to consistently maintain this volume level. As suggested, DR started playing the Wii gaming system with his father who chose the volume of the gaming. Currently, the gaming was at a soft level, and DR was comfortable. The types of games they played included sudden explosive sounds, as well as car and truck engine noises.

The next goal was to introduce a sound generator at bedtime and to work to increase the volume after routine had been established. DR had not been able to tolerate the sound in order to get to sleep even though he picked the sound stimulus. His mother used a sound simulation app on her iPad, and he tended to choose airplane cabin sound.

52.6 Assessment

In order to quantify the impact of treatment on DR's symptoms, the Sound Effects Recognition Test (SERT) was administered to the child. The SERT was developed as a tool for the assessment of identification of environmental sounds. The test consists of recorded materials and pictorial representations of various environmental sounds. A sound is presented to the patient, and the patient is required to identify the picture corresponding to the sound from a four-choice closed set. In the assessment of the effects of treatment for hyperacusis, however, this test was chosen to provide cognitive loading while the child listened to potentially distressing sounds in order to provide loudness judgments. The test has the added benefit of providing frequency information about the spectral location of the sound simulations, which can be useful in targeting particularly noxious sound stimuli for the child to habituate to.

DR was placed in the sound booth at a zero-degree azimuth, 3 feet away from a free-field speaker with an assistant in the booth with him. The clinician asked the child to choose a comfortable volume for her voice level, using monitored live voice. At his last visit approximately 5 weeks prior to the second session, he felt her voice was most comfortable at 35 dB HL. At the second session, he felt her voice was most comfortable at 40 dB HL. The clinician presented the SERT CD through a speaker in sound field set to 40 dB HL. He was then provided with closed-set choices to identify various environmental sounds. The identification of the environmental sounds was to draw his attention to a different task, and after identifying the sound, he was told to perform a loudness judgment on a scale of 6. The scale consisted of six different emoticons with varying levels of comfort, beginning with extremely comfortable, and ending with tears from discomfort. The faces were numbered from 1 to 6, with "6" causing the most discomfort and "1" being the most comfortable (▶ Fig. 52.5). His judgments were consistent and repeatable over time.

At 40 dB HL, DR judged the following environmental sounds as the most comfortable (rating of 1): toilet flush, landline phone ring, saw, church bells, and fire truck. At 40 dB HL, he judged the following sounds to be comfortable with a rating of 2: vacuum cleaner, kids playing on a playground, and dog barking. The final presentations at 40 dB HL were rated as a 3/6 for the following environmental sounds: train noise and a person whistling. The SERT was then presented at 50 dB HL, and he continued identifying the environmental sound and consistently rating it as a "6." The following stimuli were rated as most comfortable: bird song,

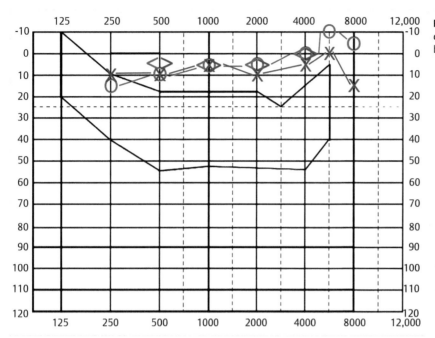

Fig. 52.2 DR's audiogram. O, right ear air conduction; X, left ear air conduction; <, right ear bone conduction; >, left ear bone conduction.

Table 52.1 Frequency-specific loudness discomfort levels

	500 Hz	1,000 Hz	2,000 Hz	4,000 Hz
Right ear	50 dB HL	50 dB HL	50 dB HL	55 dB HL
Left ear	50 dB HL	50 dB HL	55 dB HL	40 dB HL

loud coughing, a mother calling a child, children singing, dishes breaking, piano notes running a scale, water running, and a whistle being blown. He judged knocking/hammering sounds as 2/6. He judged car starting noise as 3/6. The presentation level was then increased to 60 dB HL, and he judged the following and prior mental sounds to be comfortable 1/6 on the rating scale: a kitten meowing, a clock ticking, alarm clock ringing, a door bell, and a hand bell. He judged the following environmental sounds to be 2 on a scale of 6: a baby crying, a male voice, and a base drum. He judged the following and prior mental sounds as 3/6 on the loudness judgments scale: airplane takeoff, water running, and gunshot noise.

The clinician reviewed the results with DR's mother, and explained that the goal was to be able to ultimately present these environmental sounds at realistic loudness levels and have the child rate them no higher than 3 on a scale of 6 loudness judgments. She explained that at his next visit, they would begin the assessment by presenting sounds at 50 dB HL and determine if the stimuli could be gradually increased to 70 dB HL, a more realistic loudness level for many of the sounds.

52.7 Recommendations

The following action plan was implemented as a result of Session #2:

1. DR's mother would request the teacher to complete a sound aversion diary before the next appointment.
2. DR would continue to listen to pink noise two times a day for 15 minutes at 60 to 75% of the dynamic range of the iPad.
3. DR would use headphones when playing the Wii in order to bring the sounds of the gaming system closer to him, and to be able to start to increase the volume to encourage habituation.
4. Instead of the sound generator at bedtime, parents would introduce white noise either via a radio in between stations or a fan noise. It was recommended that DR's mother start the sound before he entered the room, rather than having him choose the level of the sound, thus drawing attention to it. She would then increase the loudness level of the static noise slightly each night before he entered the room.

52.8 Additional Testing

52.8.1 Session #3

DR's mother reported that the teacher had not responded, and she had not had a chance to follow up with her. DR continued to listen to pink noise, and was able to approximate 75% of the dynamic range. They did not have headphones yet for the gaming system, but he was able to tolerate higher sound levels from the gaming system over the past week as compared to the levels he would tolerate prior to treatment. DR continued to have difficulty falling asleep with sounds being generated in his bedroom, and so his mother turned the television in the living room louder than usual, so that he would hear it in his bedroom.

Name: DR	Provider Name:
Parent/Caregiver name: Ms. R	Jenne Tunnell, AuD
DOB: 01/01/2010	Phone: xxx-xxx-xxxx
MRN: 123456	Treatment Plan Date: 12/02/2015

Other Agencies Involved:	Plan to Coordinate Services:
Dr XXXXX Behavioral Health Provider	Phone contact during the first month of treatment, then as needed, but at least 1 time every 3 months.
School XX Elementary School Mrs. X, Kindergarten teacher	Request teacher to complete sound aversion diary 1 time during the first month of treatment. Continued contact by phone as needed.

Medication(s):	Dose:	Frequency:	Indication:
Multivitamin		daily	

Fig. 52.3 Treatment plan for DR. (*continued*)

1. Problem/Symptom: Hyperacusis

Long Term Goal: Symptoms of hyperacusis will be significantly reduced and will no longer interfere with DR's functioning. This will be measured by parent report and significant change in post-treatment questionnaires at the time of discharge.

Anticipated completion date: TBD

Short Term Goals/Objectives:	**Date Established**	**Projected Completion**	**Date Achieved**
1. Understanding of Hyperacusis by all Carers	12/2/2015	12/10/2015	
2. Maintain a journal of aversion behaviors associated with different sounds and places for a typical week (including weekend and home and school hours).	12/2/2015	Before next appointment	
3. DR will listen to Pink noise 2-3 times a day for 15 minutes at a comfortable listening level with headphones. (Free mp3 at www.audiocheck.net). Level will be increased as he will allow over time.	12/2/2015	ongoing	
4. Carers will learn how to deal with DR's distress by exposure to sounds by moving him away from the sound source and reassuring and comforting him as well as explaining the source of the sound.	12/2/2015	12/10/2015	
	12/2/2015	12/24/2015	
5. DR will practice control over sounds by parent		ongoing	

Fig. 52.3 (continued)

producing a range of different sounds in a play situation.	12/2/2015	
DR will clap his hands to stop/start the sounds. (Eg. New Wii gaming system)		
6. DR will listen to a soothing sound generator at bedtime (eg. Waves, rain noise, etc.) at a comfortable volume. Once new bedtime routine is established and tolerated, volume will be slowly increased.		
Intervention/Action Individual sound therapy to help DR with desensitization and habituation of sound aversions.	Responsible Person(s) Carers Teacher	1. Jenne Tunnell, AuD

Fig. 52.3 (*continued*)

52.8.2 Assessment

DR was placed in a sound booth with supra-aural headphones. The SERT test CD was presented at 60 and 70 dB HL. As before, DR was provided with a closed set of choices to identify the various environmental sounds to help with cognitive loading. Directly after identifying the sounds, he was told to perform a loudness judgment with the scale consisting of the six different emoticons. DR's judgments were consistent and repeatable over time.

At 60 dB HL, he judged the following environmental sounds as 1 out of 6 on the comfort scale: a telephone for the right ear, a car starting, birds singing, mother's voice, piano scale, splashing water, police whistle, and hammer for the left ear. The following were judged 2 out of 6 on the comfort scale at 60 dB HL: a man whistling for the right ear and children singing for the left ear. At the same loudness level, he judged the following at 3 out of 6 on a comfort scale for the right ear: a train and toilet flush; for the left ear, man coughing and dishes breaking. He scored the following as 4 out of 6 on the comfort scale for the right ear: dog barking and sawing; for the left ear, there were no responses above 3 out of 6. For the right ear, he judged the following to be 5 out of 6 on the loudness scale: children playing and a vacuum. The following two

sounds were intolerable, scoring 6 out of 6, for the right ear: church bells and fire engine noise at 60 dB HL. Since the right ear appeared to be more sensitive than the left, only the left ear was tested at 70 dB, and he judged the following to be 1 out of 6 on a comfort scale: cat meowing, baby cry, father's voice, alarm clock, gunshots, and a small bell. He judged drum noise at 3 out of 6 and a water faucet at 5 out of 6. The sound of an airplane taking off and doorbell when presented to the left ear at 70 dB HL were 6 out of 6.

The results were reviewed with DR's mother. The clinician explained that the treatment goal was to be able to present environmental sounds at realistic loudness levels and to have DR rate them no higher than 3 on a scale of 6 loudness judgments. The third session's assessment revealed more realistic loudness levels to the environmental sounds, and DR appeared to be less sensitive to many of the sounds.

52.8.3 Recommendations

The following action plan was implemented as a result of Session #3:
1. DR's mother would request the teacher to complete a sound aversion diary before the next appointment.

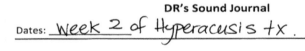

DR's Sound Journal

Fig. 52.4 Sample from DR's sound aversion diary.

Dates: <u>Week 2 of Hyperacusis tx.</u>

Day 1

Sound aversions: Loud voices while watching TV.

Context: Grown-ups watching a football game, getting rowdy. DR went to his room for a while.

Pink Noise Volume Setting:

<———|————————————>
                    ← iPad with headphones on

Day 2

Sound aversions: Choir at Church

Context: Children's Christmas play practice, consoled him and he was able to stay at church.

Pink Noise Volume Setting:

<————————|——————>

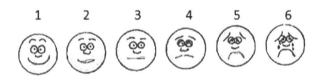

1   2   3   4   5   6

Fig. 52.5 Loudness judgment emoticons.

2. DR would continue to listen to pink noise at least two times a day for 15 minutes at 75% of the dynamic range of the iPad.
3. DR would use headphones when playing the Wii and/or watching television so that the sounds of the TV are closer to him, and he can begin to start to increase the volume to encourage habituation.
4. DR's family would continue to introduce higher levels of environmental noise at bedtime.

52.9 Additional Testing

52.9.1 Session #4

DR's mother reported that he had made significant progress. In fact, they had a fire alarm at school the day before, and he did not react negatively to this. He used headphones at home for his daily sessions with pink noise, which he listened to at 3/4 of the volume range. He also used them when gaming, and the family successfully increased the environmental background noise at bedtime.

52.9.2 Assessment

DR was evaluated in the audiometric sound booth with insert earphones. He sat at a table across from an audiologist's assistant. Under these conditions, frequency-specific LDLs were measured, as well as most comfortable levels (MCLs) and uncomfortable levels (UCLs) to live voice. His most comfortable listening level for speech on the right side was 65 dB HL, which normalized compared to his pretherapy MCL of 35 dB HL. The left ear MCL was measured at 70 dB HL, which also normalized compared to the pretherapy MCLs of 35 dB HL. UCLs were measured at 80 dB for the right ear and 85 dB for the left ear, which normalized compared to his pretreatment UCLs for speech of 50 dB HL bilaterally. The frequency-specific LDLs were measured, and the results are provided in ▶ Table 52.2.

Frequency-specific LDLs improved significantly when compared to his pretherapy judgments, which averaged 50 dB HL in sound field.

The SERT was performed at 70 dB HL under ear-specific conditions with insert earphones. The sounds that DR judged as uncomfortably loud at the right ear were dog barking, children playing, and a fire engine. At the left ear, he judged car starting, police whistle, and hammer sounds as uncomfortable. However, his behavior indicated that he was not upset by the loudness, nor did he attempt to pull the earphones out. He continued to smile and enjoy the task. When he was questioned as to why he was smiling, and if the sound was still uncomfortable, he reported that he liked being there and he liked the activity. Originally, his mother reported that his perception of hyperacusis was 4/10 on a severity scale with 10 being the most severe. Today, she reported that there was no evidence of hyperacusis.

Table 52.2 Frequency-specific listening discomfort levels

	250 Hz	500 Hz	1,000 Hz	2,000 Hz	4,000 Hz	6,000 Hz
Right ear	90 dB HL	85 dB HL	85 dB HL	80 dB HL	75 dB HL	85 dB HL
Left ear	90 dB HL	95 dB HL	80 dB HL	75 dB HL	75 dB HL	80 dB HL

52.10 Recommendations

The goals to provide individual sound therapy to help DR with desensitization and habituation of sound aversion were met successfully. DR no longer displayed symptoms of hyperacusis, and his sensitivity to sound no longer interfered with his daily functioning. This was corroborated according to parent report and child's performance on loudness judgment exercises from pre- to posttreatment.

DR was discharged from the sound therapy program, and DR's mother expressed verbal satisfaction and understanding. She was counseled to continue with the pink noise therapy for as long as she felt it to be necessary and told that there was no need to work on increasing the loudness of the headphones he wore at home.

52.11 Questions for the Reader

1. What is the definition of hyperacusis?
2. What is the prevalence of hyperacusis among school-aged children?
3. How would you evaluate a child for the presence of hyperacusis?
4. What sort of treatment would you recommend for a child whom you diagnosed with hyperacusis?
5. How would you measure the outcome of intervention for hyperacusis?

52.12 Discussion of Questions

1. **What is the definition of hyperacusis?**
   In order to better understand hyperacusis, it is helpful to understand the meaning and the distinguishing features of several terms commonly used to describe sound tolerance problems.
   Definitions
   - **Misophonia**: (Miso = hate) abnormally strong reaction to moderate-level sounds of the autonomic and limbic systems resulting from enhanced connections between the auditory and limbic system.[1]
   - **Phonophobia**: (phobia = fear) emotional fear response to a certain sound based on the type of sound, previous experiences with the sound, circumstances connected with it, and the person's psychological profile.[1]
   - **Hyperacusis**: collapsed tolerance to moderate-level environmental sounds or an abnormally strong reaction to moderate-level sound occurring within the auditory pathways.[1]
   - **Recruitment**: Rapid growth of perceived loudness for sounds located in the frequency region of the hearing loss.

2. **What is the prevalence of hyperacusis among school-aged children?**
   A study done in 2007 revealed that as many as 17 to 20% of all children with autism spectrum disorder, including those who are high functioning, have hyperacusis.[4] The researchers studied 506 children, ranging in age from 5 to 12 years, using questionnaires and LDL measurements. They defined hyperacusis as those children with lowered LDLs associated with abnormal annoyance to sounds. They selected the group with LDLs in the lowest 5%, who said "yes" to the question "Are you bothered by any kind of sounds or noise?" and were able to describe the sound, and identify at least 10 from a list of 20 sounds as "annoying." Of the children who were in lowest 5%, 42% were bothered by sounds and 3.2% were determined to have hyperacusis. The study concluded that the prevalence of hyperacusis in children is high enough to warrant including screening for it during routine clinical evaluations.

3. **How would you evaluate a child for the presence of hyperacusis?**
   At the time of this writing, there are no published guidelines or recommendations for a diagnostic protocol when evaluating hyperacusis in children. There is, however, a consensus among subject matter experts that it is important to obtain a good history in order to differentiate between hyperacusis and misophonia, as the latter would require treatment by a behavioral health professional. It stands to reason that a child with misophonia would not benefit from sound therapy treatment by an audiologist, as the underlying reason behind the adverse reactions have to do with fear, rather than abnormal sensitivity. The child should be interviewed carefully, as well as the parents/caretakers. Use of an inventory may prove helpful. ▶ Fig. 52.1 shows an example of a case history questionnaire for a child with possible hyperacusis. It is generally agreed that it is important to rule out hearing loss as a contributing factor in a child's sensitivity to sound. Finally, it is important to quantify the degree of sensitivity by measuring a child's discomfort to loud sounds.

4. **What sort of treatment would you recommend for a child whom you diagnosed with hyperacusis?**
   The goal for treatment of hyperacusis is to identify three different factors relating to the child's unusual or extreme reactions to sounds. The first is to categorize the type of sounds that are bothersome, the second to document the behaviors observed during the child's abnormal reactions, and the third to identify coping mechanisms that can help. The following is a suggested clinical pathway for management of hyperacusis in children, based on this author's review of the literature:
   1. Obtain a profile of hyperacusis in the child's everyday life:
      a) Questionnaires (▶ Fig. 52.1), case history, inventories, behavioral health evaluation.

2. Understand the impact of problem on individual/family/others:
   a) Sound aversion diaries, interviews, inventories.
3. Ensure understanding of condition by caregivers, leading to consistency in management:
   a) Counseling, promoting self-advocacy, empowering parents.
4. Provide behavioral desensitization:
   a) Clinical psychologist should break down the learned association of fear and anxiety.
   b) Allow the child to have control over loud sounds.
   c) Gentle reintroduction of situations with potential for adverse sounds.
   d) Education of child regarding the source of the sound ("knowledge is power").
5. Provide auditory desensitization:
   a) Reduce internal gain by increasing exposure to environmental sounds.
   b) Noise/sound generators.
   c) Habituation therapy (e.g., tinnitus retraining therapy [TRT]).
6. Follow-up regime.

52.13 Why Think Pink?

People with hyperacusis are more sensitive to sound above 6,000 Hz. Pink sound creates energy that is inversely proportional to the frequency of the signal, meaning the acoustic energy is constant. This results in a perception of less "hissing" than other noise, such as white noise, where the power is constant over all frequencies.

Pink noise protocol: Dr. Marsha Johnson, an audiologist in private practice in Oregon, created a 16-week program using pink noise to help hyperacusis sufferers habituate to sound. The program is available online (http://www.pinksound.info/) and is intended for individuals with normal or near-normal hearing. Participants must have passed a medical and audiologic evaluation to rule out other treatable conditions. On her website, she describes "The Pink Sound Protocol" as "a simple, easy to use at home program, adaptable for most people without serious hearing loss, and requires a few hours per week to complete the workshop exercises."

Dr. Johnson enrolled 300 volunteers in her beta study and tested them before and after completion of the 16-week program. Improvement as a result of the program was determined by identifying those whose scores lowered at least 30% on posttesting.

Her results showed that 72% of subjects met this criterion for success. Pink noise is available for free download on various online sites and applications (e.g., www.audiocheck.net).

5. **How would you measure the outcome of intervention for hyperacusis?**
   As described in this case study, outcomes may be documented with audiological test measures (e.g., LDL, MCL), by examining changes in the SERT ratings, and through parent report/diaries.

52.14 Useful Websites

1. http://www.pinksound.info/
2. www.audiocheck.net
3. www.hyperacusis.net
4. http://www.tinnitus-audiology.com
5. http://www.audiologyonline.com/ask-the-experts/hyper-acusis-in-children-699

References

[1] Jastreboff PJ, Jastreboff MM. Tinnitus retraining therapy (TRT) as a method for treatment of tinnitus and hyperacusis patients. J Am Acad Audiol. 2000; 11 (3):162–177

[2] Stiegler LN, Davis R. Understanding sound sensitivity in individuals with autism spectrum disorders. Focus Autism Other Dev Disabl. 2010; 25(2):67–75

[3] Koegel RL, Openden D, Koegel LK. A systematic desensitization paradigm to treat hypersensitivity to auditory stimuli in children with autism in family contexts. Res Pract Persons Severe Disabl. 2004; 29(2):122–134

[4] Coelho CB, Sanchez TG, Tyler RS. Hyperacusis, sound annoyance, and loudness hypersensitivity in children. Prog Brain Res. 2007; 166:169–178

Suggested Readings

[1] Finitzo-Hieber T, Gerling IJ, Matkin ND, Cherow-Skalka E. A sound effects recognition test for the pediatric audiological evaluation. Ear Hear. 1980; 1 (5):271–276

[2] Jastreboff PJ, Jastreboff MM. Treatments for decreased sound tolerance (hyperacusis and misophonia). Semin Hear. 2014; 35(2):105–120

[3] Jastreboff MM, Jastreboff PJ. Components of decreased sound tolerance: hyperacusis, misophonia, phonophobia. ITHS News Lett. 2001; 2:5–7

[4] Johnson M. A tool for measuring hyperacusis. Hear J. 1999; 52:3

[5] Tyler RS, Pienkowski M, Roncancio ER, et al. A review of hyperacusis and future directions: part I. Definitions and manifestations. Am J Audiol. 2014; 23(4):402–419

[6] Pienkowski M, Tyler RS, Roncancio ER, et al. A review of hyperacusis and future directions: part II. Measurement, mechanisms, and treatment. Am J Audiol. 2014; 23(4):420–436

53 Cochlear Implantation in a Child with Single-Sided Deafness

Kristi Reed

53.1 Clinical History and Description

HN was born full term with the complication of maternal hemorrhage. He required a 4-day neonatal intensive care unit (NICU) stay and was diagnosed with bicuspid aortic valve and dilated ascending aorta. He passed his newborn hearing screen in the right ear and referred twice in the left. There was no reported family history of hearing loss. There were no concerns about speech and language development as HN was scoring above average on standardized speech evaluations. From age 2 to 3 years, HN had significant issues with chronic otitis media and was referred to an ear, nose, and throat (ENT) physician for pressure equalizing (PE) tubes. PE tubes were inserted when the patient was 4 years old.

53.2 Audiological Testing

At 2 months of age, auditory brainstem response (ABR) testing was performed using unmasked click stimuli in each ear. Thresholds were determined to be within normal limits (15 dB) bilaterally, and no further testing was recommended. Immediately following HN's PE tube surgery at the age of 4 years, a diagnostic ABR was performed. The ABR revealed normal auditory sensitivity in the right ear, and no responses to the output limits of the equipment in the left ear to click, tone burst, and masked bone conduction stimuli. Distortion product otoacoustic emissions (DPOAEs) were present in the right ear and absent in the left.

Behavioral booth testing was completed at the age of 4.3 years using conditioned play audiometry. In the left ear, no responses were obtained to the output limits of the equipment to either pure tone or speech stimuli. Speech recognition testing was completed in the sound field. At a + 5 dB SNR, patient's speech understanding was fair and at a 0 dB SNR, his understanding was poor (▶ Table 53.1).

53.3 Additional Testing

Magnetic resonance imaging (MRI) and computed tomography (CT) were also completed. The MRI revealed normal auditory nerve structures, bilaterally. The CT indicated HN had left enlarged vestibular aqueduct (EVA) and cochleovestibular dysplasia without a well-formed modiolus or apical turn. An auditory-verbal therapist completed a formal speech and language evaluation. HN was found to have receptive and expressive language scores in the normal range, but some articulation errors and hypernasal resonance were noted.

53.4 Intervention

HN's family was thoroughly counseled regarding all amplification options available to treat single-sided deafness (SSD), including contralateral routing of signal (CROS) hearing aids, bone conduction devices, and cochlear implant (CI). HN's parents chose a CI. HN was implanted with a Cochlear Nucleus CI24RE Contour Advance electrode. Intraoperative testing was conducted during implantation. Impedances were within normal limits for all electrodes, and AutoNRT responses were obtained for 9 out of the 12 electrodes. HN experienced no complications during surgery or recovery.

53.5 Outcomes

HN's CI was activated 3 weeks after surgery. At his 1-month follow-up appointment, aided testing was completed in the booth. In the CI-only condition (normal hearing ear occluded), HN responded within normal limits to all Ling 6 sounds, and his speech reception threshold was 20 dB HL (hearing level). His speech recognition scores were slightly worse than the scores prior to implantation. Over the next few months, however, his speech recognition scores continued to improve, and he was able to perform more difficult tests at each follow-up appointment (▶ Table 53.2). Subjectively, parents reported HN was hearing better at home and was asking for repetition less frequently. HN was putting the processor on himself and he was wearing it all waking hours without concern. Parents reported HN was enrolled in a mainstream kindergarten classroom and was doing very well in school.

Table 53.1 Thresholds in the left ear using conditioned play audiometry, and speech perception in sound field on the Lexical Neighborhood Test (LNT)

125 Hz	250 Hz	500 Hz	2,000 Hz	4,000 Hz	Speech perception in the sound field
NR	NR	NR	NR	NR	72%: + 5 dB SNR 32%: 0 dB SNR

Abbreviations: SNR, signal-to-noise ratio.

Table 53.2 Postactivation test results

Frequency-specific thresholds (dB HL) CI only (right ear occluded)							Speech reception threshold (dB)	Recorded speech perception in noise (50 dB HL)
	250 Hz	500 Hz	1,000 Hz	2,000 Hz	4,000 Hz	6,000 Hz	CI only (right ear occluded)	Binaural
1 mo	20	20	20	20	20	20	20	64% LNT (+ 10 dB SNR)
3 mo	5	5	10	10	10	15	15	84% LNT (+ 10 dB SNR)
6 mo	15	10	10	10	15	15	15	84% PBK (+ 10 dB SNR) 80% PBK (+ 5 dB SNR)
1 y	15	10	15	15	15	20	20	100% PBK (+ 10 dB SNR) 88% PBK (+ 5 DB SNR) 99% pediatric AZBio (+ 10 dB SNR)
1.6 y	15	10	10	15	15	15	15	80% PBK (+ 10 dB SNR) 99% pediatric AZBio (+ 10 dB SNR)

Abbreviations: CI, cochlear implant; LNT, Lexical Neighborhood Test; PBK, phonetically balanced kindergarten word lists; SNR, signal-to-noise ratio.

53.6 Questions for the Reader

1. When would you consider cochlear implantation in a child with SSD?
2. What patient or family factors would contraindicate cochlear implantation in a child with SSD?
3. What information should be provided to the patient and/or caregivers prior to making a decision about cochlear implantation?
4. Do you think progress with the implant could be affected by the child's age? If so, what would the impact be?
5. What other interventions or accommodations could benefit this child in his day-to-day life function?
6. What additional measures could be performed to evaluate benefit?

53.7 Discussion of Questions

1. **When would you consider cochlear implantation in a child with SSD?**
   CI should be a consideration for every child with SSD, but especially in cases where the hearing loss will likely progress in the contralateral ear. Aided testing with traditional amplification and bone conduction device may be helpful in determining whether the child is receiving benefit from other types of amplification before moving forward with CI. Aided testing should include speech recognition testing in noise and localization tasks, if possible. Bone conduction and CROS aids may not adequately address issues with localization and understanding in background noise.

2. **What patient or family factors would contraindicate cochlear implantation in a child with SSD?**
   Patient contraindications could include absence of the auditory nerve, malformations of inner ear anatomy that hinder electrode insertion, and medical complications that prevent the child from being a good surgical candidate. Family factors that could contraindicate cochlear implantation may include inappropriate expectations for their child's outcomes and

lack of consistent follow-through with audiology and speech therapy.

3. **What information should be provided to the patient and/or caregivers prior to making a decision about cochlear implantation?**
   Caregivers and patients (as age appropriate) should be fully informed about all of their amplification choices. They should be given information about how all of the different devices work within the auditory system and the benefits and drawbacks of each treatment option. They should be fully informed about the risks of surgery. It is critical that they understand the factors that influence outcomes and have appropriate expectations for their child, taking into account the child's history and any complicating medical issues.

4. **Do you think progress with the implant could be affected by the child's age? If so, what would the impact be?**
   Length of deafness can affect the level of benefit the child receives from the CI. Studies have shown that the earlier a child is implanted, the greater the chances of achieving true binaural hearing. A lack of auditory stimulation results in reorganization of the cortex very early in life. If intervention is delayed in a child with congenital SSD, the child may not perform as well as he would have had he been implanted earlier. Research suggests that implantation during the sensitive period of development correlates with better outcomes.[1,2]

5. **What other interventions or accommodations could benefit this child in his day-to-day life function?**
   Preferential seating and an FM (frequency modulation) system in the classroom, reduced background noise, and amplification that offers streaming capabilities.

6. **What additional measures could be performed to evaluate benefit?**
   Outcome measures such as the Children's Home Inventory for Listening Difficulties (CHILD) and the Speech, Spatial, and Qualities of Hearing Scale (SSQ) for children with impaired hearing would provide additional information about subjective benefit with the CI.

References

[1] Gordon K, Henkin Y, Kral A. Asymmetric hearing during development: the aural preference syndrome and treatment options. Pediatrics. 2015; 136 (1):141–153

[2] Kral A, Hubka P, Heid S, Tillein J. Single-sided deafness leads to unilateral aural preference within an early sensitive period. Brain. 2013; 136(Pt 1):180–193

Suggested Readings

[1] Erbele ID, Bernstein JG, Schuchman GI, Brungart DS, Rivera A. An initial experience of cochlear implantation for patients with single-sided deafness after prior osseointegrated hearing device. Otol Neurotol. 2015; 36(1):e24–e29

[2] Lieu JE. Speech-language and educational consequences of unilateral hearing loss in children. Arch Otolaryngol Head Neck Surg. 2004; 130(5):524–530

[3] Mertens G, Kleine Punte A, De Bodt M, Van de Heyning P. Binaural auditory outcomes in patients with postlingual profound unilateral hearing loss: 3 years after cochlear implantation. Audiol Neurootol. 2015; 20 Suppl 1:67–72

[4] van Zon A, Peters JP, Stegeman I, Smit AL, Grolman W. Cochlear implantation for patients with single-sided deafness or asymmetrical hearing loss: a systematic review of the evidence. Otol Neurotol. 2015; 36(2):209–219

[5] Vincent C, Arndt S, Firszt JB, et al. Identification and evaluation of cochlear implant candidates with asymmetrical hearing loss. Audiol Neurootol. 2015; 20 Suppl 1:87–89

[6] Vlastarakos PV, Nazos K, Tavoulari EF, Nikolopoulos TP. Cochlear implantation for single-sided deafness: the outcomes. An evidence-based approach. Eur Arch Otorhinolaryngol. 2014; 271(8):2119–2126

[7] Zeitler DM, Dorman MF, Natale SJ, Loiselle L, Yost WA, Gifford RH. Sound source localization and speech understanding in complex listening environments by single-sided deaf listeners after cochlear implantation. Otol Neurotol. 2015; 36(9):1467–1471

54 Unilateral Auditory Neuropathy Spectrum Disorder

Katherine Schaars

54.1 Clinical History and Description

At the age of 3 years, JW was brought in by his mother for a hearing test. His mother reported that JW passed his newborn hearing screen and had no family history of hearing loss. She stated that he had had normal overall growth and development. She further stated that JW used to use his right ear when listening on a telephone and had never complained of hearing issues, until 3 months prior. His mom reported that 3 months ago she started noticing that JW would not use his right ear anymore on the phone and instead insisted he needed to use his left ear. JW told his mother that he could not hear out of the right ear due to "rats" that were scratching in his ear. She reported that she started having concerns as she started noticing these consistent behaviors. Prior to being seen by a pediatric audiologist, JW had a hearing test at an ear, nose, and throat (ENT) doctor's office, where testing revealed normal hearing in the left ear and a hearing loss in the right ear. However, additional information regarding the degree or type of loss was unavailable at that time. While going over the initial case history, she was very upset and reported that she knew something was wrong with JW's hearing but that she had been unable to get any answers. While observing his mother become upset, JW told his mother that he would be able to hear again if the rats in his ear would just go away.

54.2 Audiologic Findings

Otoscopy revealed nonoccluding cerumen bilaterally. Tympanometry tracings were type A and suggested normal tympanic membrane movement, bilaterally on the day of test. Acoustic reflexes were not tested at this appointment. Distortion product otoacoustic emissions (DPOAEs) were robustly present, bilaterally, for all tested frequencies, 2,000 to 8,500 Hz, indicating normal outer hair cell function of the cochlea (▶ Fig. 54.1). A speech reception threshold (SRT) was obtained at 15 dB in the left ear, and pure-tone thresholds were obtained within normal limits for the left ear indicating normal auditory sensitivity. JW was very cooperative during the appointment. He was able to condition to the task using play audiometry and provide reliable responses when stimuli were presented to his left ear. However, when testing was attempted in his right ear, JW became very unreliable and was unable to condition to the task. He provided many false-positives in the right ear and none in the left ear. Fatigue was not suspected to be a factor, as JW's reliability was continuous throughout the appointment and only changed in response to the ear being tested. Speech, pure-tone, and narrowband stimuli were presented to the right ear; however, JW was unable to condition to the task and did not provide reliable responses. A reliable response was obtained in the right ear at 100 dB at 1,000 Hz; however, because masking was not used, the response may not represent JW's true threshold.

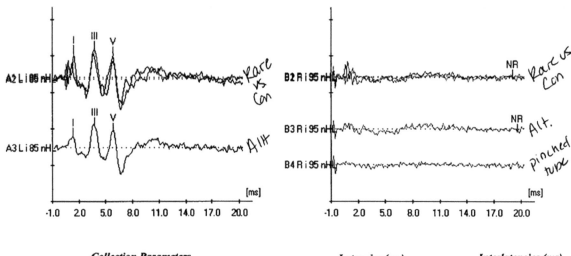

		Collection Parameters				Latencies (ms)					Interlatencies (ms)		
Wave	Transducer	Ear	Intensity	Type	Frequency	I	II	III	IV	V	I-III	III-V	I-V
A1	Insert Earphones	Left	85dB nHL	Click	N/A	1.45		3.78		5.87	2.33	2.08	4.42
A2	Insert Earphones	Left	85dB nHL	Click	N/A								
A3	Insert Earphones	Left	85dB nHL	Click	N/A	1.37		3.78		5.87	2.42	2.08	4.50
B1	Insert Earphones	Right	95dB nHL	Click	N/A								
B2	Insert Earphones	Right	95dB nHL	Click	N/A								
B3	Insert Earphones	Right	95dB nHL	Click	N/A								

Fig. 54.1 ABR tracings for click stimuli.

Additional information was not obtained due to time constraints.

Due to JW's inability to condition to the task in the right ear, along with the presented case history and inconsistent behavioral responses, it was recommended that an auditory brainstem response (ABR) test be completed. Family was given the option to attempt an unsedated ABR first, but his mom did not believe that JW would be able to remain quiet and still long enough to obtain accurate results. Therefore, a sedated ABR was scheduled.

54.3 Sedated ABR

Two days after initial behavioral testing was completed, a sedated ABR was performed (▶ Fig. 54.2). Results revealed synchronous neural responses to suprathreshold click stimuli in the left ear with no evidence of inversion of the waves to change in polarity, indicating an absence of auditory neuro-

pathy spectrum disorder (ANSD). Estimated threshold responses to tone-burst stimuli were consistent with normal peripheral auditory sensitivity in the left ear. No response to any presented stimuli, click or tone burst, was obtained in the right ear to the limits of the equipment. To evaluate ANSD, a suprathreshold click stimuli is presented to determine if reversal is noted in the waves with change in polarity. Should this occur, it may suggest a dyssynchronous auditory system. Due to the output limits of the equipment, responses of the waveforms to change in polarity were unable to be evaluated as the equipment was unable to produce suprathreshold stimuli. However, if present, the cochlear microphonic can also be evaluated. The cochlear microphonic represents response from the hair cells, while the ABR waveforms are generated by the auditory nerve. Reversal in the cochlear microphonic with change in polarity of the stimulus is considered normal. While small, a stimulus-following cochlear microphonic was observed to both condensation and rarefaction stimuli and was absent to a pinched tube with no stimuli, to rule out the possibility of

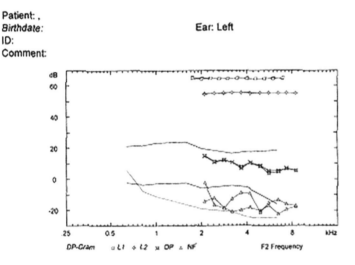

BIO-LOGIC OTOACOUSTIC EMISSIONS (OAE) REPORT - Page 1 of 2

Fig. 54.2 DPOAEs from first appointment.

Patient: ,
Birthdate:
ID:
Comment:

Ear: Left

Left: 26-Feb-14: -: 2-8.5 kHz Diagnostic Test: 14B26D02.OAE

L1(dB)	L2(dB)	F1(Hz)	F2(Hz)	GM(Hz)	DP(dB)	NF(dB)	DP-NF(dB)
65.0	55.1	6984	8531	7719	5.3	-17.8	23.1
64.8	55.5	6047	7359	6671	6.7	-19.5	26.2
64.6	55.4	5297	6469	5854	5.1	-22.5	27.6
64.7	55.4	4594	5625	5083	5.2	-17.0	22.2
64.7	55.4	4031	4922	4454	8.5	-20.5	29.0
64.9	55.3	3469	4219	3825	10.4	-18.4	28.8
64.7	55.3	3000	3656	3312	6.7	-20.0	26.7
64.6	55.5	2625	3188	2893	10.4	-21.1	31.5
84.8	55.2	2297	2813	2542	12.0	-18.8	30.8
64.8	55.2	2016	2438	2217	10.9	-12.2	23.1
65.3	54.7	1734	2109	1913	14.7	-14.6	29.3
65.0	55.0	6984	8531	7719	5.2	-17.2	22.4
64.7	55.5	6047	7359	6671	7.0	-16.1	23.1
64.6	55.4	5297	6469	5854	4.7	-13.5	18.2
64.6	55.4	4594	5625	5083	3.6	-15.5	19.1
64.6	55.3	4031	4922	4454	8.1	-21.6	29.7
64.8	55.2	3469	4219	3825	10.3	-9.6	19.9
64.6	55.3	3000	3656	3312	7.8	-9.1	16.9
64.6	55.5	2625	3188	2893	10.5	-12.9	23.4
64.8	55.3	2297	2813	2542	12.1	-19.1	31.2
64.6	55.2	2016	2438	2217	11.1	-16.9	28.0

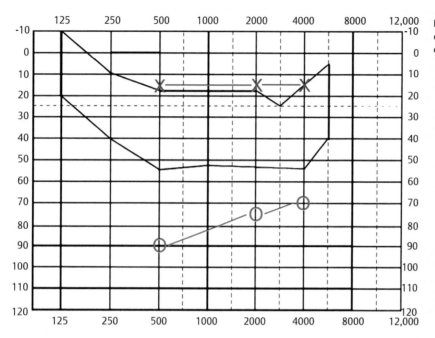

Fig. 54.3 Pure-tone thresholds from hearing aid exam and select appointment. O, right ear air conduction; X, left ear air conduction.

the response as artifact, suggesting outer hair/cochlear contribution and preservation. These findings may suggest ANSD.

54.3.1 Question: What is the Probable Diagnosis? What Recommendations/Referrals Should Be Made?

The family was counseled that, based on the sedated ABR results in conjunction with the present DPOAEs obtained at JW's last appointment, responses suggest a neural/retrocochlear pathology. JW's mom was informed that based on the ABR testing, imaging, such as a magnetic resonance imaging (MRI), may be useful in establishing a differential diagnosis. She was encouraged to schedule an appointment with JW's ENT to set up a referral to radiology. The ENT ordered a computed tomography (CT) scan, which came back normal, but never ordered an MRI despite multiple recommendations by his audiologist. The family was also referred to genetics, and a hearing aid evaluation was set up to discuss amplification options.

54.3.2 Hearing Aid Exam and Select

The family did not return for 5 months. At that time, JW's mom reported that she was having difficulty accepting his hearing loss and expressed concern that she did not have any answer to why this was happening. Booth testing was completed to obtain information regarding how JW responded behaviorally to sound.

Testing Completed at Hearing Aid Evaluation

Otoscopy revealed clear canals bilaterally. Tympanometry tracings were type A and revealed normal middle ear function bilaterally on the day of test. An SRT was obtained at 85 dB in the right ear and 15 dB in the left ear. Pure-tone thresholds revealed normal hearing sensitivity in the left ear and a severe rising to moderately

severe hearing loss in the right ear. Bone conduction was unable to be tested due to patient fatigue (▶ Fig. 54.3).

54.4 Outcomes

JW has since been fitted with a behind-the-ear hearing aid with a custom mold for his right ear. The hearing aid was programmed to his behavioral audiogram threshold responses and verified using simulated real-ear measures. Once fitted with the hearing aid, JW stated that it sounded wonderful, and he loved wearing it. He now wears the hearing aid consistently and daily at home and at school. Aided testing in the monaural condition, with his better, left ear plugged, revealed thresholds within normal limits and SRT at 25 dB HL. Word recognition in quiet is excellent (92%) for average speech and fair (72%) for soft speech. Since being fitted with amplification, he has become more reliable in booth testing. Prior to being fitted with amplification, JW fatigued quickly and had difficulty completing speech testing in the right ear. Since being fitted with amplification, he is now able to complete a full audiogram, 250 to 8,000 Hz, unaided and complete aided testing in one appointment (▶ Fig. 54.4). He no longer demonstrates a significant difference in his ability to perform tasks in the right versus left ear. JW reported that he no longer hears "rats" and is making appropriate progress in school. It is possible that the hearing aid was able to mask tinnitus, which he perceived as tinnitus.

54.5 Questions for the Reader

1. What methods, beyond testing in the booth, could be used to monitor JW's hearing aid benefit?
2. What testing would you want to complete during an aided appointment?
3. How often would you monitor JW's hearing?
4. What is another intervention that may be considered if amplification no longer provides adequate benefit?
5. What testing is needed to diagnose ANSD?

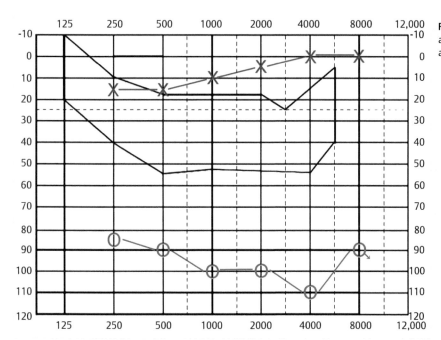

Fig. 54.4 Pure-tone thresholds from most recent audiogram. O, right ear air conduction; X, left ear air conduction; Arrows, no response.

54.6 Discussion of Questions

1. **What methods, beyond testing in the booth, could be used to monitor JW's hearing aid benefit?**

   Booth testing provides significant data regarding thresholds at different frequencies and the ability to understand speech in a controlled setting. However, it is possible that the controlled nature of booth testing may fail to identify every problem a child has in other daily listening environments. For example, a child may perform well in speech testing due to the limited amount of time he/she has to pay attention, yet struggle throughout a longer school day, suggesting that a remote-microphone system may be needed to reduce listening fatigue. Questionnaires can provide useful subjective information to determine where the family, teacher, or patient is encountering daily communication difficulties. By providing questionnaires before and after amplification, the audiologist can obtain a better idea of where amplification is beneficial and what areas still need to be addressed. Questionnaires are developed to provide different benefits. The SIFTER (Screening Instrument for Targeting Educational Risks) focuses on educational risk and may help the audiologist make beneficial referrals to other professionals (i.e., speech therapists or tutoring services) as well as ensure that all appropriate classroom accommodations, such as priority seating, are being utilized. The COW (Children's Outcome Worksheet) allows families to specify five situations where improved hearing is desired, thus allowing the audiologist to focus on personalized results. Finally, questionnaires can facilitate a teamwork approach that allows parents and teachers to become more involved in the child's success.

2. **What testing would you want to complete during an aided appointment?**

   In any individual where monaural amplification is being used in the presence of a better ear, it is important to perform testing in both the monaural and binaural conditions. Standard aided testing should include SRTs, word or sentence recognition in quiet and noise, aided thresholds using narrowband noise or warble tones, and Ling 6 stimuli when appropriate. As aided testing is completed in the sound-field, pure-tone stimuli cannot be used, as it creates standing waves; therefore, narrowband noise or warble tones must be used instead. Word recognition should be completed in quiet at soft and normal conversational levels. Testing in the monaural condition should be completed with the better, nonaided ear plugged. This allows for the hearing aid to be tested without the benefit of the other ear. Testing in the binaural condition should be completed with the hearing aid on and the better ear unplugged. It is important to monitor that the aided responses in the monaural condition are better than in the monaural condition unaided in the same ear. Testing completed in the binaural condition allows the audiologist to check that aiding the ANSD ear is not negatively impacting performance for the better hearing ear. Binaural testing should reveal responses that are better than the monaural condition of the amplified ear alone and similar to, if not better than, the monaural condition of the better, unaided ear. If responses in the binaural aided condition are worse than the monaural condition of the better, unaided ear, then amplification may need to be discontinued due to the negative impact. Questionnaires would be beneficial in this situation to help determine the patient's perceived benefit of amplification is consistent with behavioral testing.

3. **How often would you monitor JW's hearing?**

   In pediatric patients, it is more difficult to get an accurate, complete audiogram and aided thresholds in one appointment, so more frequent follow-up is necessary. After the initial hearing aid fitting, follow-up testing should be completed after 1 month, which allows the brain to have time to adapt the new hearing aid. For all patients, but especially for those with ANSD, it is important to counsel the family of possible negative reactions to the hearing aid and to encourage the family to call if they notice any negative responses to the hearing aid. If so, an appointment may be set up sooner. Aided testing should be completed at the 1-month follow-up, or over the course of a few weeks should the patient be unable to complete testing during one appointment. JW was initially followed up every 3 months to determine if he had any fluctuation in hearing and to monitor aided benefit. Once his hearing appeared stable over a year, it was determined that we would monitor his hearing every 6 months going forward. It is important that the family understands that fluctuating hearing loss may occur in children with ANSD and the importance of calling when JW reports that his hearing aid is too soft or too loud, as this may be a sign of fluctuation.

4. **What is another intervention that may be considered if amplification no longer provides adequate benefit?**
Another option for children with ANSD may be a cochlear implant (CI). It is important that any child considered for a CI be evaluated by a CI surgeon and an audiologist who specializes in CI to determine if he or she is a candidate. In JW's case, there was normal speech and language development and his mother was strongly opposed to a CI. However, a CI evaluation should be completed in children who are not making appropriate progress in speech recognition and language development. Once it has been determined that the child is not making progress, even with appropriately programmed hearing aids, they should be referred for a CI evaluation as soon as possible. In children identified with ANSD under the age of 1 year, especially those who were born premature, a repeat ABR is recommended at 6 months of age

to monitor ABR waveforms. In children in whom improvement is seen, several ABRs may be needed to monitor these changes.

5. **What testing is needed to diagnose ANSD?**
In order to establish a diagnosis of ANSD, it is important to evaluate the function of the cochlear hair cells and the auditory nerve. The minimum battery would include OAEs, either transient-evoked or distortion product, and a click ABR. The ABR should be performed at suprathreshold level, 80 to 90 dB nHL, evaluating the cochlear microphonic for inversion with the change in polarity. It is important to run a rarefaction-leading and condensation-leading polarity wave separately to truly evaluate the nerve. Other tests, such as acoustic reflex thresholds, should be utilized if possible; however, these tests may be difficult to obtain in very young infants.

Suggested Reading

[1] American Academy of Audiology Clinical Practice Guidelines. Pediatric Amplification. June 2013

[2] Guidelines Development Conference on the Identification and Management of Infants with Auditory Neuropathy. International Newborn Hearing Screening Conference; June 19–21, 2008; Como, Italy. Available at: http://www.thechildrenshospital.org/conditions/speech/danielscenter/ANSD-Guidelines.aspx

[3] Madell JR, Flexer C, eds. Pediatric Audiology: Diagnosis, Technology, and Management. New York, NY: Thieme; 2008

[4] Katz J, Medwetsky L, Burkard R, Hood L, eds. Handbook of Clinical Audiology. Baltimore, MD: Lippincott Williams & Wilkins; 2009

55 Cochlear Implantation for Enlarged Vestibular Aqueduct

Jane Burton and Meredith Holcomb

55.1 Clinical History and Description

William, age 10 years, presented to the clinic with complaints of decrease in hearing sensitivity following a head trauma incident during baseball practice.

William was previously followed at another site for a history of sensorineural hearing loss in the right ear, with normal hearing sensitivity in the left ear. He reportedly passed his newborn hearing screening in the left ear and referred in the right ear. Previous ENT work-up did not include radiographic imaging.

William was evaluated at our clinic for a hearing evaluation at 10 years of age. Six weeks prior to the visit, William was struck in the head with a pitch while playing baseball. This resulted in complaints of increased hearing difficulty and increased bilateral tinnitus. He denied symptoms of dizziness.

55.2 Audiologic Testing

Results from initial audiological assessment revealed normal hearing sensitivity from 250 to 2,000 Hz, sloping to a moderately severe sensorineural hearing loss in the left ear, and a severe to profound sensorineural hearing loss in the right ear (▶ Fig. 55.1). Speech reception thresholds (SRTs) were 5 dB HL in the left ear and 75 dB HL in the right ear. Word recognition scores using recorded NU-6 (Northwestern University Auditory Test Number Six) materials were 100% for the left ear (tested at 40 dB HL) and 8% for the right ear (tested at 100 dB HL, the patient's most comfortable level). Type A tympanograms were obtained bilaterally. Results indicated a significant decrease in hearing sensitivity, bilaterally, and a decrease in word recognition in the right ear compared to previous records.

55.3 Questions for the Reader

1. What diagnosis does the patient's history and audiological presentation suggest? Are any hallmark symptoms of this diagnosis missing?
2. What additional testing could be recommended due to the suspected diagnosis?
3. What recommendations for aural rehabilitation might you consider for this patient?

55.4 Discussion of Questions

1. **What diagnosis does the patient's history and audiological presentation suggest? Are any hallmark symptoms of this diagnosis missing?**

The sudden decrease in hearing and increase in tinnitus following a blow to the head as well as the marked congenital asymmetrical hearing loss are suggestive of enlarged vestibular aqueduct (EVA). EVA is characterized by congenital hearing loss, often asymmetric, ranging in severity from normal hearing sensitivity to profound hearing loss.[1,2,3] For cases of EVA, at least 40%[3] and up to 90 to 100% are bilateral.[2,4,5] Hearing loss is often progressive or fluctuating,[2] with annual decreases of 4 to 25 dB HL measured in some studies.[1,6] Head trauma is often associated with decreases in hearing, as well as onset or increase in tinnitus or balance symptoms. These symptoms are thought to be a result of physical or chemical damage from a rush of endolymph into the cochlea, causing either physical damage to the hair cells or a toxic chemical imbalance in the inner ear.[1]

William does not exhibit low-frequency air–bone gaps often present in patients with EVA. Conductive components

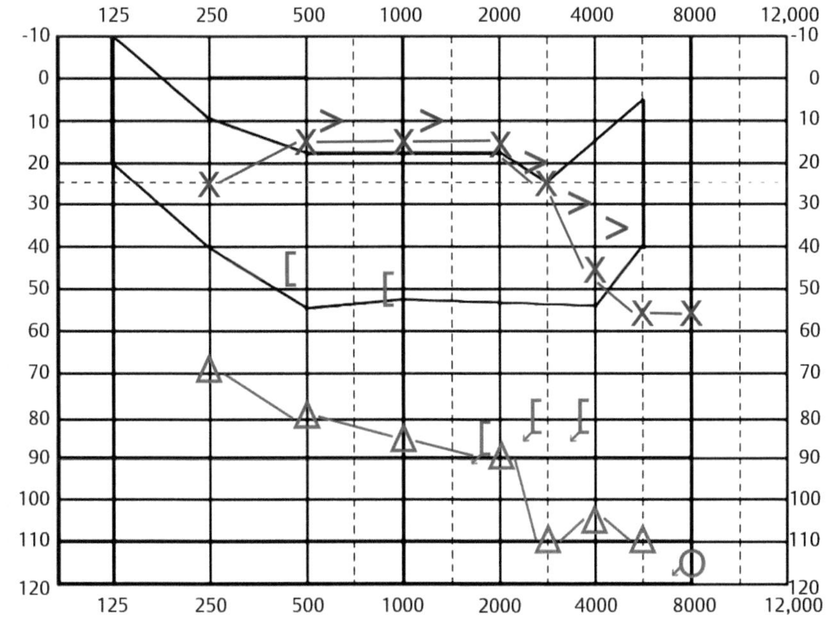

Fig. 55.1 Initial audiogram obtained at 10 years of age. O, right ear air conduction; X, left ear air conduction; >, left ear bone conduction; △, right ear air conduction masked; [, right ear bone conduction masked; Arrows, no response.

are observed in as few as 11 to 28%[2,3] and in as many as 80 to 100% of patients with EVA,[4,7,8,9,10] in the presence of normal tympanograms. The third window theory suggests that the enlarged endolymphatic duct acts as a third window in addition to the oval and round windows.[11] Sound pressure from the stapes may be directed away from the basilar membrane into the aqueduct, causing an increase in air conduction thresholds and, thus, a discrepancy between air and bone conduction not otherwise due to middle ear dysfunction.[8,9] Because of the severity of hearing loss in William's right ear, bone conduction thresholds could not be obtained beyond 50 dB HL, at which level William indicated vibrotactile responses. Thus, it is possible an air–bone gap was present in this ear, but could not be measured.

2. **What additional testing could be recommended due to the suspected diagnosis?**

EVA is diagnosed by temporal bone computed tomography (CT) scan or magnetic resonance imaging (MRI). The patient should be referred to an otologist or a pediatric otolaryngologist with expertise in pediatric hearing loss with recommendation of medical work-up for suspected EVA. In order to further confirm suspicions prior to completion of recommended imaging, multifrequency tympanometry can be used to identify patients with EVA. The resonant frequency of the middle ear system will be lower due to the large endolymphatic duct and sac.[5] Recent studies have also suggested that wide-band acoustic immittance will identify third window disorders, including EVA and semicircular canal dehiscence (SCD). A characteristic notch is observed at 1,000 Hz in patients with SCD[12] or EVA.[13] Additionally, vestibular evoked myogenic potential (VEMP) testing is an appropriate option for older children or adult patients who were not previously diagnosed at a younger age. VEMPs will be present at lower presentation levels and higher amplitudes in patients with EVA and normal immittance measures due to the third window effect.[10] If a true conductive component is present, VEMPs will be absent; therefore, this testing would assist with differential diagnosis.

3. **What recommendations for aural rehabilitation might you consider for this patient?**

- Traditional hearing aid: A traditional hearing aid could be considered for the left ear. When fitting hearing aids on patients with EVA who would benefit from amplification, there are two special considerations the audiologist should remember. First, the selected instrument should allow for extra gain headroom because EVA is often associated with progressive hearing loss. Second, following confirmation of the EVA diagnosis, bone conduction thresholds should be omitted in the fitting to avoid overamplification. A remote microphone system could be used with the left hearing aid in the classroom to facilitate better audibility of the teacher's instruction. While a power hearing aid is available for the right ear, it is not recommended due to the severity of the hearing loss and the extremely poor word recognition score.
- Contralateral-routing-of-signal (CROS) hearing system or an osseointegrated (OI) device: While both options route sound from the right ear to the left ear, an OI device is

more invasive and requires surgery. Because of William's academic success and his risk for progressive hearing loss in the left ear, the family was not interested in either option.
- Cochlear implant (CI): The severity of hearing loss and poor word recognition in the right ear certainly fit the candidacy criteria for a CI, but the better hearing left ear would be a contraindication per FDA criteria. A CI is a possible recommendation for the right ear if the hearing loss in William's left ear progresses. Though current FDA pediatric CI candidacy requires severe-to-profound hearing loss in both ears, off-label cochlear implantation may be considered before William's left ear progresses to that degree. Off-label cochlear implantation is a decision to be made between the patient and provider. Counseling regarding risks, alternatives, and insurance coverage should be completed with the patient and family before moving forward with surgery. Patients with EVA are known to have excellent outcomes with CIs,[14,15] with better outcomes observed for EVA patients without additional cochleovestibular anomalies.[4]
- No Intervention: Some clinicians will forgo intervention in this case as hearing in the left ear is adequate for William to communicate successfully. However, it is well documented that children with unilateral hearing loss perform worse in noise and exhibit more academic delays as compared to their normal-hearing peers.

55.5 Diagnosis and Recommended Treatment

CT scan of the temporal bones without contrast revealed EVAs bilaterally (▶ Fig. 55.2; ▶ Fig. 55.3). William continued to receive frequent audiological monitoring due to this diagnosis. Over the course of 1 year, the left ear decreased slightly, with normal hearing sensitivity from 250 to 1,500 Hz, sloping to a high-frequency sensorineural hearing loss, fluctuating between moderate and severe degrees of severity (▶ Fig. 55.4). His left ear was then fitted with a behind-the-ear hearing aid.

Approximately 15 months after William initially presented to the clinic, he returned with complaints of decreased hearing in the left ear following several days of sinus pressure and congestion. Hearing loss in the left ear had progressed to a moderate mixed hearing loss from 250 to 750 Hz, sloping to a severe-to-profound sensorineural hearing loss from 1,000 to 8,000 Hz. An SRT was obtained at 65 dB HL. Word recognition score using recorded NU-6 materials revealed a decline from 100 to 44% for the left ear (tested at 90 dB HL, the patient's most comfortable level). Type A tympanogram was recorded in the left ear (▶ Fig. 55.5).

The rapid decrease in left ear hearing sensitivity prompted initial recommendation for a CI evaluation for the right ear. William was initially prescribed systemic steroids and later received intratympanic steroid injections to improve the left ear hearing sensitivity. Serial audiograms over the next month indicated fluctuating left ear hearing loss (▶ Fig. 55.6; ▶ Fig. 55.7).

William completed an evaluation for CI candidacy in the right ear where he scored 32% for aided speech perception testing

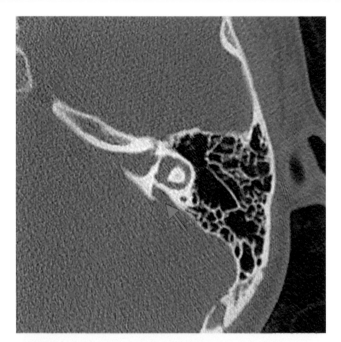

Fig. 55.2 Left ear CT scan (*arrow* identifies enlarged vestibular aqueduct).

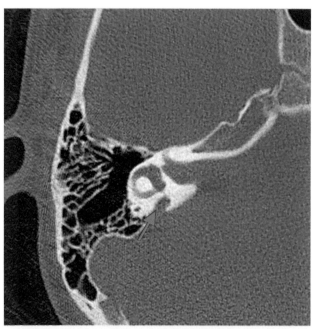

Fig. 55.3 Right ear CT scan (*arrow* identifies enlarged vestibular aqueduct).

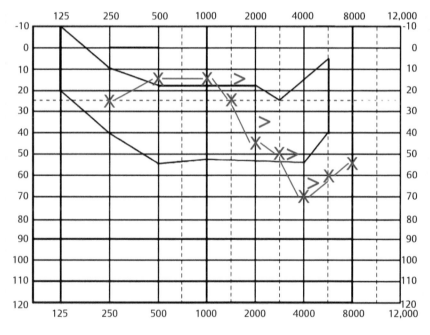

Fig. 55.4 Audiogram obtained approximately 1 year after initial visit. X, left ear air conduction; >, left ear bone conduction.

using AzBio sentences in a quiet test condition. CI surgery for the right ear was subsequently scheduled.

Immediately prior to surgery, William experienced yet another significant decrease in left ear hearing thresholds (▶ Fig. 55.8), and both ears met FDA criteria for CI candidacy. The audiologist, surgeon, and family elected to implant the poorer hearing right ear first.

William was successfully implanted, and at his initial activation, he displayed improved articulation of the /s/ sound when wearing his CI processor. He was also able to distinguish different speakers' voices at activation using the CI alone. His most recent CI audiogram (5 years post-op) revealed aided sound-field detection thresholds of 25 to 30 dB HL for the frequencies of 250 to 8,000 Hz and an SRT of 25 dB HL (▶ Fig. 55.9). Speech perception scores using AzBio sentence testing with presentation level of 60 dB SPL were 82% in quiet, 84% in + 10 SNR (signal-to-noise ratio) noise condition, and 46% in + 5 SNR noise condition using his CI alone at his most recent evaluation (▶ Table 55.1). His right CI speech perception score has improved 50% since surgery (AzBio Quiet Condition).

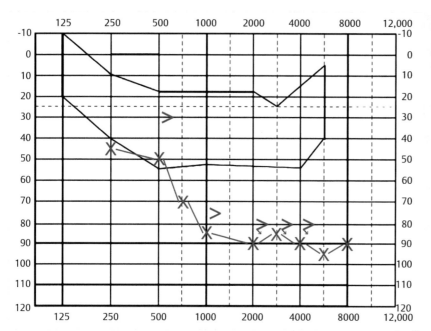

Fig. 55.5 Audiogram obtained approximately 15 months after initial visit. X, left ear air conduction; >, left ear bone conduction; Arrows, no response.

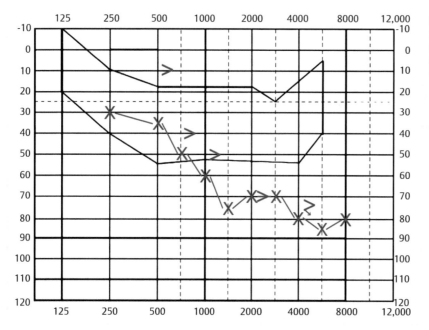

Fig. 55.6 First audiogram obtained after intra-tympanic steroids were administered following abrupt decrease in hearing sensitivity. X, left ear air conduction; >, left ear bone conduction; Arrows, no response.

55.6 Outcome

William is now 17 years old, and he uses a CI in the right ear. He no longer uses a hearing aid in the left ear due to yet another decrease in hearing sensitivity and no perceived benefit with the hearing aid (▶ Fig. 55.10).

He does not use a personal remote microphone system in the classroom. He trialed a remote microphone system for a few months, but he did not like it. He is on the A honor roll in the academically gifted program, and performs well in his advanced placement classes. He is also a terrific athlete and recently received a full athletic college scholarship and will pitch on the baseball team. He is aware of the risks of head trauma, but he chooses to pursue his dream of becoming a Major League baseball player.

To date, William has not pursued a CI evaluation or surgery for the left ear, as he is concerned with the possible postoperative vestibular side effects that could interfere with baseball. According to his most recent audiograms, William continues to experience fluctuations in left ear hearing sensitivity, ranging from a mild-to-severe mixed hearing loss to a flat severe sensorineural hearing loss. Cochlear implantation was a successful intervention for this case. William quickly improved his speech understanding with his right CI and continues to enjoy and benefit from his device.

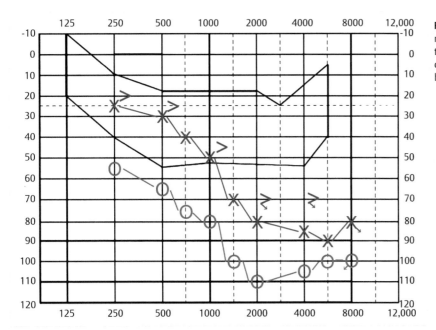

Fig. 55.7 Second audiogram obtained approximately 1 month after the initiation of intratympanic steroid treatment. O, right ear air conduction; X, left ear air conduction; >, left ear bone conduction; Arrows, no response.

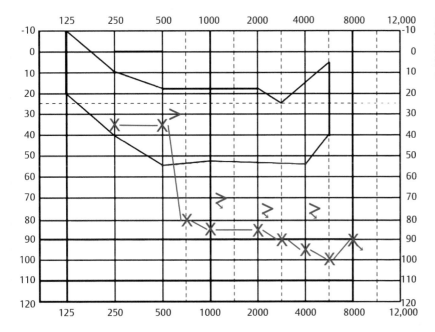

Fig. 55.8 Audiogram obtained immediately prior to cochlear implant surgery for the right ear. Note an additional decrease in hearing sensitivity for the left ear. X, left ear air conduction; >, left ear bone conduction; Arrows, no response.

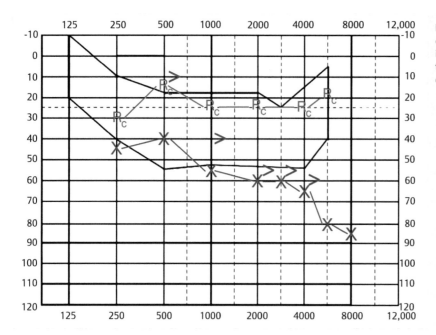

Fig. 55.9 Audiogram showing aided sound-field detection thresholds with use of the cochlear implant for the right ear and unaided thresholds for the left ear. X, left ear air conduction; >, left ear bone conduction; RC, right cochlear implant.

Table 55.1 Speech recognition results obtained with use of cochlear implant for the right ear alone. This testing was completed 5 years after he received his cochlear implant

Test	List #	Score
CNC: words	9	72%
CNC: phonemes	9	86%
AzBio sentences: quiet	1	82%
AzBio sentences: + 10 SNR	2	84%
AzBio sentences: + 5 SNR	3	46%

Abbreviations: CNC, consonant-nucleus-consonant; SNR signal-to-noise ratio.

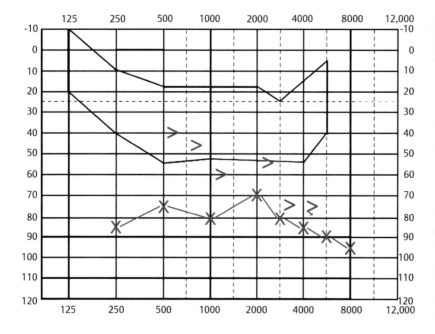

Fig. 55.10 Audiogram with unaided hearing thresholds for the left ear obtained at 17 years of age. X, left ear air conduction; >, left ear bone conduction; Arrows, no response.

References

[1] Jackler RK, De La Cruz A. The large vestibular aqueduct syndrome. Laryngoscope. 1989; 99(12):1238–1242, discussion 1242–1243

[2] Madden C, Halsted M, Benton C, Greinwald J, Choo D. Enlarged vestibular aqueduct syndrome in the pediatric population. Otol Neurotol. 2003; 24 (4):625–632

[3] Arjmand EM, Webber A. Audiometric findings in children with a large vestibular aqueduct. Arch Otolaryngol Head Neck Surg. 2004; 130(10):1169–1174

[4] Pritchett C, Zwolan T, Huq F, et al. Variations in the cochlear implant experience in children with enlarged vestibular aqueduct. Laryngoscope. 2015; 125 (9):2169–2174

[5] Sato E, Nakashima T, Lilly DJ, et al. Tympanometric findings in patients with enlarged vestibular aqueducts. Laryngoscope. 2002; 112(9):1642–1646

[6] Govaerts PJ, Casselman J, Daemers K, De Ceulaer G, Somers T, Offeciers FE. Audiological findings in large vestibular aqueduct syndrome. Int J Pediatr Otorhinolaryngol. 1999; 51(3):157–164

[7] Nakashima T, Ueda H, Furuhashi A, et al. Air-bone gap and resonant frequency in large vestibular aqueduct syndrome. Am J Otol. 2000; 21(5):671–674

[8] Mimura T, Sato E, Sugiura M, Yoshino T, Naganawa S, Nakashima T. Hearing loss in patients with enlarged vestibular aqueduct: air-bone gap and audiological Bing test. Int J Audiol. 2005; 44(8):466–469

[9] Merchant SN, Nakajima HH, Halpin C, et al. Clinical investigation and mechanism of air-bone gaps in large vestibular aqueduct syndrome. Ann Otol Rhinol Laryngol. 2007; 116(7):532–541

[10] Zhou G, Gopen Q. Characteristics of vestibular evoked myogenic potentials in children with enlarged vestibular aqueduct. Laryngoscope. 2011; 121 (1):220–225

[11] Seo YJ, Kim J, Choi JY. Correlation of vestibular aqueduct size with air-bone gap in enlarged vestibular aqueduct syndrome. Laryngoscope. 2016; 126 (7):1633–1638

[12] Merchant GR, Röösli C, Niesten ME, et al. Power reflectance as a screening tool for the diagnosis of superior semicircular canal dehiscence. Otol Neurotol. 2015; 36(1):172–177

[13] Smith BA, McCaslin DL. Audiovestibular findings in children with enlarged vestibular aqueduct. ENT Audiol News. 2015; 24(5):73–76

[14] Miyamoto RT, Bichey BG, Wynne MK, Kirk KI. Cochlear implantation with large vestibular aqueduct syndrome. Laryngoscope. 2002; 112(7, Pt 1):1178–1182

[15] Lee KH, Lee J, Isaacson B, Kutz JW, Roland PS. Cochlear implantation in children with enlarged vestibular aqueduct. Laryngoscope. 2010; 120(8):1675–1681

Suggested Reading

[1] Vestibular Disorders Association. Enlarged vestibular aqueduct (EVA). Available at: http://vestibular.org/enlarged-vestibular-aqueduct-syndrome-evas

[2] National Institute on Deafness and Other Communication Disorders. Enlarged vestibular aqueducts and childhood hearing loss. Available at: https://www.nidcd.nih.gov/health/enlarged-vestibular-aqueducts-and-childhood-hearing-loss#treat

56 Does Stimulation Rate Matter?

Bari Pham

56.1 Clinical History and Description

In 2016, a 16-year-old bimodal patient transferred services to an outpatient children's hospital facility to manage hearing aid and cochlear implant (CI) services. This patient originally passed his newborn hearing screen. His medical history was significant for chronic otitis media with insertion of multiple sets of pressure equalization tubes. According to chart notes, the hearing loss was first identified at age 4, and soon after, he was fitted with monaural amplification due to the results indicating a mild to profound sensorineural loss in the right ear and a profound sensorineural hearing loss in the left ear. Magnetic resonance imaging (MRI) revealed enlarged vestibular aqueduct for the left ear and a normal temporal bone anatomy for the right ear. The otologist suspected that the hearing loss in the right ear was related to a structural abnormality not visible on MRI; however, computed tomography (CT) was not ordered at the time. Because of progression of hearing loss in right ear and ongoing speech concerns, CI candidacy was sought when the child was 6 years old. At age 6 years, he was implanted with a Cochlear Nucleus 24 Freedom CI in the left ear, and he used a Freedom external sound processor system. At age 12, he was upgraded to the Cochlear Nucleus 5 sound processor system.

Because of insurance problems and family custodial issues, the patient had been using a loaner hearing aid for the right ear for over a year. Once insurance was obtained and services were transferred, the patient was scheduled for an audiological evaluation.

56.2 Audiologic Testing

At the first appointment at the children's hospital outpatient facility, hearing levels in the right ear and maintenance map settings were evaluated. His mother expressed interest in a hybrid CI for the right ear and an upgrade in the left ear. The patient reported a preference of his hearing aid over his CI. His CI MAP parameters included Advanced Combination Encoder (ACE) strategy, MP1 + 2 mode, stimulation rate at 2,400 pps, maxima at 10, and pulse width at 12. The MAP stimulation levels (i.e., T and C levels) were set with a flat profile with an electrical dynamic range of 50 clinical units.

Remapping was completed after detection responses were obtained in the sound field (▶ Fig. 56.1, ▶ Fig. 56.2). AutoNRT was performed on nine electrodes and imported into maintenance MAP settings. Using a discrimination task (i.e., count the beeps), T levels were measured, and C levels were adjusted to provide an electrical dynamic range of 40 clinical units across the electrode array. Overall, T levels were reduced 10 to 20 clinical units as compared to his original MAP, possibly due to the higher than expected T levels with the previous MAP (▶ Fig. 56.1).

The patient was instructed to try new MAP settings for 1 month and return for complete CI evaluation to assess speech perception skills for possible bilateral CI candidacy. In the meantime, the patient returned for fitting of a Resound Linx 2 7–88 behind-the-ear hearing aid in the right ear using real-ear measures. The patient returned 1 month later, and speech perception scores were obtained using recorded

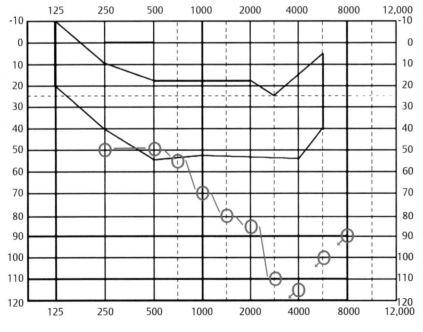

Fig. 56.1 Unaided hearing thresholds in right ear at initial evaluation. O, right ear air conduction.

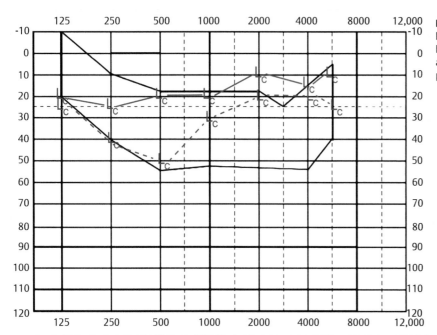

Fig. 56.2 LC, left cochlear implant; short dashed lines, initial evaluation with left cochlear implant before mapping; long dashed lines, initial evaluation after mapping left cochlear implant (no parameter changes).

stimuli for low-level speech and for speech in noise conditions (▶ Table 56.1; ▶ Table 56.2).

Based on the overall test results, bilateral candidacy was not recommended due to poor speech understanding in noise with the CI. The patient reported that he preferred his hearing aid over his CI. Aural rehabilitation recommendations were made along with a follow-up mapping appointment with a representative from Cochlear Americas to further review the patient's MAP settings to determine if more specific parameters should be adjusted that would improve overall understanding.

which was not previously detected, and he noticed sound at further distances. The patient was provided three different programs with various dynamic ranges from 30 to 40 clinical units, to allow him the ability to modify volume based on the environment.

The patient returned 1 month later, now at age 17, and reported improved hearing and understanding. He did not vary program settings, and remained on program 1, which had a 35 clinical unit dynamic range. His mother stated she could now call his name at greater distances, and he would respond. Testing with the implant alone revealed the following results (▶ Fig. 56.3).

Follow-up fine tuning to T and C levels was conducted using a discrimination task (i.e., count the beeps) along with loudness balancing. The majority of T levels remained stable, but some were increased by 5 to 10 clinical units. The dynamic range was also evaluated, and the patient preferred 40 clinical units.

Table 56.1 Speech perception scores 1 month following remapping

Recorded stimuli	SRT	Quiet NU-6 @55 dB HL	AzBio +5 SNR	NU-6 +5 SNR
Binaural	20 dB HL	72%	75%	36%
Right (HA)	30 dB HL	58%	58%	40%
Left (CI)	25 dB HL	64%	23%	0%

Parameters that were specifically unusual were the high stimulation rate and reduced pulse width. A new map was created with default parameters including the ACE coding strategy, a stimulation rate of 900 pps/channel, maxima at 8, and a pulse width of 25. To save time and ensure that changing the stimulation rate was a good direction to start with this patient, T and C levels were found on one electrode and all others interpolated based on recommendation by the representative from Cochlear. Typically, T and C levels would be checked on several electrodes, but due to the significant adjustments made with various MAP parameters, interpolation was pursued based on middle electrode responses. A dynamic range of 35 clinical units was set, and the implant was activated. The patient immediately reported improved understanding. He was asked to repeat back open-set sentences without visual cues, and he obtained 100% correct. He also noticed that he could hear snapping at ear level,

Table 56.2 Hearing thresholds (dB HL) 1 month following remapping

	250 Hz	500 Hz	1 KHz	2 KHz	4 KHz	6 KHz
Binaural	30	25	30	20	25	25
Right (HA)	35	30	40	40	45	50
Left (CI)	25	25	25	20	15	25

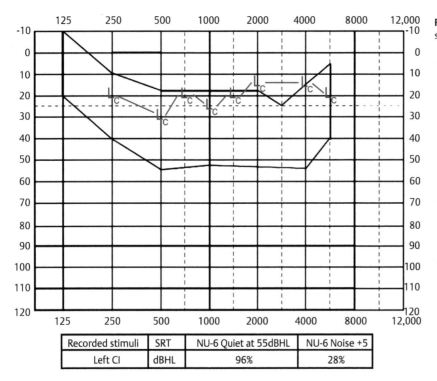

Fig. 56.3 Follow-up results following reduced stimulation rate. LC, left cochlear implant.

Recorded stimuli	SRT	NU-6 Quiet at 55dBHL	NU-6 Noise +5
Left CI	dBHL	96%	28%

56.3 Diagnosis and Recommended Treatment

The patient will continue using his device with the new maintenance MAP setting and return for a repeat comprehensive CI evaluation. He reported satisfaction with his hearing aid and CI settings.

56.4 Questions for the Reader

1. If speech perception scores were better initially with the CI, would the patient have been a good bilateral implant candidate with the goal of using an *external hybrid processor system* in the right ear?
2. Should you consider changing stimulation rate based on patient complaints, anatomy, and performance or hearing history?
3. Could changing the stimulation rate improve the patient's performance?

56.5 Discussion of Questions

1. **If speech perception scores were better initially with the CI, would the patient have been a good bilateral implant candidate with the goal of using an *external hybrid processor system* in the right ear?**
   Yes; because the hearing loss is severe-to-profound in the high frequencies, it is reasonable to consider a CI. The surgeon may consider a lateral wall electrode array, which may allow for preservation of the low-frequency acoustic hearing. If low-frequency hearing was preserved, the patient may benefit from an electric-acoustic external sound processor. Access to low-frequency acoustic hearing may allow for preservation of fine temporal structure.

2. **Should you consider changing stimulation rate based on patient complaints, anatomy, and performance or hearing history?**
   Those who suffer from neurological impairments, such as cytomegalovirus, auditory neuropathy spectrum disorder, and dementia may have difficulty processing high

stimulation rates. Another population to consider stimulation rate changes includes meningitic patients who have cochlear ossification and long-term deafened individuals. Any patient who is not doing well with the given stimulation rate may benefit from a trial with a different rate.

3. **Could changing the stimulation rate improve the patient's performance?**

It is often thought that an increase in stimulation rate will improve a user's overall speech recognition performance, though there is no evidence to support this theory. As CIs have advanced and the number of electrodes have increased with the goal to improve the quality of speech, there are still acoustic qualities of speech that cannot be mimicked. Those most notably difficult to mirror are the spectral resolution of speech and limited access to temporal cues. In an attempt to improve fine temporal structure cues, implant manufacturers have recommended high stimulation rates (above 1,800 pps/channel). Higher rates of electrical stimulation theoretically allow for the representation of more information in the temporal envelope, which should, in turn, improve speech recognition.

Higher stimulations may also reduce T levels, which would have the effect of increasing the electrical dynamic range (because C levels are less likely to change with increases in stimulation rate as compared to T levels). Despite the larger electrical dynamic range with high stimulation rates, intensity resolution is similar between low and high rates. High sampling rates can also offer better temporal sampling of the input acoustic signal.[1]

A review of studies revealed no consistent difference in overall speech recognition abilities between low and high stimulation rates.[2]

In a 2012 study of Nucleus CI24 users, moderate (900 pps/channel) and high (2,400 pps/channel) rates were evaluated to determine if a difference in speech recognition performance existed in quiet and noisy environments.[2] In quiet, performance was better with 900 pps/channel though no significant difference in noise was revealed. Subjectively, users preferred the 900 pps/channel especially in quiet.

References

[1] Shannon RV, Cruz RJ, Galvin JJ, III. Effect of stimulation rate on cochlear implant users' phoneme, word and sentence recognition in quiet and in noise. Audiol Neurootol. 2011; 16(2):113–123

[2] Park SH, Kim E, Lee HJ, Kim HJ. Effects of electrical stimulation rate on speech recognition in cochlear implant users. Korean J Audiol. 2012; 16(1):6–9

Suggested Reading

[1] Arora K, Vandali A, Dowell R, Dawson P. Effects of stimulation rate on modulation detection and speech recognition by cochlear implant users. Int J Audiol. 2011; 50(2):123–132

[2] AudiologyOnline. Cochlear implant hybrids: who is a candidate? You may be surprised. 2006. Available at: http://www.audiologyonline.com/articles/cochlear-implant-hybrids-who-candidate-990. Accessed July 24, 2017

[3] Srinivasan AG, Padilla M, Shannon RV, Landsberger DM (2013). Improving speech perception in noise with current focusing in cochlear implant users. Hearing research, 299: 29-36.

[4] Pelosi S, Rivas A, Haynes DS, Bennett ML, Labadie RF, Hedley-Williams A, et al. (2012). Stimulation rate reduction and auditory development in poorly performing cochlear implant users with auditory neuropathy. Otology and Neurotology: Official Publication Of The American Otological Society, American Neurotology Society [And] European Academy Of Otology And Neurotology, 33(9): 1502-1506.

[5] Friesen LM, Shannon RV, Cruz RJ. (2005). Effects of stimulation rate on speech recognition with cochlear implants. Audiology and Neuro-Otology, 10(3): 169-184.

57 Cochlear Implantation for Children with Single-Sided Deafness

David R Friedmann, Janet Green, Laurel Mahoney, William Shapiro, and J. Thomas Roland, Jr.

57.1 Clinical History and Description

Anna, a 3-year-old girl, was a product of a full-term pregnancy without complications. She passed newborn hearing screening in the right ear and was referred in the left ear prior to discharge from the nursery. She was subsequently seen for a diagnostic auditory brainstem response (ABR) evaluation, which was consistent with hearing within normal limits in the right ear and a severe to profound sensorineural hearing loss in the left ear. Etiology of this hearing loss was unknown. She did undergo genetic testing, which did not identify any known mutations.

Shortly after her diagnosis, Anna was fitted with a hearing aid in the left ear that she wore until recently and subsequently rejected. English is not her primary language, but she is exposed to it at home. Anna is otherwise in good general health. There were no cognitive issues suspected from her evaluations.

57.2 Audiologic Testing

Pure tone testing was performed under insert earphones with good reliability via conditioned play audiometry. Results were consistent with hearing within normal limits from 125 to 8,000 Hz in the right ear, and a profound hearing loss in the left ear with no measurable hearing to the limits of the audiometer. Tympanometric results were consistent with normal (type A) middle ear function bilaterally. Distortion product otoacoustic emissions were present in the right ear and absent in the left ear.

Speech perception testing was performed, in sound field, at 60 dBA in noise with a bone anchored implant. Given Anna's young age and limited knowledge of English, testing was limited to single words and closed-set speech perception. Speech perception scores and signal-to-noise ratio are listed in ▶ Table 57.1.

57.3 Surgical Assessment

Given the profound hearing loss with no measurable hearing, a magnetic resonance imaging (MRI) of the brain was performed with particular attention to the presence of a cochlear nerve innervating the cochlea. Since there is a significant incidence of cochlear nerve insufficiency in congenital single-sided deafness (SSD), this is an important step in the candidacy evaluation. The MRI did raise suspicion of a hypoplastic cochlear nerve on the left but it was felt there was an adequate nerve from the cochlea. There were no cochlear abnormalities.

Table 57.1 Pre-op testing

Pre-op testing	Quiet	Speech right/ noise left	Speech left/ noise right
MLNT words (+ 5 dB SNR)	DNT	58%	50%

Abbreviation: MLNT, Multisyllabic Lexical Neighborhood Test.

57.4 Impressions

The paradigm for treatment of unilateral hearing loss has undergone significant changes. While minor hearing asymmetries may be observed and supported with preferential seating and remote microphone units, studies reveal that more significant unilateral hearing impairment may negatively impact language development and academic performance.

With newborn screening programs, early detection of hearing loss has improved drastically. The prevalence of unilateral sensorineural hearing loss is estimated to be 13 per 1,000 newborns, with true SSD less frequent in this population, and 3% of school-aged children. Because of difficulty in detection and the progressive nature of some types of hearing loss, the recorded prevalence of unilateral hearing impairment in children actually increases with age, underlying the importance of monitoring patients over time.

SSD refers to a special case of a unilateral hearing loss in which a patient has one ear with severe-profound sensorineural hearing loss, with normal hearing in the contralateral ear. The most common causes for unilateral hearing loss are related to temporal bone anomalies including enlarged vestibular aqueduct, cochlear dysplasias, or cochlear nerve hypoplasia/aplasia.

Most rehabilitative options for SSD route sound to the contralateral cochlea, resulting in only unilateral auditory stimulation (i.e., CROS, bone anchored implant). Cochlear implantation is the only treatment modality that may restore bilateral auditory input to patients with SSD. The benefits of true binaural hearing including improved hearing in difficult listening situations and the ability to localize sound are currently only available with a cochlear implant (CI). In children with an etiology that may be progressive such as enlarged vestibular aqueduct, "threatening" the normal hearing contralateral ear, consideration should be given to the potential of the better ear to have progressive hearing loss over time as well. Further studies in the pediatric SSD population will help us better understand who will benefit most from this technology.

57.5 Questions for the Reader

1. What developmental issues should be discussed with parents regarding the role for rehabilitation of SSD children?
2. What rehabilitative options are there for SSD and how do they work?
3. What advantage does cochlear implantation have over other treatment options for SSD?
4. What diagnostic information must be ascertained before planning cochlear implantation in children with congenital profound hearing loss?

57.6 Discussion of Questions

1. **What developmental issues should be discussed with parents regarding the role for rehabilitation of SSD children?**

   Longitudinal data have emerged on social and academic issues with unilateral hearing loss compared to normal hearing siblings and peers. These should be discussed in counseling parents as should the potential for a child with an otherwise "invisible" disability to become labeled by classmates if assistive devices are used.

2. **What rehabilitative options are there for SSD and how do they work?**

   CROS and bone anchored implants work through different mechanisms to transfer sound from the poorer hearing ear to the better hearing ear. They provide some but not all of the benefits of binaural hearing. They can actually make listening more difficult when noise is incident on the poorer hearing ear and routed to the better hearing ear.

3. **What advantage does cochlear implantation have over other treatment options for SSD?**

   Cochlear implantation for SSD offers potential for improved hearing in noise, especially with sound incident on the poorer hearing ear and noise in the better hearing ear. Additionally, data show improved localization abilities, an impossible task with only a single hearing ear or with routing of sound to the only hearing ear as with a CROS or bone anchored implant.

4. **What diagnostic information must be ascertained before planning cochlear implantation in children with congenital profound hearing loss?**

   As there is a significant rate of absent cochlear nerves in patients with congenital SSD, the presence of a nerve should be confirmed before considering cochlear implantation. In the absence of any true behavioral auditory responses with the poorer ear appropriately isolated, neuroimaging can be used to confirm the presence of a cochlea and cochlear nerve.

57.7 Diagnosis and Recommended Treatment

Behavioral testing was consistent with hearing within normal limits in the right ear and a profound hearing loss in the left ear, consistent with the prior ABR. From an audiological perspective, Anna was felt to be an appropriate candidate for a CI in the left ear.

Because of the presence of a profound hearing loss in the left ear, it was discussed Anna will likely have more difficulty in some listening situations, such as in noisy environments (e.g., classroom). Although outcomes cannot be predicted, a CI in the left ear may provide some of the benefits of binaural hearing, such as localization and improved speech understanding in noise. We would also expect that she would derive some degree of word recognition ability in the left ear alone. The parents were extensively counseled regarding CIs as a treatment for SSD and the team felt they demonstrated realistic expectations for

Table 57.2 Speech testing 1 year postimplant

1 year evaluation	Bimodal	Left CI alone	Right ear alone
LNT words (quiet)	92%	92%	100%
LNT phonemes	95%	97%	100%
Common phrases (+ 10 dB): speech front/ noise front	100%	90%	100%
Common phrases (+ 10 dB): speech front/ noise right	100%	100%	100%
Common phrases (+ 10 dB): speech front/ noise left	100%	100%	100%
LNT words (quiet) Mini-Mic to CI alone	–	80%	–
HINT sentences (quiet) Mini-Mic to CI alone	–	74%	–

Abbreviation: HINT, Hearing in Noise Test; LNT, Lexical Neighborhood Test.

outcomes. Anna underwent successful left cochlear implantation at the age of 3. Intraoperative testing and X-ray confirmed device functionality and proper location.

57.8 Outcome

At her 1-year evaluation, Anna has 22 active electrodes. Speech perception was performed using both "plug and muff" technique and manufacturer's specific Direct Connect software to isolate the implanted ear. Testing was also performed with noise incident from right left and front as indicated in ▶ Table 57.2 from her evaluation. Anna does quite well with her CI including the speech in noise conditions. Anna and her family report she enjoys wearing her CI and uses it in school.

Suggested Reading

[1] Lieu JE, Tye-Murray N, Fu Q. Longitudinal study of children with unilateral hearing loss. Laryngoscope. 2012; 122(9):2088–2095

[2] Bess FH, Tharpe AM. Performance and management of children with unilateral sensorineural hearing loss. Scand Audiol Suppl. 1988; 30:75–79

[3] Arndt S, Aschendorff A, Laszig R, et al. Comparison of pseudobinaural hearing to real binaural hearing rehabilitation after cochlear implantation in patients with unilateral deafness and tinnitus. Otol Neurotol. 2011; 32(1):39–47

[4] Vermeire K, Van de Heyning P. Binaural hearing after cochlear implantation in subjects with unilateral sensorineural deafness and tinnitus. Audiol Neurootol. 2009; 14(3):163–171

[5] Arndt S, Prosse S, Laszig R, Wesarg T, Aschendorff A, Hassepass F. Cochlear implantation in children with single-sided deafness: does aetiology and duration of deafness matter? Audiol Neurootol. 2015; 20 Suppl 1:21–30

[6] Friedmann DR, Ahmed OH, McMenomey SO, Shapiro WH, Waltzman SB, Roland JT, Jr. Single-sided deafness cochlear implantation: Candidacy, evaluation and outcomes in children and adults. Otol Neurotol. 2016; 37(2):e154–e160

[7] Young NM, Kim FM, Ryan ME, Tournis E, Yaras S. Pediatric cochlear implantation of children with eighth nerve deficiency. Int J Pediatr Otorhinolaryngol. 2012; 76(10):1442–1448

58 Family Not Following Up with Audiological Recommendations

Joni Alberg

58.1 Clinical History and Description

CJ failed his newborn hearing screening in both ears. His parents were not able to return for a rescreen within the 1-month window recommended by the hospital. CJ did receive well-baby checkups at the local health department, but the parents do not remember anyone telling them they needed to have his hearing rescreened. When CJ was assessed for kindergarten enrollment, he failed the hearing screening and was referred to a local audiologist for a diagnostic evaluation.

According to the audiologist, the parents were very concerned about CJ's hearing loss and expressed guilt for not having followed through earlier. Because he is their firstborn, they did not realize that his delay in speech and language development was cause for concern. The parents appeared to be very committed to doing "whatever it takes" to help CJ.

58.2 Audiologic Testing

CJ was found to have moderate to severe, bilateral, sensorineural hearing loss. The audiologist explained the hearing loss to the parents using a picture audiogram. He also told them about free services available from a local program providing support for parents of children who are deaf or hard-of-hearing and offered to make an immediate referral. The parents expressed gratitude.

At the end of the diagnostic evaluation, the audiologist made ear mold impressions and told CJ's parents he would order hearing aids. Because CJ qualified for Medicaid, the cost of the hearing aids would not be a problem for the parents. The audiologist also told the parents he would call them when the hearing aids were ready for CJ. He explained it could be as long as 3 to 4 weeks because he would have to receive Medicaid approval prior to purchasing the hearing aids. The parents left the appointment, a bit overwhelmed, but agreed to return when the hearing aids were ready to be fitted.

58.2.1 Follow-up

The local support program received the referral for CJ and his family the day following the diagnosis of his hearing loss. A parent educator was assigned to provide support for the family. Two days later, the parent educator contacted the audiologist to obtain background information about the family, including the audiological report. Information about the family and the report were sent to the parent educator via secure email. The parent educator called the parents right away, but did not reach them. She left a voice message stating who she was and why she had called. After leaving two subsequent messages, she finally reached the mother and scheduled a home visit for the following week.

58.3 One Month Later

The hearing aids have arrived at the audiology office. The parents are called and a message is left telling them to call to schedule a hearing aid fitting appointment. Three more messages were left over the course of the next 3 weeks. No response was received from the parents.

58.4 Questions for the Reader

1. What should the audiologist do as the family is not responding?

58.5 Discussion of Questions

1. **What should the audiologist do as the family is not responding?**
   Frustrated, the audiologist calls the parent educator to ask if she could please try to contact the parents and encourage them to come in to pick up the hearing aids. He expresses that he thought the parents were "on board" with putting hearing aids on CJ, but now figures they only appeared to understand the hearing loss and what it will take to help CJ.

58.5.1 Follow-up

The parent educator calls the mother and reaches her the same day. The parent educator asks the mother how she and the family are doing. This is what she learns:
- The father lost his job.
- The family is being evicted from their apartment.
- There is a new baby in the family who needs diapers.
- The mother knows the hearing aids are waiting to be picked up.
- She knows CJ needs them, and she feels badly they have not been able to get to the audiologist's office.
- She does not know when they will be able to get there because at the moment, money, food, diapers, and a place to live are more urgent for the family.

58.6 Additional Questions for the Reader

1. What can the parent educator and the audiologist do to assist this family and arrange for services for CJ?

58.7 Discussion of Additional Questions

1. **What can the parent educator and the audiologist do to assist this family and arrange for services for CJ?**

   The family situation is currently overwhelming. The parents are dealing with basic survival issues at the same time as their son is having problems that will affect his lifelong language, literacy, and education. How can the audiologist and parent educator help?

   If there is a social worker at either facility, could he or she assist the family in contacting and obtaining local social services? Social services might be able to assist the father in obtaining unemployment insurance, provide diapers, and possibly find housing.

   Would the family be able to come to the clinic if transportation could be arranged? Can Medicaid provide transportation? Can the social worker, parent educator, or school provide transportation?

- Is CJ attending school? How is he managing?
- Is there a speech-language pathologist, a teacher of the deaf, or an auditory-verbal therapist at the school who could assist in providing services to CJ?
- Is a school or home visit possible by the audiology clinic?
- Both the audiologist and parent educator have a responsibility to follow up with this family. How can they do that?

Responsibilities do not end with making a diagnosis. All the professionals involved have some responsibility for follow-up.

If families do not return for necessary follow-up, we cannot immediately conclude that they are irresponsible. While hearing loss may be the only thing we are thinking about when working with a child, we can provide better services to the child if we can look at the whole family, understand their issues, and try and arrange for additional assistance.

59 Child with Severe Profound Hearing Loss Born to Parents with Deafness

Michael Douglas

59.1 Clinical History and Description

Baby Jonathan was born full term. His parents reported the following case history with the assistance of a sign language interpreter. He had five newborn hearing screenings and only passed one ear on one screening. There is a strong family history of hearing loss as both of Jonathan's parents and his older sister have profound hearing loss. Jonathan's older sister uses a cochlear implant and is currently enrolled in a listening and spoken language (LSL) preschool for children with hearing loss. Jonathan's grandmother and many more of his immediate family do not have hearing loss.

59.2 Audiologic, Medical and Auditory-Speech-Language Testing

At 3 months of age, Jonathan received a complete diagnostic assessment. Auditory brainstem response (ABR) testing was first completed with a high-frequency click stimulus (condensation and rarefaction). At 90 dB nHL, no response was observed for either ear. Testing was then completed with tone bursts from 500 to 4,000 Hz. No response was observed for either ear at 95 dB nHL. Bone conduction testing was completed at 500 and 2,000 Hz, and no response was observed at the limits of the equipment. Tympanograms were obtained with a 1,000-Hz probe tone and showed normal middle ear pressure and compliance, bilaterally. Distortion product oto-acoustic emissions were absent from 2,000 to 6,000 Hz bilaterally. Overall, results indicated at least a severe to profound sensorineural hearing loss bilaterally. Results were discussed with Jonathan's parents through the sign language interpreter. The parents were interested in pursuing a cochlear implant workup for Jonathan and were subsequently referred to the cochlear implant team.

At 4 months of age, Jonathan received medical testing, hearing aids, and was enrolled in Part C early intervention services. He also received a speech and language evaluation at the cochlear implant center by a t/LSL specialist.

59.2.1 Medical Testing Results

A computed tomography (CT) scan without contrast indicated the anatomy of the inner ear structures is within normal limits bilaterally with suspicion of dehiscence of the right posterior and superior semicircular canals and normal temporal bone. A magnetic resonance imaging (MRI) of the brain with contrast indicated no focal lesions or visualized acute process.

59.2.2 Hearing Aid Fitting

Jonathan's hearing aids were programmed to Desired Sensation Level (DSL) 5.0 Child targets using a measured real-ear-to-coupler difference (RECD). The best possible match to targets was obtained while not exceeding the maximum power output (MPO) targets of the hearing aids. Jonathan received the following hearing aids:
- *Right hearing aid.* Make: Oticon Model: Safari 300 SP.
- *Left hearing aid.* Make: Oticon Model: Safari 300 SP.

59.3 Auditory-Speech-Language Evaluation

According to parent report and clinical observation using the Rosetti Infant-Toddler Language Scale, and an auditory development checklist, Jonathan's language comprehension skills were scattered at the 0- to 3-month level, while language expression was solid at 0 to 3 months with emerging skills at 3 to 6 months. Overall, his performance indicated delayed receptive and expressive language skills when compared to children with typical hearing at his chronological age. The family indicated they would like to enroll him in private individual therapy with the LSL specialist.

59.4 Questions for the Reader

1. If the parents are deaf and require a sign language interpreter, why would they pursue a cochlear implant and listening and spoken language?
2. Will the presence of sign language in his life truncate his ability to learn spoken language?
3. What kind of intervention environment will allow this child to develop adequate listening and spoken language skills comparable to children with typical hearing?

59.5 Discussion of Questions

1. **If the parents are deaf and require a sign language interpreter, why would they pursue a cochlear implant and listening and spoken language?**
   Questions like this are best answered by asking the family. During a semi-structured interview, the parents indicated that they want their children, first and foremost, to be able to communicate with everyone in their family, neighborhood, and school. Second, the parents reported they wanted him "to have better work opportunities" than they have experienced.

2. **Will the presence of sign language in his life truncate his ability to learn spoken language?**
   Jonathan's spoken language learning would certainly be at risk if Jonathan did not receive a cochlear implant and did not receive appropriate intervention. If a child cannot receive and perceive the full range of speech sounds of a language, the chances of developing satisfactory spoken language abilities are remote. This requires all children with hearing impairments in spoken language programs (regardless of their linguistic backgrounds) to have access to soft conversational speech (ideally 20–25 dB HL) across all frequencies

within the speech spectrum. For dual language competency to occur, intervention needs to be designed to provide detailed information to the brain in both languages with the ultimate goal of fluent and accurate expression in both languages. There is an emerging body of research concerning the learning of two spoken languages for children with hearing loss, demonstrating little to no evidence that acquiring the two spoken languages from birth causes severe language delays.[1]

However, for children who are deaf and raised with bimodal languages (with one being spoken language and the other being sign language), the acquisition of proficient spoken language is much more complicated. First, children have restricted access to spoken language as a result of their hearing loss. A child who is deaf and whose brain does not have access to intelligible speech/spoken information via a cochlear implant must acquire spoken languages mainly through the visual channel, for example, through speech reading. For these children, learning a spoken language tends to be a slow process that requires exceptional efforts by the child and his or her parents. As a consequence, the spoken language development of children who are deaf and who do not receive a cochlear implant is usually very deficient when compared to hearing children. Second, many children who are deaf have limited sign language input, because their parents, family members, and teachers usually do not have fluent signing skills. Hearing parents often start to learn sign language themselves, only when the deafness of their child has been detected and are limited in their ability to respond intuitively to children who are deaf due to their limited signing skills. It is this lack of quality in sign language interactions in the early ages that result in deficient sign language abilities of children who are deaf and born to parents with normal hearing who do not know sign language. In other words, setting up a bimodal system is much more difficult for children who are deaf. Many of them will not acquire nativelike skills in one of the languages.

However, in this case, Jonathan has a potentially unique advantage. Both of his parents are fluent signers, and his grandmother is willing to be an active participant in his spoken language learning. Considering Jonathan's age with no other medical or cognitive concerns, Jonathan has a potentially favorable bimodal language prognosis with an appropriate and mutually agreed upon language development plan, particularly if he is able to receive extensive exposure to an enriched spoken language model via his grandmother.

3. **What kind of intervention environment will allow this child to develop adequate listening and spoken language skills comparable to children with typical hearing?**
In this case, the professionals could implement a family-centered coordination of services approach. Initially, a deaf educator would provide services in the home language for the parents so they could learn and become comfortable with the hearing technology and language learning techniques. In individual therapy, the LSL specialist could work with Jonathan's familial spoken language models (with the parents as they are able) to learn the same ideas, strategies, and techniques from a spoken language perspective. As Jonathan becomes old enough for the toddler immersion program, the coordinated service model could continue. The deaf educator would continue to work with him and his parents at home in sign language with a focus on coordinating lesson plans alongside the LSL professionals who work with him and his spoken language models at the implant center. Regular assessment could be conducted in both languages at 6-month intervals and his treatment plan changed according to his developing needs.

59.6 Outcome

At 10 months of age, Jonathan received bilateral cochlear implant devices. He was enrolled in Part C early intervention home-based services where a teacher of the deaf worked with his parents on language teaching strategies in sign language, and he attended individual LSL services at the cochlear implant center with his parents and grandparent. At 18 months of age, he was enrolled in a half-day toddler program run by LSL professionals 3 days a week. By age 3, he achieved the language results in both languages provided in ▶ Table 59.1.

At age 3, Jonathan continued his LSL training in a special preschool for children with hearing loss, but his time in the program increased to 5 days a week for 8 hours a day with 1 hour of speech-language therapy with an LSL professional each week. Coordinated services through Part C ended, and Jonathan's home language was supported by his parents and encouraged by the LSL professionals. Parents would attend school functions with an interpreter, and they would implement the strategies taught by the deaf educator in their primary language at home. Formal and informal assessment continued at 6-month intervals. By age 4, Jonathan achieved the language results in Spoken English provided in ▶ Table 59.2.

Table 59.1 Language testing results in both languages at age 3 years

37 mo	Articulation (AAPS)	Language quotient (TELD)	Exp. vocab (EVT)	Recep. vocab (PPVT)	Talking (TASL)
Standard scores	93	86	101	91	Level 2
Signing skills		Prefers to sign with certain people	Talks more than signs	Understands more than uses	Strings 2–3 Occasional 6 or more

Table 59.2 Language test results in Spoken English at age 4 years

48 mo	Articulation (AAPS)	Omnibus language (CELF-P)	Exp. vocab (EVT)	Recep. vocab (PPVT)	Talking (TASL)
Standard scores	118	110	124	110	Level 3

Jonathan will continue one more year in the program with a split placement between his LSL preschool and a mainstream setting with deaf education support. Jonathan had the honor of saying the pledge of allegiance at his preschool class graduation ceremony.

Suggested Reading

[1] Bunta F, Douglas M, Dickson H, Cantu A, Wickesberg J, Gifford RH. Dual language versus English-only support for bilingual children with hearing loss who use cochlear implants and hearing aids. Int J Lang Commun Disord. 2016; 51(4):460–472

[2] Douglas M. Dual Language Learning for children with Hearing Loss: Assessment, intervention and Program Development. Innsbruck, Austria: MED-EL; 2014

[3] Herman D, Knoors H, Ormel E, Verhoeven L. Modeling reading vocabulary learning in deaf children in bilingual education programs. J Deaf Stud Deaf Educ. 2008; 10(1093):1–19

60 Why Is JS Not Making Progress?

Jane R. Madell

60.1 Clinical History and Description

JS failed newborn hearing screening bilaterally. Auditory brain-stem response (ABR) testing confirmed a bilateral, severe to profound hearing loss. He was fit with hearing aids at 2 months of age and began auditory-verbal therapy, immediately. Both mother and his therapist did not believe that JS was making sufficient progress, and at 6 months of age, he received bilateral cochlear implants. According to the parents, JS used his cochlear implants during all waking hours. The family attended auditory-verbal therapy regularly. JS's mother continued to be concerned that he was not making progress. JS was not speaking and did not seem to understand spoken information, so the mother decided to get a second opinion.

JS came to the center for evaluation at 18 months of age, after wearing his cochlear implants for 12 months. Previous reports and tests were reviewed. Evaluations and family did not indicate any other conditions that might contribute to JS's delay. One of the first questions I always ask a family is, *"What do you think your child is hearing with and without technology?"* When I asked this question, the family reported that they were not sure what JS was hearing, and they did not observe a significant difference, with or without technology. The auditory-verbal therapist was contacted and was also unable to identify what JS was hearing. She assumed that the family was not having JS use technology consistently, and was not deliberately working with JS to facilitate the development of his spoken language. She considered the possibility that JS might have autism spectrum disorder. The cochlear implant audiologist who had been following JS had not performed behavioral testing.

60.2 Audiologic Testing

JS was tested with the technology, and testing indicated sound-field detection thresholds at –5 to –10 dB HL with use of cochlear implants (▶ Table 60.1).

60.3 Questions for the Reader

1. Should we be concerned that the parents and auditory-verbal therapist do not know what JS is hearing with his cochlear implants?
2. What do you think about JS's implant thresholds? Are they appropriate?

60.4 Discussion of Questions

1. **Should we be concerned that the parents and auditory-verbal therapist do not know what JS is hearing with his cochlear implants?**
   Not having any audiologic evidence about what auditory information is getting to JS's brain is clearly a RED FLAG. We expect families and therapists to know what phonemes a child is hearing with technology. Ideally, they should be able to report what a child is hearing with technology on the right and left ears separately, and bilaterally. Unless we have this information, we cannot tell if technology is set appropriately, and if changes in settings are required.

2. **What do you think about JS's implant thresholds? Are they appropriate?**
   Technology thresholds should be at 20 to 25 dB HL. Thresholds at –5 or –10 dB HL are overstimulating the auditory system and may be causing a decrease in performance by distorting the signal.

60.5 Diagnosis and Recommended Treatment

JS's cochlear implants were mapped inappropriately. Once JS's cochlear implants were reprogrammed, behavioral implant thresholds were obtained at 20 to 25 dB HL (▶ Table 60.2). JS appeared to be comfortable with the new settings.

Table 60.1 Soundfield detection thresholds (dB HL) with cochlear implants (CI) at initial evaluation

	500 dB	1,000 dB	2,000 dB	3,000 dB	4,000 dB	6,000 dB
Right CI	–5	–5	–10	–10	–5	–10
Left CI	–5	–5	–10	–10	–10	–5

Table 60.2 Implant thresholds in dB HL with reprogrammed cochlear implants (CI)

	500 dB	1,000 dB	2,000 dB	3,000 dB	4,000 dB	6,000 dB
Right CI	20	25	20	25	25	20
Left CI	25	25	20	20	15	20

Follow-up with family and the auditory-verbal therapist indicated that JS was beginning to develop spoken language and was attending to sound in the environment. JS was significantly delayed in his spoken language development because he did not have access to clear auditory information until he was 18 months of age; but now, JS was making good progress.

60.6 Additional Questions for the Reader

1. Should the audiologist who was managing JS, and his auditory-verbal therapist, have recognized that something was wrong? What should they have done about it?
2. Is cochlear implant programming alone sufficient for monitoring performance or is behavioral testing also essential?

60.7 Discussion of Additional Questions

1. **Should the audiologist who was managing JS, and his auditory-verbal therapist, have recognized that something was wrong? What should they have done about it?**
It should not have taken 12 months for the professionals who were working with JS to recognize that his lack of progress was a problem. Both the cochlear implant audiologist and the auditory-verbal therapist should have recognized that something was wrong and should not have blamed it on parents or other disorders, without first verifying technology programming and function.

2. **Is cochlear implant programming alone sufficient for monitoring performance or is behavioral testing also essential?**
The audiologist should have obtained soundfield detection thresholds with use of each implant. If she had, she would have recognized that JS was being overstimulated. The auditory-verbal therapist should have requested cochlear implant thresholds to be certain that JS's brain was receiving auditory information at appropriate levels throughout the frequency range.

60.8 Outcome

Once JS's cochlear implants were appropriately remapped, JS continued to make good progress in his development of spoken language skills.

Suggested Reading

[1] Davidson LS, Geers AE, Nicholas JG. The effects of audibility and novel word learning ability on vocabulary level in children with cochlear implants. Cochlear Implants Int. 2014; 15(4):211–221

[2] Davidson LS, Skinner MW, Holstad BA, et al. The effect of instantaneous input dynamic range setting on the speech perception of children with the nucleus 24 implant. Ear Hear. 2009; 30(3):340–349

[3] Firszt JB, Holden LK, Skinner MW, et al. Recognition of speech presented at soft to loud levels by adult cochlear implant recipients of three cochlear implant systems. Ear Hear. 2004; 25(4):375–387

[4] Holden LK, Finley CC, Firszt JB, et al. Factors affecting open-set word recognition in adults with cochlear implants. Ear Hear. 2013; 34(3):342–360

[5] Skinner MW. Optimizing cochlear implant speech performance. Ann Otol Rhinol Laryngol Suppl. 2003; 191:4–13

61 Progressive Hearing Loss

Jackie L. Clark

61.1 Clinical History and Description

TK's prenatal medical history was unremarkable, with hospital delivery records indicating a gestation age of 40 weeks (i.e., full term), following a prolonged labor. Immediate postpartum delivery records indicated 9/9 APGARS (Appearance, Pulse, Grimace, Activity, Respiration Score) recorded at 1- and 5-minute intervals, respectively. However, TK experienced intermittent anoxic episodes during the delivery process, and had to be placed on mechanical ventilation briefly while he was a newborn well-baby nursery resident. Parental report included a positive family history of hearing loss from a paternal uncle who was described as "deaf." After passing the initial newborn hearing screen, TK's parents continued to believe the screening results were incorrect and pursued audiological testing throughout his infancy.

Due to parental concern, TK also was followed by an otolaryngologist who diagnosed the infant with chronic otitis media. His parents reported that at 12 months of age, TK had a vocabulary of 17 words, but by 18 months of age, speech acquisition seemed to have significantly stalled. Despite pressure equalization tubes placed bilaterally at 18 months of age, his parents became more concerned about his inability to produce sibilant phonemes and an apparent heavy reliance upon speech reading.

Eventually, a diagnostic auditory brainstem response (ABR) testing was ordered by his otolaryngologist and completed at another facility when he was 3 ½ years old. Since the ABR findings suggested a borderline mild to moderate conductive loss in the right ear, and moderate sensorineural hearing loss (SNHL) for the left ear, and subsequently was provided a medical clearance, he was referred for hearing aid fitting at our clinic.

61.1.1 Audiologic Findings at Our Center

TK's audiological management through our clinic began at 39 months of age. Behavioral audiometric results completed on his first visit were consistent with minimal response levels when using visual reinforcement audiometry. Responses indicated, at worst, a mild to moderate conductive hearing loss in the right ear, and moderate to borderline severe SNHL for the left ear (▶ Fig. 61.1). Cursory otoscopic inspection revealed clear canals bilaterally. Tympanometric results were consistent with limited mobility (right ear), and essentially normal mobility (left ear) of the tympanic membrane (TM). In light of TK's medical diagnoses of chronic otitis media coupled with "good to fair" audiometric response reliability, the tympanometric and pure tone audiometric thresholds supported the findings of a conductive (right ear) and sensorineural (left ear) etiology. It was recommended that TK return to his otolaryngologist to rule out active conductive pathology.

TK's otolaryngologist's audiologist conducted a three-frequency pure tone measure for both ears, another sedated click-evoked ABR, immittance measures, and transient evoked (TE) otoacoustic emission (OAE) measures when TK was 45 months of age. ABR results revealed synchronous neural responses to click stimuli consistent with mild peripheral impairment for the left ear and moderate peripheral impairment for the left ear. His TE OAE results and TM mobility were within normal limits for the right ear; poorly formed TE OAE with tympanometry results reflecting significant negative middle ear pressure were found for the left ear. Unfortunately, TK awoke before bone conduction and tone burst ABRs could be completed. The three-frequency pure tone thresholds obtained at the otolaryngologist's office

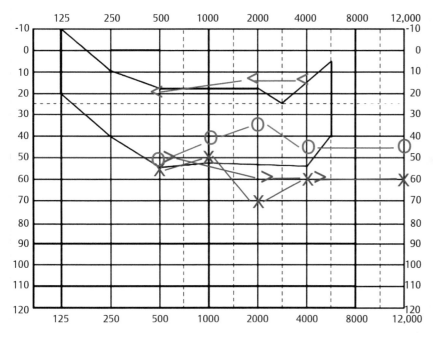

Fig. 61.1 Initial pure tone behavioral results: TK at 39 months. O, right ear air conduction; X, left ear air conduction; <, right ear bone conduction; >, left ear bone conduction.

were in agreement with those obtained at the Callier Center when TK was 39 months old (▶ Table 61.1). With this information, TK returned to the Callier Center for hearing aid evaluation and fitting.

Choice of hearing aids was determined from the audiological information gathered from his behavioral results at our center as well as from the other facility. It is important to keep in mind that best practice for dispensing hearing aids dictates the necessity of not only obtaining an audiologic examination no more than 6 months before hearing aids are dispensed, but also receiving medical clearance and conducting appropriate verification measures (e.g., real ear measures and/or functional gain). The aim, when measuring real ear measures for real ear insertion gain (REIG) or real ear aided response (REAR), is to match as closely as possible a validated prescriptive target (e.g., DSL v.5 or NAL-NL2) at the time of hearing aid dispensing. In the case of TK, the subsequent verification using simulated probe microphone measures of appropriate hearing aid function demonstrated a match of DSL prescription targets, and the maximum output (SSPL 90) was below the predicted uncomfortable loudness (UCL) target. In addition, behavioral functional measures while wearing both hearing aids demonstrated improved soundfield thresholds when compared to his unaided/ear-specific air conduction thresholds (▶ Table 61.2). TK's hearing status was monitored on a regular basis so that any hearing aid programming and/or ear mold modifications could be completed on a timely basis until stable thresholds were confirmed.

Table 61.1 Initial pure tone behavioral results: TK at 39 months

		250	500	1,000	2,000	3,000	4,000	8,000	SAT
Right ear	AC	NT	50	40	35	NT	45	-	45
	BC	NT	20	NT	15	NT	15		
Left ear	AC	NT	55	50	70	NT	60	-	60
	BC	NT	50	NT	60	NT	60		

Abbreviation: AC, air conduction; BC, bone conduction.

Table 61.2 Sequential air conduction pure tone and aided behavioral results (45 months–8 years old)

		250	500	1,000	2,000	3,000	4,000	6,000	8,000	SAT/SRT
45 mo old	Right ear	65	60	50	45	60	55	75	55	55
	R aided – SF	NT	25	15	25	25	30	NT	NT	30
	Left ear	60	65	60	75	85	70	80	75	70
	L aided – SF	NT	30	35	45	45	45	NT	NT	35
5 y old	Right ear	NT	65	55	65	50	55	80	NT	65
	Left ear	NT	85	90	80	70	65	NT	NT	90
	L aided – SF	45	35	40	40	40	40	NT	NT	45
6 y old	Right ear	55	60	55	65	50	55	80	80	60
	Left ear	90	85	90	80	70	50	80	90	85
8 y old	Right ear	70	70	75	75	85	85	90	NR/90	75
	R aided – SF	NT	15	15	30	35	45	NT	NT	20
	Left ear	90	85	95	85	85	80	95	90	90
	L aided – SF	NT	40	40	40	30	30	NT	NT	40
	L-CI (3-mo post)	NT	35	25	30	NT	30	NT	NT	40

Over a 5-year period, TK continued to have chronic middle ear condition, which resulted in multiple sets of pressure equalization tubes bilaterally. Unfortunately, in addition to the chronicity of middle ear pathology, TK's air and bone conduction pure tone thresholds deteriorated for both ears over time (see ▶ Table 61.2). Consequently, after genetic testing was ordered by the otolaryngologist, the findings confirmed *GJB2* (Connexin 26) mutation in TK's genes.

61.2 Diagnosis and Recommended Treatment

Both tympanometry with acoustic reflexes and pure tones, over time, supported a middle ear condition. However, long-term audiological monitoring of air and bone conduction thresholds (▶ Table 61.2) allowed a clearer definition of the etiology of the hearing loss as not being solely a middle ear condition, but also a progressive SNHL due to a genetic trait.

61.3 Additional Audiologic Testing

Once TK reached school age and after a considerable amount of negotiation with the school, a personal, ear-level, remote microphone (RM) system was provided by the school. The RM system was coupled to his hearing aids for schooltime use. His parents indicated that TK was performing well in the classroom setting, especially when wearing his RM system. As a consequence of progressively deteriorating hearing loss, more extensive testing was included within the monitoring protocol as well as an investigation of cochlear implantation candidacy. In addition to ear-specific audiometric speech and pure tone behavioral threshold quantification, there was also aided late cortical (P1) evoked potentials investigation to assess synaptic transmission efficiency and maturation of the thalamocortical portions of the auditory pathway.[1] TK's aided P1 response latencies were considered grossly within the expected range for a normal hearing age matched child when he was 5 and 8 years old (▶ Fig. 61.2), thus supporting the adequacy of the hearing aid fitting.

Despite the severity and progressive nature of his hearing loss, parental report, aided soundfield and probe microphone measures, as well as pediatric speech perception tests (Meaningful Auditory Integration Scale [MAIS]; Multisyllable Lexical Neighborhood Test [MLNT]; and Lexical Neighborhood Test [LNT]) provided a viable means of monitoring TK's hearing status (▶ Table 61.2, ▶ Table 61.3). Reportedly, his academic performance was on track for his age.

However, as TK was beginning the third grade, his parents became increasingly alarmed that, despite school-based speech therapy, his expressive language as well as academic performance began to significantly deteriorate, and his fatigue at the end of the school day was unusually high. Though the critically necessary RM system was operational, and pure tone thresholds did not significantly change, TK was struggling more than previously in the classroom setting. As a consequence, TK was referred to another facility for determination of cochlear implantation candidacy (▶ Table 61.3).

61.4 Questions for the Reader

1. What is the Newborn Hearing Screening Program?
2. What is the difference between fluctuating and progressive hearing loss?
3. What is happening to the auditory system with *GJB2*?
4. Would you recommend amplification and/or hearing assistance technology when a progressive hearing loss is present? If so, what would you recommend?
5. What other recommendations would you suggest for this family?

61.5 Discussion of Questions

1. **What is the Newborn Hearing Screening Program?**
Over 23 years ago, the National Institutes of Health recommended that all babies within the borders of the United States be screened at birth for hearing loss prior to discharge from the hospital. Currently, there are 43 states with some form of regulatory language related to newborn hearing screening. While legislation specifies a minimum expectation for state policy, there is no clear-cut definition of how hearing screenings should be implemented.[2] Just because many states have legislation for newborn hearing screening, it does not mean that there is a mandated protocol. There are some statewide programs that have been implementing screenings without any legislation, with protocols determined through determination of best practices. Despite the disparate protocols across facilities, almost 98% of newborns were screened for hearing loss by 2010.[2]

With the advent of universal newborn hearing screening, many babies are identified with hearing loss, which eventually over time will be resolved or remediated with amplification. Unlike the other identified conditions during newborn screenings, the hearing screening does not depend solely upon medical intervention. Rather, newborn hearing screening programs depend heavily upon effective follow-up audiological testing and intervention often paired with the medical evaluation. Ultimately, depending upon etiology, the otologic and audiologic diagnoses will identify the type (i.e., SNHL, conductive or mixed) and nature (stable, fluctuating, or progressive) of the hearing loss. Of those infants correctly referred for diagnostic evaluation, many will be audiologically diagnosed with SNHL; the remaining newborns were identified with conductive sequelae. Not all hearing loss in children is congenital, but acquired. As a consequence, Joint Commission on Infant Hearing[3] also recommends monitoring of infants and children who are at risk for delayed hearing loss.

2. **What is the difference between fluctuating and progressive hearing loss?**
Approximately, 1 to 4 out of 1,000 infants will be identified at birth with permanent hearing loss.[4] It is expected that an additional 16% of children will be identified with permanent hearing loss in the postnatal years.[5] Fluctuating hearing loss in childhood is most frequently attributed to a conductive component at the outer or middle ear system, and often is considered a remediable condition through pharmacological or surgical intervention. Some of the outer and middle ear

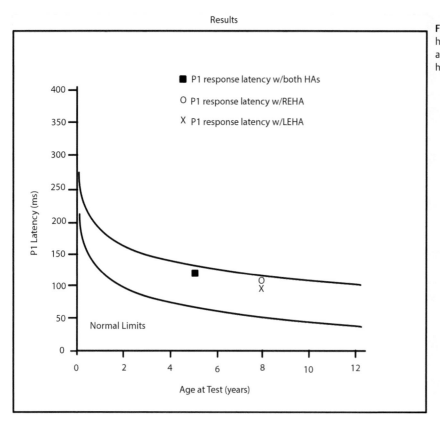

Results

Fig. 61.2 P1 values at 5 and 8 years of age with hearing aids (note P1 values for normal hearing age children are designated as solid lines in a horizontal orientation).

conditions that often create a fluctuating hearing loss include the following: otitis media with effusion, complications of otitis media with effusion, excessive cerumen, or otitis externa, in early childhood or much later in adolescence/ early adulthood with hearing loss of which will be attributed as acquired.

Far more concerning to the audiologist and the family of child identified with hearing loss is the realization that the nature of the hearing loss is not only irresolvable, but also progressive. As the term implies, a progressive SNHL becomes increasingly worse over time with an unpredictable and varied speed, configuration, and degree of threshold deterioration. When the progression of hearing loss is slow, the child may have no awareness of any changes in hearing status, but the more obvious sign would eventually be delay or deterioration in speech and language development or deterioration in academic performance. Causes for progressive SNHL include cytomegalovirus, congenital syphilis, inner ear aplasia and abnormalities, toxoplasmosis acquired in-utero, autoimmune inner ear disease, and numerous genetic causes.

3. **What is happening to the auditory system with *GJB2*?**
A number of nonsyndromic hearing loss and deafness traits that are considered congenital (i.e., at birth) occur in the absence of other associated medical etiology, and may present audiometrically as mild to profound degree of SNHL. Since nonsyndromic hearing loss is inherited, identification of those genetic traits depends on genetic testing as well as ascertainment about familial hearing and hearing loss history. Different family members may be affected by the same genetic trait, but degree of hearing and hearing loss will vary.

It is estimated that almost one half of childhood hearing has a genetic etiology, with the most significant cause by mutations in the *GJB2* gene.[6] There are a number of *GJB2* gene mutations known to occur in humans that will cause nonsyndromic hearing loss. *GJB2* gene, also known as *CX26, DFNA3, DFNB1*, gap junction protein, or *NSRD1*, are critical in producing specific proteins called Connexin. Connexin are found throughout the human body, and are especially instrumental in maintaining the proper potassium ions within the inner ear. As a consequence of a "loss of function" for the cochlea to maintain potassium levels within the cochlea, it is not unusual for an individual to have a progressive hearing loss over time.

4. **Would you recommend amplification and/or hearing assistance technology when a progressive hearing loss is present? If so, what would you recommend?**
Of course, amplification is called for when measureable audiometric thresholds are found outside of the range of normal. Once an audiological remediation pathway has been determined for a child with progressive hearing loss, the onus is upon the hearing health care team to aggressively monitor all aspects of auditory performance over time. Choice of amplification is mitigated upon the amount of programmability and flexibility offered in case the need to increase gain arises over a short or prolonged period of time. Not only is aggressive monitoring of the auditory system necessary, but also frequent assessments of auditory function are called for in the instance of a progressive hearing loss. It is also important to encourage ongoing patient and family counseling should any changes in auditory performance change.

Table 61.3 Speech perception results: pre–cochlear implant and 3 months post–cochlear implant

| | Pre–cochlear implant | | 3 mo post–cochlear implant |
	Right	Left	Left
MAIS	34/40		
MLNT	79% (h)	67% (h)	50% (e)
MLNT: phonemes	92%	81%	72%
LNT	52% (h)	56% (h)	68% (e)
LNT: phonemes	76%	79%	81%
HINT (no noise)	76%	80%	NT
HINT (+ 10 SNR)	72%	58%	NT

Abbreviations: e, easy words; h, hard words; LNT, Lexical Neighborhood Test; MAIS, Meaningful Auditory Integration Scale; MLNT, Multisyllable Lexical Neighborhood Test.

It is well recognized that background noise has a negative impact (though with great variability) on speech understanding/recognition performance, especially within a classroom setting.[7] In addition to amplification, it was also recommended that TK use an RM system during the school day so that he would be able to reap a clearer message from the instructor. Though amplification and remote-microphone systems stand at the core of the technology recommendations,[7] it was also important to include strategic seating/placement along with other accommodations in his Individualized Education Plan.

5. **What other recommendations would you suggest for this family?**
Due to the progressive nature of TK's hearing loss, it is important to counsel the family on the possible next audiological steps if the personal hearing aids no longer offer adequate benefit. The family should be counseled on the importance of identifying changes in academic performance, as well as the daily emotional and stress level of the child.

61.6 Outcome

When the personal hearing aids no longer provide adequate benefit, a referral for cochlear implantation is imperative. In the case of TK, he received cochlear implant for the left ear while he was in the third grade. He continued to use traditional hearing aid in the right ear as well as the RM system. TK was discharged from the care of our facility so that his hearing function could be more closely monitored by a cochlear implant team at another facility. This case is a good demonstration of the importance of long-term collaborative relationships between facilities in order to ultimately obtain stable audiological thresholds.

References

[1] Sharma A, Martin K, Roland P, et al. P1 latency as a biomarker for central auditory development in children with hearing impairment. J Am Acad Audiol. 2005; 16(8):564–573

[2] National Center for Hearing Assessment and Management. Universal Newborn Hearing Screening: Summary Statistics of UNHS in the United States. www.infanthearing.org/legislation. Accessed June 21, 2016

[3] Joint Committee on Infant Hearing. Year 2000 position statement: principles and guidelines for early hearing detection and intervention programs. Am J Audiol. 2000; 9:9–29

[4] National Center for Hearing Assessment and Management. Issues & Evidence of Congenital Hearing Loss. http://www.infanthearing.org/summary/prevalence.html. Accessed June 21, 2016

[5] Fortnum HM, Summerfield AQ, Marshall DH, Davis AC, Bamford JM. Prevalence of permanent childhood hearing impairment in the United Kingdom and implications for universal neonatal hearing screening: questionnaire based ascertainment study. BMJ. 2001; 323(7312):536–540

[6] Lafferty KA, Hodges R, Rehm HI. Genetics of hearing loss. In: Madell JR, Flexer C. eds. Pediatric Audiology. 2nd ed. New York: Thieme; 2014;22–35

[7] Crandell C, Smaldino J. Room acoustics and auditory rehabilitation technology. In: Katz J, ed. Handbook of Clinical Audiology. 5th ed. Philadelphia, PA: Lippincott Williams & Wilkins; 2002:607–630

62 Use of LENA to Explore Classroom Listening Concerns for Student with Auditory Neuropathy Spectrum Disorder

Lori A. Pakulski and Katherine Anderson

62.1 Clinical History and Description

Farouk, a 10-year-old male twin, was diagnosed with auditory neuropathy spectrum disorder (ANSD) at 3 months of age. His twin brother does not have an auditory disorder. ANSD is a type of hearing loss that can be congenital or acquired and typically impacts synchronous neural transmission in the auditory pathway while the outer hair cells function normally. Although the site of lesion for ANSD is often unknown, it may occur in the inner hair cells, the cochlear synapse, the cochlear spiral ganglia, or the auditory nerve. Intact outer hair cell function is indicated by normal otoacoustic emissions (OAEs) and/or a present cochlear microphonic but an absent or abnormal auditory brainstem response (ABR) result. The audiogram may show a wide range of findings with hearing thresholds falling anywhere within the normal to a profound hearing loss range. However, persons with ANSD typically have poorer speech recognition than would be expected based on audiometric findings, especially in challenging listening environments such as background noise.

Later, Farouk was diagnosed with attention deficit hyperactivity disorder, for which he is currently taking medication.

62.1.1 Farouk's Birth History

During her pregnancy with twins, his mother reportedly developed gestational diabetes. Farouk was twin B and donor of a twin–twin transfusion, necessitated by a disease of the placenta that affects identical twin pregnancies. The twin boys were born prematurely at 34 weeks by cesarean section. Farouk reportedly weighed 4 pounds 9 ounces at birth. Also at birth, he was jaundiced, had severe anemia, a condition in which the body does not have enough healthy red blood cells, and had difficulty breathing, which was treated with mechanical ventilation. He remained in the neonatal intensive care unit for 2 weeks.

62.2 Audiologic Testing and Related Assessments

As an infant, abnormal ABR waveforms were obtained, and middle ear dysfunction was ruled out during newborn ABR assessment (▶ Fig. 62.1). The audiogram in ▶ Fig. 62.1 also shows conditioned auditory responses in the profound hearing loss range. These responses were obtained over several testing sessions using an operant, visually reinforced behavioral response technique referred to as visual reinforcement audiometry.

By age 2, Farouk had repeated bouts of otitis media and underwent an adenoidectomy and myringotomy. It was not until close to 2 years of age that OAE testing and results from behavioral testing led to diagnosis of ANSD. Farouk was fitted with bilateral hearing aids at age 2.2.

Because of lack of spoken language development with hearing aids, Farouk received a cochlear implant (CI) in his right ear at age 2 years 11 months, and he received his second implant in his left ear at age 5 years 6 months, marking the first time Farouk's brain could receive auditory information through both of his ears.

Farouk currently uses Cochlear Nucleus 6 CI sound processors. He attends his neighborhood grade school, where he uses a remote microphone (RM) system coupled to his CIs. While Farouk strives to be an oral communicator, his spoken communication skills are severely delayed. He has an Individualized Education Program (IEP) for language arts, math, speech-language therapy, and occupational therapy. He is mainstreamed for social studies, science, and attends "specials" (art, physical education, etc.) with his peers. He is encouraged to voice for himself, but his school has also assigned him a sign language interpreter in the classroom. The interpreter uses Signing Exact English (SEE) syntax. Farouk's mother is concerned with the slow rate at which he is learning new sounds and words in the classroom and with his lack of progress in reading.

In recent testing at age 10, an otoscopic examination was unremarkable. Immittance testing revealed normal middle ear functioning. Results of the audiometric evaluation (▶ Fig. 62.2) showed CI sound-field detection thresholds indicating good access, across the speech frequency spectrum, to low-level sounds (15–30 dB across all test frequencies). Additional results showed that Farouk responded to all Ling 6 sounds at 30 dB binaurally with his CIs. He achieved 88% for closed-set word recognition at 50 dB for the NU-CHIPS test form 1. He achieved 90% accuracy on the Lexical Neighborhood Test Easy Words, although unclear articulation affected the scoring of his responses.

Farouk's severe-profound impairment in communication, socialization and pragmatics, and academic learning is likely due to combined effects of the auditory disorder, speech/language delay (secondary to the hearing loss), lack of opportunity for spoken communication, and a challenging family environment. In school, Farouk does not have much of an opportunity to interact with classmates, as he largely works alone within the classroom setting with his interpreter. However, in the small-sized intervention room (five students) and during mainstream specials, Farouk does not take opportunities to interact with other peers. His parents and teachers comment that he does not understand what his peers are saying to him, and his peers do not understand his speech, so communication is difficult. Thus, a classroom-based evaluation was warranted to examine the possible classroom listening factors that may further compound Farouk's compromised communication system.

In order to gain an ear-level perspective of what Farouk experiences in the classroom and across his school day, he was asked to wear a **L**anguage **E**nvironment **Ana**lysis (LENA) System digital language processor (DLP). His twin also wore a DLP on the same day for comparison. The LENA DLP provides a day-long, high-quality digital recording, or snapshot, of the auditory environ-

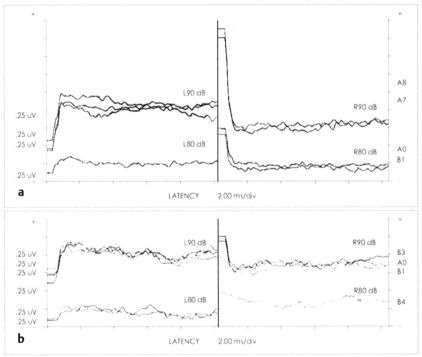

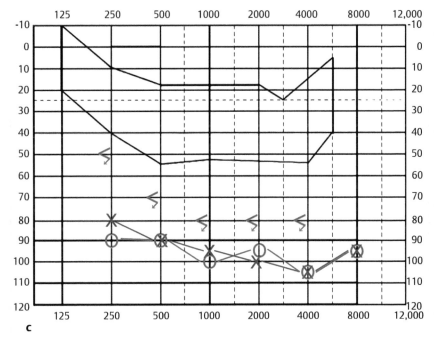

Fig. 62.1 Farouk's early audiometric results (6 months of age), characterized by normal otoacoustic emissions, abnormal auditory brainstem responses, and severe-to-profound sensorineural hearing loss, as shown on the audiogram. The thresholds on the audiogram were obtained, over multiple test sessions, via visual reinforcement audiometry (VRA). O, right ear air conduction; X, left ear air conduction; <, right ear bone conduction; Arrows, no response.

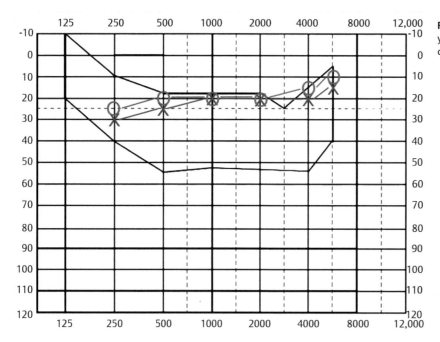

Fig. 62.2 Cochlear implant thresholds at age 9 years. O, right ear air conduction; X, left ear air conduction.

ment, in this case on a typical school day. His teachers completed a journal of instructional and other school activities to provide context for the LENA findings. Recordings were analyzed using the LENA Pro computer software, and types of distant noise and dB levels were obtained through LENA Advanced Data Extractor software. Segments were randomly selected to ascertain descriptive information and to compare the language-learning environments with teacher journals.

62.2.1 LENA Findings and Classroom Acoustics

Classroom acoustics are a common concern for language-learning of students, particularly those with auditory disorders. The acoustics are influenced by ambient (in-room noise), internal and external background noise, speech-to-noise ratio (SNR) of the listener, and reflected or reverberated sounds.[1,2] Yet, it can be difficult to describe a student's daily listening experience, or "noise-scape," and even more challenging to understand how the noise-scape impacts daily learning and well-being.

In an effort to better understand how the acoustic environment might contribute to Farouk's slow progress in communication development, the authors of this case study obtained a snapshot of Farouk's daily noise-scape at school, using the LENA technology. Klatte and her colleagues provide recent and comprehensive evidence of the importance of studying the noise-scape in the regular education classroom.[1,2,3,4] Noise, reverberation, and other classroom environmental factors have the potential for a profound, but not completely understood, impact on teacher–student dialogue as well as student learning because listeners must extract messages from highly variable acoustic signals. Further, there is still much to be learned about the impact of unfavorable noise-scapes on teacher talk, teacher instruction, and student talk, particularly when auditory disorders exist.

Farouk's language-learning environment is highly variable and includes many factors. ▶ Fig. 62.3 provides sample snapshots of the range of experiences across his school day (approximately 20–35 minutes for each language-learning environment). Specifically, the acoustic environment is described relative to the LENA analysis variables and includes structured classroom learning (general education and the intervention room) and unstructured learning and socialization (represented by physical education and lunch/recess). Teacher and student talk is also provided as average words spoken within a 5-minute interval.

▶ Fig. 62.4 provides a sample of adult words and student vocalizations as determined by averages of 5-minute intervals within the hour, according to Twin A's recording. Bear in mind the logarithmic scale along the y-axis. ▶ Fig. 62.5 provides a sample of the noise-scape levels in the language-learning environments analyzed in ▶ Fig. 62.3. In full-scale root mean square, the closer a sound is to 0 (scale minimum), the louder it is perceived, and the closer a sound is to –90 (scale maximum), the quieter it is perceived. The minimum and maximum levels provided for each language-learning environment represent the extreme sound levels during the time frame analyzed for ▶ Fig. 62.3.

62.3 Conclusions and Clinical Implications

Farouk's acoustic experiences were highly variable in both structured and unstructured environments. Nevertheless, some trends can be identified from the data:

- Teacher talk far outweighed student talk in his classes. This may be in part due to frequent disruptions in the "flow of instruction" necessitated by repetitions and efforts to control noise through classroom management. Similar findings were found in the recording of the twin brother in his classes.

Fig. 62.3 Snapshot of Farouk's daily sound-scape.

General education classroom: Twin A

- Coughing
- Clothes/papers rustling
- Tapping on desk
- Teacher-student talk (dialogue)
- Clapping
- Coughing

Average adult words: 565
Average student words: 0.5

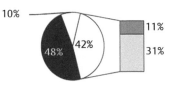

Lunch/Recess: Twin A

- Footsteps
- Multiple students talking
- Slaming locker doors

Average adult words:7
Average student words:8

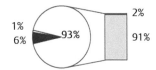

Intervention classroom: Twin B

- Furniture moving
- Clothes rustling
- Markers squeaking on whiteboard
- Teacher- student talk (dialogue)

Average adult words: 221
Average student words: .05

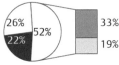

Physical education: Twin B

- Multiple students talking/yelling
- Speech echoes
- Balls bouncing
- Teacher instruction (monologue)

Average adult words: 153
Average student words: 3

■ Meaningful speech   ▢ Background speech   ▨ Distant speech
⊔ Silence/background noise   ⊙ Overlaping vocalizations

Key Discriptions[13]:
Meaningful speech: Vocalizations from key child and nearby adults and children
Background speech: Overlaping noise and distant speech
Overlaping vocalizations: More than one person talking at a time
Distant speech: Vocalizations from adults not readily near key child
Silence/background noise: no sound, non-vocal distant sounds, or sounds not matched to LENA models
Adult/student words: Estimated count of words spoken by nearby adult (teacher) and student (Twin A orB)

- Overall, average levels of noise were louder in unstructured environments when compared to structured environments.
- Language-learning and social environments were noticeably different: academic teaching in both structured and unstructured classrooms were primarily oral instruction with little child talk.
- The general education teacher talked more than twice as much as other teachers; child words were consistent and represented only a fraction of total talk.
- Extraneous noise had common, overlapping features, including speech not directed at the target students, as well as some unique issues (e.g., marker squeaking on whiteboard in intervention room). The overlapping speech is particularly notable because it may lead to the "café effect" (a manifestation of the Lombard effect in social situations whereby everyone talks louder because of the reverberation/noise level). During these times, a target student was working in the same room on entirely different content with a paraprofessional while the teacher and groups of students talked about other subjects. While *least restrictive environment* is desirable, measures could be taken to reduce the café effect and improve listening for individuals, including acoustic partitions and use of an RM system.
- Interestingly, student talk was the same for both twins; hearing loss did not make a difference in this snapshot.

Other noticeable concerns for Farouk: He may not be receiving all instructional information because of background noise—potentially impacting learning. Without an RM system, he likely will not hear his teacher or classmates clearly when they are

Adult and Farouk's words

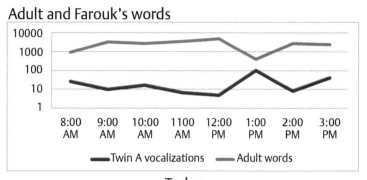

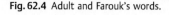
Fig. 62.4 Adult and Farouk's words.

Today
Maximum:- 16.62 Minimum: -40.88 Average: -27.88

Acoustic variability across the day

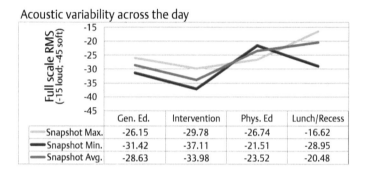

Fig. 62.5 Acoustic variability across the day.

talking from across the room during relevant discussions. Listening becomes more effortful, and noise makes concentration and mental work more difficult.[5]

Although LENA data logging described in this article represents only a snapshot in a single school day, this type of exploration holds much potential for better understanding the language-learning environments and potential impact of the noise-scape on learning of children with auditory disorders. With these data, professionals can make the necessary changes to the environment, better define a student's needs and *least restrictive environment*, and determine the appropriate technology and other important teaching and learning factors.

62.4 Outcome

To date, Farouk has shown improvement of his listening skills, but he is reluctant to use them at school. Parents and school personnel have been supportive of using sign-assisted communication. Farouk's academic and communication skills have not yet improved at this time.

62.5 Questions for the Reader

1. What causes ANSD, and why is this diagnosis particularly challenging?
2. What are some of the potential challenges or ways in which ANSD impacts a school-aged child?
3. Why is it important that more professionals do the type of daily noise-scape analysis that was completed using the LENA?

4. What is the impact of higher intensity noise in unstructured environments when compared to structured environments for a child with auditory disorders?
5. What is the impact of classroom acoustics on a child with ANSD?

62.6 Discussion of Questions

1. **What causes ANSD, and why is this diagnosis particularly challenging?**
   The exact cause may not be known, but risk factors associated with ANSD include (1) hyperbilirubinemia ranging from just above normal to quite high, including infants that have gone through exchange transfusions, (2) prematurity (25–36 weeks' gestational age), and (3) perinatal asphyxia. ANSD is also associated with both recessive and dominant inheritance patterns.[6] If infant testing is conducted with OAEs only, ANSD can go undiagnosed; it can also occur later in life. Even when diagnosis is made, it is a challenging disorder because of the great associated variability. According to Anderson, "If you've seen one child with ANSD, you've seen one child with ANSD."[7] The child's long-term functionality will vary greatly depending on the cause/location of the disorder, how quickly it is diagnosed, and the nature of the intervention. Further, ANSD is often unpredictable. Additionally, hearing thresholds can be deceiving because speech perception is typically far worse than seen in children with comparable degrees of hearing loss, and speech perception is particularly impacted by background noise.

2. **What are some of the potential challenges or ways in which ANSD impacts a school-aged child?**

Because it is difficult to know whether a child is understanding spoken language, particularly in noise and/or across the distance, children with ANSD may miss significant parts of instruction and peer interaction, and these missed opportunities may go completely unnoticed, or may be blamed on other issues such as attention or motivational concerns.

3. **Why is it important that more professionals do the type of daily noise-scape analysis that was completed using the LENA?**

Noise is everywhere and frequently overlooked. Few recognize the serious impact our daily noise-scapes have on both well-being and academic learning. Even when professionals and parents recognize that noise may have a negative impact on a child or a class, it is difficult to quantify. The noise experience may be different from the front to the back of the classroom, and varies across a day. Further, noise can be insidious, and without specific data, it is difficult to know where to begin to improve the daily experience of a certain child. Lastly, the LENA also provides data including how much talking adults and children may be doing. For example, a well-intentioned teacher may strive to provide instruction despite the café effect and other noise-related issues, and in doing so, talk an entire period. Yet, children need opportunities to talk and share ideas as well in order to develop literate language. Describing these daily experiences can help professionals and parents address individual needs.

4. **What is the impact of higher intensity noise in unstructured environments when compared to structured environments for a child with auditory disorders?**

As briefly discussed, the louder the noise, the louder people talk in order to be heard. Consequently, the overall noise floor can be quite high at times. In an unstructured environment, there may be little control, and people may sometimes find themselves shouting to be heard. In a more structured classroom, teachers may command attention or use an RM to be heard. However, little research has examined whether teacher's voices exceed comfortable listening levels in an attempt to be heard over a noisy class/classroom.

5. **What is the impact of classroom acoustics on a child, including those with ANSD?**

Classroom acoustics are generally known to create listening challenges because of noise, but the impacts on general well-being and learning are not often recognized or are underestimated. According to researchers:

- Facilitating listening is necessary for successful learning because classroom instruction is typically delivered orally.[1]
- Optimal acoustical conditions for instruction are essential to learning facilitation.[6]
- School children, especially those with ANSD, are negatively affected by poor SNR because their communication and listening skills are not fully developed and are compromised.[3,5]

Additionally, negative outcomes for school children in unfavorable noise-scapes have been documented, including reduced cognitive performance, annoyance, altered social-emotional school attitudes, compromised language and reading acquisition, poor execution of oral instructions, poorer performance on phonological discrimination tasks, differences in teacher and student vocalizations, difficulty categorizing speech sounds, and decreased speech intelligibility.[6]

References

[1] Klatte M, Bergström K, Lachmann T. Does noise affect learning? A short review on noise effects on cognitive performance in children. Front Psychol. 2013; 4:578

[2] Klatte M, Hellbruck J. Effects of classroom acoustics on performance and well-being in elementary school children: A field study. Paper presented at: Proceedings of the 39th International Congress and Exposition on Noise Control Engineering; June 2010; Lisbon, Portugal. Available at: toc.proceedings.com/10940webtoc.pdf

[3] Klatte M, Lachmann T, Meis M. Effects of noise and reverberation on speech perception and listening comprehension of children and adults in a classroom-like setting. Noise Health. 2010; 12(49):270–282

[4] Klatte M, Meis M, Sukowski H, Schick A. Effects of irrelevant speech and traffic noise on speech perception and cognitive performance in elementary school children. Noise Health. 2007; 9(36):64–74

[5] Talarico M, Abdilla G, Aliferis M, et al. Effect of age and cognition on childhood speech in noise perception abilities. Audiol Neurootol. 2007; 12(1):13–19

[6] Yang W, Bradley JS. Effects of room acoustics on the intelligibility of speech in classrooms for young children. J Acoust Soc Am. 2009; 125(2):922–933

[7] Anderson K. Auditory neuropathy/auditory dyssynchrony spectrum disorder – in brief. 2016. Available at: http://successforkidswithhearingloss.com/ansd/

Suggested Reading

[1] Hood LJ. Auditory neuropathy/dys-synchrony disorder: diagnosis and Management. Otolarygol Clin North Am. 2015; 48(6):1027–1040

[2] LENA Research Foundation. Available at: www.lenafoundation.org

[3] Shield BM, Dockrell JE. The effects of environmental and classroom noise on the academic attainments of primary school children. J Acoust Soc Am. 2008; 123(1):133–144

[4] Uhler K, Heringer A, Thompson N, Yoshinaga-Itano C.. A tutorial on auditory neuropathy/dyssynchrony for the speech-language pathologist and audiologist. Semin Speech Lang. 2012; 33(4):354–366

63 Management of Hearing Loss in a Case of Vestibular Aqueduct Syndrome

Patricia Roush

63.1 Clinical History and Description

Georgia, an 11-year-old girl, was identified with left unilateral hearing loss following a failed newborn hearing screen. She has received pediatric audiology care in the same medical center for the past 11 years. This case study reviews the comprehensive audiologic, otologic, and educational follow-up needed when an infant is diagnosed with unilateral hearing loss.

Georgia was born at 37 weeks' gestation following an uncomplicated pregnancy and delivery. She weighed 8.8 lbs at birth and had Apgar scores of 8 and 9. She passed her initial newborn hearing screen with automated auditory brainstem response (AABR) in the right ear but did not pass in the left. A similar result was obtained at the time of an outpatient re-screen 1 month later. A diagnostic auditory brainstem response (ABR) evaluation at 2 months of age was consistent with normal hearing sensitivity in the right ear and a moderate sensorineural hearing loss in the left ear. The results were discussed with her family and the implications of unilateral hearing loss and potential benefits and limitations of hearing aid use for the left ear were discussed. Georgia's parents indicated they preferred to delay hearing aid fitting until they had an opportunity to see how her speech and language developed. A return appointment was scheduled for otologic examination, and with the family's permission, a referral was made for early intervention services. Two weeks later, an otologic examination was completed and magnetic resonance imagining (MRI) and electrocardiogram (EKG) tests were ordered. In addition, cytomegalovirus (CMV) and Connexin 26 and 30 tests were performed using the blood sample obtained to screen for metabolic disorders in the newborn period (Guthrie's test). The EKG, CMV, and Connexin tests all came back negative. At 3 months of age, Georgia was enrolled in the state's birth-to-three early intervention program and a teacher of the deaf and hard of hearing provided monthly in-home visits.

At 4 months of age, MRI was performed and the results showed bilateral enlargement of the vestibular aqueducts and endolymphatic sacs resulting in a diagnosis of enlarged vestibular aqueduct (EVA). EVA is one of the most common inner ear malformations associated with sensorineural hearing loss.[1,2] It is estimated that between 1 and 12% of children with sensorineural hearing loss have EVA.[3,4] Hearing loss resulting from EVA is often progressive, may fluctuate, and may be conductive, sensorineural, or mixed. Conductive hearing loss with EVA may be present even in the presence of normal tympanometry.[1,5] Because EVA can be associated with Pendred's syndrome, an autosomal recessive genetic disorder that is caused by a mutation in the *SLC26A4* gene,[6] Georgia was referred for a genetics consultation. At 5 months of age, the genetics consultation was completed, and lab results confirmed that Georgia had two copies of the *SLC26A4* gene that causes Pendred's syndrome. In addition to hearing loss, some individuals with Pendred's syndrome develop an enlarged thyroid gland (goiter), so it was recommended that Georgia's health care provider monitor her thyroid growth.

63.2 Audiologic Testing Including Assessment of Auditory and Speech and Language Abilities

Since the MRI showed bilateral EVA, Georgia's parents received extensive counseling about the possibility of hearing loss developing in the right ear as well as further progression to the hearing loss in the left ear. It was recommended that she return for behavioral audiometry to obtain frequency-specific hearing thresholds for each ear.

At 8 months of age, Georgia returned for behavioral hearing assessment using visual reinforcement audiometry (VRA). Tympanometry was normal in the right ear and showed negative middle ear pressure in the left ear. Distortion product otoacoustic emissions (DPOAE) testing was completed and showed present DPOAEs for the right ear and absent DPOAEs for the left ear. A complete audiogram was obtained for the right ear showing normal hearing sensitivity. Georgia became fatigued before a left ear audiogram could be obtained (▶ Fig. 63.1).

Georgia returned for further behavioral audiologic assessment with VRA at 12 months of age. A query of Georgia's parents regarding her communication development indicated she was responding to a variety of sounds and beginning to understand and respond to simple commands. A complete audiogram was obtained for each ear using VRA with insert earphones and results confirmed normal hearing for the right ear and a mild to moderate hearing loss for the left ear (▶ Fig. 63.2). These findings were in good agreement with the ABR completed at 2 months of age. It was recommended that the family continue to participate in early intervention services and return for follow-up assessment in 3 months.

Unfortunately, the family did not return until 9 months later at age 17 months. At that time, tympanometry was consistent with normal middle ear function bilaterally. As expected, Georgia was more difficult to test at age 17 months than she was at a younger age; testing could only be completed for the right ear and thresholds obtained were significantly poorer than during previous tests (▶ Fig. 63.3). The family was advised of our concern regarding progression of the hearing loss in the right ear and a return appointment for reevaluation was scheduled 1 month later.

The family returned as scheduled; however, Georgia would not tolerate insert earphones. Testing was completed in sound field using VRA and repeatable head turn responses were obtained, suggesting a moderate hearing loss for at least the better ear (▶ Fig. 63.4).

After consultation with Georgia's parents and an otolaryngologist, it was recommended she have a repeat ABR under sedation. At 19 months of age, the results of the ABR confirmed

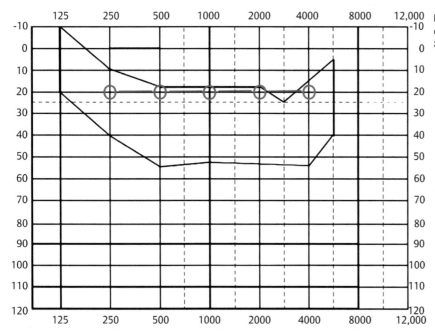

Fig. 63.1 Audiogram obtained for the right ear with visual reinforcement audiometry at 8 months of age. O, right ear air conduction.

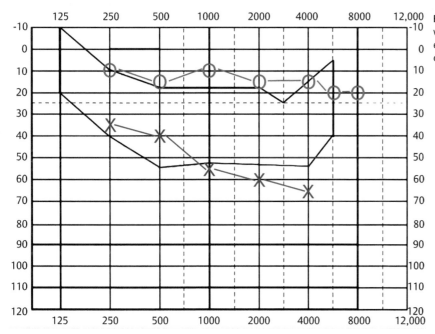

Fig. 63.2 Audiogram obtained for both ears with visual reinforcement audiometry and insert earphones at 12 months of age. O, right ear air conduction; X, left ear air conduction.

that Georgia's hearing loss in the right ear had progressed and that she now had a mild-to-moderate bilateral sensorineural hearing loss (see ▶ Fig. 63.5 for estimated hearing level [eHL] thresholds based on the ABR). Binaural hearing aid use was recommended and Georgia returned 2 weeks later for hearing aid fitting. Real ear to coupler difference measurements (RECDs) were obtained for each ear and hearing aids were programmed using desired sensation level (DSL) prescriptive targets. Hearing aid verification was completed using an Audioscan Verifit to ensure that the maximum power output did not exceed prescriptive targets and that targets were met for soft, average, and loud conversational speech inputs. In addition to binaural hearing aids, a personal remote microphone (RM) system was also

dispensed for the family to use in noisy environments or when there was increased distance between Georgia and the speaker's voice. The family was counseled extensively on the importance of hearing aid use during waking hours and it was recommended that she return for repeat testing on a monthly basis.

Return testing at 23 and 24 months of age (▶ Fig. 63.6) showed significantly more progression to the hearing loss with thresholds in the moderate to severe range. Due to the significant decrease in hearing thresholds and the inability to provide adequate high-frequency audibility with conventional signal processing, new hearing aids with nonlinear frequency compression were dispensed. In addition, due to the rapid decrease in Georgia's hearing thresholds, it was recommended that a speech and language

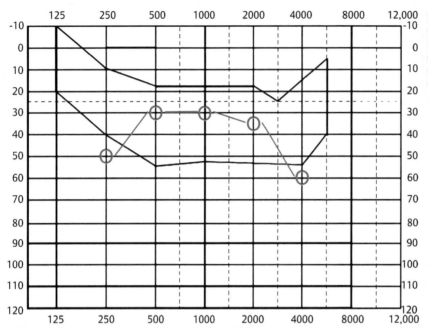

Fig. 63.3 Audiogram obtained for the right ear using visual reinforcement audiometry with insert earphone at 17 months of age. Note decrease in thresholds as compared to audiogram obtained at 8 months of age. O, right ear air conduction.

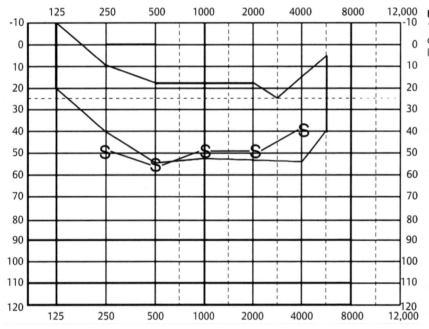

Fig. 63.4 Audiogram obtained in sound field at 18 months of age showing hearing thresholds consistent with a moderate hearing loss for at least the better ear. S, soundfield air conduction.

evaluation be completed by a speech language pathologist on the cochlear implant (CI) team to obtain baseline speech and language information and to review Georgia's current services.

Despite the rapid progression to her hearing loss, Georgia continued to make significant gains in her speech and language development and the results of the speech and language evaluation indicated Georgia had age-appropriate speech and language skills and no significant concerns were noted. It was recommended that she continue to receive services and that she return for reevaluation of her speech and language in 1 year. Her family followed recommendations regarding the need for frequent monitoring of hearing thresholds and full-time hearing aid use. These frequent follow-up visits allowed her audiologist to make adjustments to the hearing

aids as needed to ensure she had adequate audibility of speech even as her hearing thresholds decreased.

Despite these proactive measures, Georgia's hearing loss continued to progress and by 3.5 years of age, testing with play audiometry showed hearing thresholds in the moderate to profound range bilaterally, with left ear thresholds significantly poorer than the right ear (▶ Fig. 63.7a). Although a significant air–bone gap is evident, tympanometry was consistent with normal middle ear function (▶ Fig. 63.7b), not an unusual finding in cases of EVA. Unaided speech recognition testing with phonetically balanced kindergarten (PBK) words presented via monitored live voice at a comfortable loudness above threshold were 24 and 16% for the right and left ears, respectively, and a score of only 52% was obtained in the

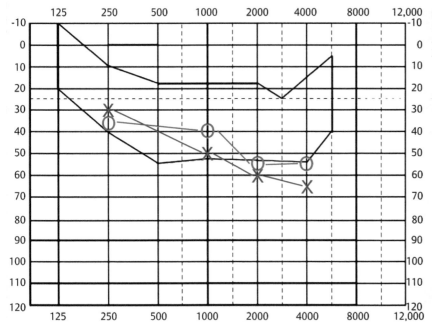

Fig. 63.5 Estimated hearing levels in dBeHL based on sedated auditory brainstem evaluation at 20 months of age. O, right ear air conduction; X, left ear air conduction.

binaural aided condition for speech presented at 55 dbHL. Both parents were in the sound booth during Georgia's aided speech recognition testing and were able to observe the difficulty she had repeating single words presented at an average conversational loudness. Despite this demonstration and extensive counseling about the potential benefits of cochlear implantation for children with this degree of hearing loss, the parents remained reluctant to schedule an appointment to learn more about cochlear implantation. A repeat speech and language evaluation was completed as recommended and the evaluation showed that Georgia was not making appropriate progress with test scores showing a moderate language delay. Recommendations included increased therapy and a cochlear implantation consultation.

A few days following the speech and language evaluation, Georgia's teacher of the deaf called and said that Georgia's mother had been overwhelmed by the results of the speech and language evaluation and with the possibility cochlear implantation. She stated that she thought Georgia was doing better than the results of the evaluation indicated and she felt Georgia had not performed at her best on the day of the evaluation. She did indicate she was willing to arrange additional therapy and it was agreed that a repeat evaluation should be completed in 6 months.

Six months later, the mother was called to schedule the follow-up evaluation and she declined to schedule an appointment. The family did return for their regularly scheduled audiology follow-up visit as planned 3 months later. Although pure-tone thresholds remained stable, Georgia's unaided word recognition scores were 30 and 26% for the right and left ears, respectively, and her binaural aided speech recognition score at 55 dBHL was only 36%. After a lengthy discussion, the family agreed to proceed with further assessment to determine her candidacy for CI.

63.3 Questions for the Reader

1. Given the test results obtained at 3.5 years of age (▶ Fig. 63.7a), do you think Georgia would benefit from CI? If yes, would you recommend unilateral or bilateral CI for her?
2. Why do you think the family cancelled the 6-month follow-up speech and language evaluation?
3. What measures might the pediatric audiologist and speech pathologist take to assist the family with their decision regarding CI for Georgia?

63.4 Discussion of Questions

1. **Given the test results obtained at 3.5 years of age (▶ Fig. 63.7a), do you think Georgia would benefit from CI? If yes, would you recommend unilateral or bilateral CI for her?**

Although Georgia still had a significant amount of residual hearing at 3.5 years of age, in the right ear she only had aidable residual hearing through 2,000 Hz, while in the left ear, aidable residual hearing was limited to the 250 to 1,000 Hz range. Thus, even with the use of nonlinear frequency compression technology in her hearing aids, the left ear in particular remained a challenging hearing loss to fit and to provide sufficient access to high-frequency sounds. Furthermore, Georgia's unaided and aided word recognition abilities were very poor in both ears and she was beginning to show significant delays in speech and language development. For these reasons, Georgia was deemed to be a CI candidate. Given the significantly poorer high-frequency thresholds in the left ear, a left CI was recommended. At the time Georgia was being considered for CI, electric acoustic stimulation (EAS) technology was not avail-

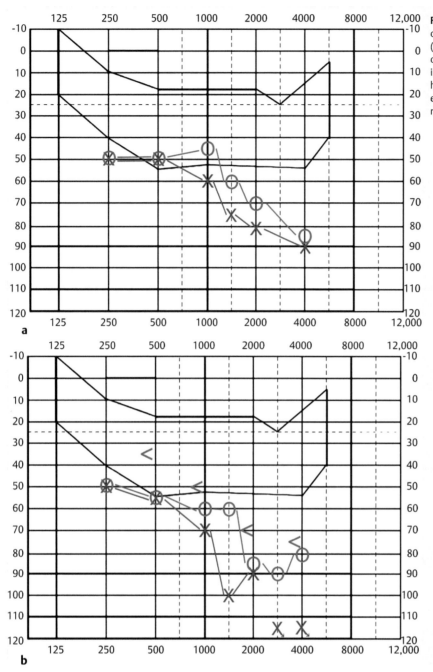

Fig. 63.6 (a) Audiogram obtained at 23 months of age using visual reinforcement audiometry (VRA) with insert earphones. **(b)** Audiogram obtained at 24 months of age using VRA with insert earphones. Note further progression to hearing loss, particularly in the left ear. O, right ear air conduction; X, left ear air conduction; <, right ear bone conduction; Arrows, no response.

able for children so this option was not discussed. In regard to bilateral CI, see current speech recognition scores for each ear in ► Table 63.1 and further discussion regarding bilateral CI in the "Outcome" section below.

2. **Why do you think the family cancelled the 6-month follow-up speech and language evaluation?**
   Parents of children with hearing loss face many difficult decisions not only at the time of diagnosis, but also for many years as they try to meet their child's changing needs. In this case, the family initially thought their child had normal hearing in one ear but then were faced with

the need to accept not only the fact that she had bilateral hearing loss, but also that the hearing loss was progressing over time. It is not unusual for families to struggle with acceptance of changes in hearing as well as the need to move forward with new treatment recommendations. In addition, at those times, parents may have differing opinions regarding decisions to move forward with management recommendations. In this case, fear of more bad news regarding their child's speech and language development and the family's fear of cochlear implantation may have influenced their decision to cancel the speech and language evaluation.

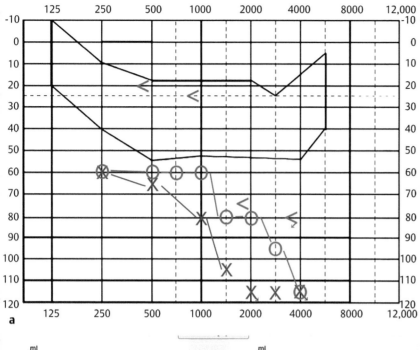

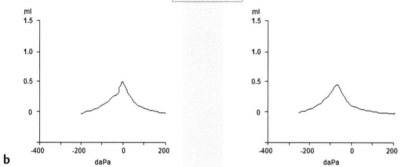

Fig. 63.7 (a) Audiogram obtained at 3.5 years of age showing moderate to profound bilateral hearing loss with air bone gap at 500 and 1,000 Hz. **(b)** Tympanometry consistent with normal middle ear function obtained on same day as audiogram showing conductive component to hearing loss. O, right ear air conduction; X, left ear air conduction; <, right ear bone conduction; Arrows, no response.

3. **What measures might the pediatric audiologist and speech pathologist take to assist the family with their decision regarding cochlear implantation for Georgia?**
Following the initial diagnosis of hearing loss when both parents are present, it is not unusual for only one parent (often the mother) to attend the child's frequent follow-up visits. This allows that parent to participate in testing and therapy sessions and to adjust to changes over time. Often, the parent who is not able to attend hears the information second hand and has not had the opportunity to hear the information presented by the professional and to ask questions along the way. Audiologists and speech pathologists may be able to assist families with moving forward with decision making by encouraging the parent who does not usually attend the visit to come to an upcoming appointment. In addition to allowing the other parent to ask questions directly, the audiologist can also set up a demonstration of the child's aided listening abilities with both parents in the sound booth so they are better able to understand the difficulties the child is having in a controlled listening environment.

In many cases, it is helpful to connect families with other families of children with hearing loss who are ahead of them in the process and who may be of support to the family. The audiologist can facilitate this once the necessary permissions from both families have been obtained. Many cities also have organized group parent support programs that can be very beneficial to families as well.

63.5 Recommended Treatment

After proceeding with additional CI evaluation and speaking with the audiologist, otologist, and speech and language pathologist, the family decided to move forward with a CI for the left ear. At 5 years of age, Georgia received a left Nucleus CI512 cochlear implant for the left ear.

63.6 Outcome

Georgia had successful CI surgery for her left ear. At age 11 years (5 years post CI surgery), she continues to be a successful bimodal user with a CI in her left ear and a hearing aid in the right. ▶ Fig. 63.8 shows the unaided audiogram for the right ear and aided CI detection thresholds for the left ear. ▶ Table 63.1 shows her most recent speech recognition scores. She is currently mainstreamed in the fourth grade where she receives itinerant services from a teacher of the deaf and uses an RM system.

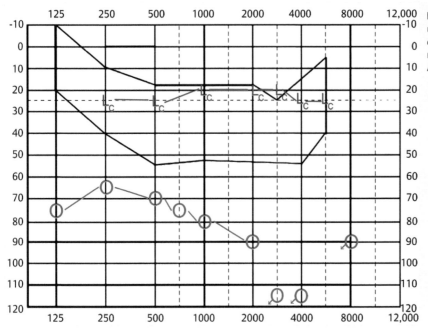

Fig. 63.8 Audiogram at age 11 years showing unaided thresholds for the right ear and aided detection thresholds with CI for the left ear. O, right ear air conduction; LC, left cochlear implant; Arrows, no response.

Table 63.1 Speech recognition scores 5 years post cochlear implant (CI) activation

Condition	Words (%)	Phonemes (%)
CNC left (CI)	88	94
CNC right (HA)	16	38
CNC binaural (HA&CI)	86	94
BabyBio right (HA), quiet	52	
BabyBio binaural (HA&CI), quiet	99	
BabyBio + 5 dB SNR (HA)	17	
BabyBio, binaural + 5 dB SNR (HA&CI)	92	

Abbreviations: CNC, consonant–nucleus vowel–consonant; HA, hearing aid; SNR, signal-to-noise ratio.

While there has been some discussion regarding the possibility of moving forward with a second CI for her right ear given her poor aided speech recognition scores in the hearing aid–only condition, Georgia's parents feel she is doing very well with her current CI and hearing aid and are not interested in moving ahead with a second device at this time.

References

[1] Mukerji SS, Parmar HA, Ibrahim M, Mukherji SK. Congenital malformations of the temporal bone. Neuroimaging Clin N Am. 2011; 21(3):603–619, viii

[2] Dewan K, Wippold FJ, II, Lieu JE. Enlarged vestibular aqueduct in pediatric sensorineural hearing loss. Otolaryngol Head Neck Surg. 2009; 140 (4):552–558

[3] Emmett JR. The large vestibular aqueduct syndrome. Am J Otol. 1985; 6 (5):387–415

[4] Arcand P, Desrosiers M, Dubé J, Abela A. The large vestibular aqueduct syndrome and sensorineural hearing loss in the pediatric population. J Otolaryngol. 1991; 20(4):247–250

[5] Madden C, Halsted M, Benton C, Greinwald J, Choo D. Enlarged vestibular aqueduct syndrome in the pediatric population. Otol Neurotol. 2003; 24 (4):625–632

[6] Koffler T, Ushakov K, Avraham KB. Genetics of hearing loss: syndromic. Otolaryngol Clin North Am. 2015; 48(6):1041–1061

64 Considerations for Hearing Technology for Minimal to Mild Hearing Loss

Andrea D. Warner-Czyz and Shawna Jackson

64.1 Clinical History and Description

The patient, Hailey, now 9 years old, was seen at an audiology clinic at age 5 years, 4 months (5;4) to determine potential underlying factors affecting progression in speech-language therapy for a phonological speech disorder with articulation and resonance difficulties.

Hailey was referred to our clinic for a speech and language evaluation at age 4 years by her early childhood interventionist. Per parent report, Hailey experienced difficulty with behavior, articulation, and language comprehension. These issues began at 8 months of age, possibly due to the presence of recurrent otitis media.

Hailey was the product of a full-term pregnancy, complicated by a diagnosis of placenta previa at 11 weeks of gestation and a nuchal cord at birth. She passed a newborn hearing screening in both ears at the hospital prior to discharge. Per parent report, Hailey exhibited delays across developmental realms. For example, Hailey achieved motor milestones later than typically developing peers, sitting alone at 10 months and walking at 16 months. Communication milestones also showed delays, with cooing and babbling emerging at 13 months and first words at 15 months of age. Other significant audiologic history included sensitivity to loud sounds plus a history of allergies (pollen), frequent colds, ear infections, and two sets of bilateral pressure equalization tubes at 8 and 32 months of age. Social and cognitive milestones, including interacting well with other children, paying attention, and overall cooperation, appeared within normal limits.

At the initial visit with a speech-language pathologist at our center, Hailey's parents reported they and Hailey's pediatrician had concerns about her speech and language development. At age 4;3, Hailey primarily expressed herself via gestures and pointing, occasionally using the 25 to 75 words in her vocabulary. Although her mother estimated she could understand 75% of what Hailey said, that value decreased for friends (25–50%) and strangers (25%). Hailey's speech and language abilities were significantly poorer when compared with expected developmental milestones such as saying all speech sounds in words and using sentences with four or more words and more than one action word.

Hailey's mother reported that her daughter responded to her voice but closely watched her face when she spoke to her. Hailey was referred to a local otorhinolaryngologist at age 2;6 for testing due to concerns about her hearing. Per parent report, hearing loss was ruled out because sound-field testing supported normal hearing sensitivity between 500 and 4,000 Hz for at least the better ear (▶ Fig. 64.1). Tympanometry at that time revealed normal middle ear pressure and tympanic membrane mobility.

Hailey's mother reported they participated in early childhood intervention services for speech and language services four times per month from age 14 months to 3 years. She attended special services in the Head Start program through the local school district. Hailey's Admission, Review, and Dismissal (ARD) meeting at age 3 years resulted in the recommendation of speech-language therapy for a phonological disorder. The disconnect between Hailey's intelligence and pretend play skills, which matched developmental age-mates, and her inability to meet expected progression in therapy lead the therapist to strongly recommended further evaluation.

64.2 Assessment of Auditory and Spoken Language Abilities

At age 4;1, Hailey completed the *Clinical Assessment of Articulation and Phonology (CAAP)*, a valid and reliable norm-referenced measure of speech production abilities in children from 2;6 to 11;11. Results indicated a consonant inventory score of 82, which corresponded to a standard score < 55, percentile rank of 4, and age equivalence of < 2.9. She consistently substituted /d/ for most initial consonants and deleted 9 out of 26 final consonants. For phonological processes, she obtained a standard score < 55 with a percentile rank < 1 and an age equivalent performance < 2.6. The most common phonological processes exhibited by Hailey included final consonant deletion (50% of occurrence), cluster reduction (100% occurrence), substitutions with vocalization (88%), fronting (50%), stopping (100%), and prevocalic voicing for assimilation (50%). In sum, Hailey exhibited a 16-month delay in consonant inventory and a 19-month delay in phonological processes. Speech therapy was initiated through a group therapy camp at our clinic. After continued lack of progress over the 6 months, combined with Hailey's embarrassment about her problem, the speech-language pathologist recommended an audiologic evaluation.

Hailey underwent a comprehensive audiologic evaluation composed of observational checklists, behavioral measures, and electrophysiological testing, at 5;4. The *Auditory Skills Checklist (ASC)* is a 35-item criterion-referenced evaluation tool that assesses auditory skill development from detection to discrimination, identification, and comprehension based on parent report and clinician observation. Hailey attained a total score of 44/70, with nearly maximum scores through level 6 of the ASC, which includes skills from awareness and detection through association of sound with objects, common phrases, and simple directions. Hailey's mom indicated that she could remember groups of words with up to four critical elements, though discrimination based on segmental features (e.g., bat versus bite or boat; Ling sounds) still was emerging.

Ear-specific responses, obtained via conditioned play audiometry using ER3A insert earphones, revealed a bilateral symmetric cookie-bite sensorineural hearing loss of minimal degree, as shown in ▶ Fig. 64.2. Tympanometry revealed normal tympanic membrane mobility and middle ear pressure in both ears. Acoustic reflexes were present at appropriate intensities bilaterally

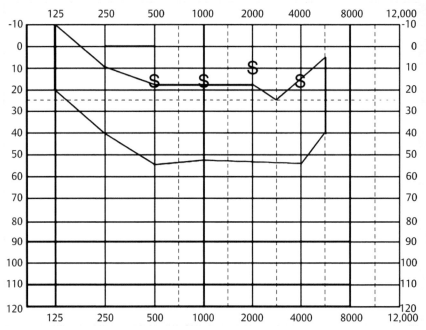

Fig. 64.1 Hearing screening obtained in the sound field using visual reinforcement audiometry at 2;6. S, soundfield air conduction.

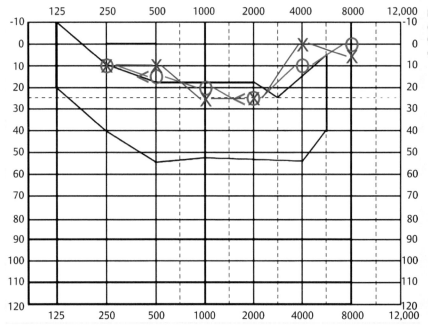

Fig. 64.2 Ear-specific pure-tone thresholds obtained via conditioned play audiometry at 5;4. O, right ear air conduction; X, left ear air conduction; <, right ear bone conduction.

with ipsilateral and contralateral stimulation. Distortion-product otoacoustic emission responses were present but abnormal. That is, the signal-to-noise ratio exceeded 10 dB, but the absolute level of the distortion product did not exceed 5 dB.

Based on concerns from both the parent and the pediatrician, we referred to an otolaryngologist for (1) medical follow-up for initial identification of hearing loss; (2) possible imaging studies to further investigate pathology of hearing loss; and (3) medical clearance for hearing aid evaluation and fitting. Additionally, we suggested Hailey continue speech-language therapy and return every 6 months for regular monitoring of her hearing sensitivity.

64.3 Questions for the Readers

1. Which additional referrals could or should you make for this child?
2. Would you recommend auditory technology for this child with a cookie-bite hearing loss of minimal to mild degree?

3. Which type of special considerations might this child need relative to her social, communication, and academic needs?

4. What could have been done earlier?

64.4 Discussion of Questions

1. **Which additional referrals could or should you make for this child?**

Clinicians should suspect a hereditary hearing loss with cookie-bite configurations, thereby supporting relevance of genetic testing and counseling. A clinical geneticist not only can confirm diagnosis of a genetic hearing loss, but also can provide appropriate guidance for further testing, construct family pedigrees, and counsel regarding future pregnancies. In addition, determination of a genetic component to the hearing loss could provide indication of progression of hearing loss and steer intervention strategies.

In Hailey's case, both the audiologist and the otorhinolaryngologist recommended genetic consultation, but test availability, insurance coverage, and financial considerations prevented completion of this recommendation. Therefore, the audiologist queried Hailey's parents on their own hearing acuity, which revealed that Hailey's father complained that Hailey's mother did not hear well. We recommended a hearing evaluation for both Hailey's mother and older sister, in line with recommendations by pediatric otorhinolaryngologists who suggest testing family members as part of the workup of prelingual sensorineural hearing loss. In fact, 30% of pediatric otorhinolaryngologists routinely recommend audiometry for parents and 54% recommend audiologic testing of siblings to provide more comprehensive knowledge of the role of genetics in pediatric hearing loss.[1] Immediate audiologic assessment of Hailey's mother revealed a previously undiagnosed cookie-bite sensorineural hearing loss of moderate degree (▶ Fig. 64.3). Hailey's older sister similarly was diagnosed with a mild

sensorineural hearing loss of cookie-bite configuration, as shown in ▶ Fig. 64.4. Within 2 weeks of Hailey's initial diagnosis, a maternal aunt also was diagnosed with a hearing loss, which Hailey's mother reported had a similar configuration. Congruence among multiple family members suggests a hereditary component to the patient's hearing loss and significant sensorineural progressive component.

The information provided through audiometric testing of Hailey's older sister and mother afforded the clinician to make an educated estimate of the possible progression of the hearing loss over time. Given the possibility for a progressive hearing loss, intervention through amplification was strongly encouraged. In addition, we recommended regular monitoring of Hailey's hearing through both audiometric and distortion product otoacoustic emissions with adjustments to hearing amplification and school intervention strategies as needed.

Although Hailey did not report peer problems or academic difficulties, her family should have access to resources to counseling through a rehabilitation specialist, psychologist, or social workers to support her well-being, social interactions, and self-advocacy skills. Additionally, families with children who have hearing loss with a genetic component should have awareness of the Hereditary Hearing Impairment Resource Registry (HHIRR), an archive established by the National Institutes on Deafness and Other Communication Disorders. The HHIRR serves as a national resource that disseminates clinical information and research updates to professionals and families about hereditary hearing loss, and matches families with research opportunities.

2. **Would you recommend auditory technology for this child with a cookie-bite hearing loss of minimal to mild degree?**

We recommended bilateral low-level amplification for Hailey's minimal hearing loss for multiple reasons.

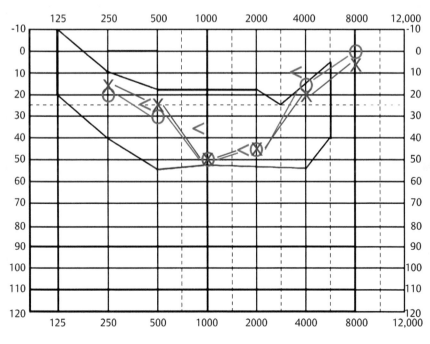

Fig. 64.3 Pure-tone audiogram of Hailey's mother obtained on the day of initial diagnosis of Hailey's hearing loss. O, right ear air conduction; X, left ear air conduction; <, right ear bone conduction.

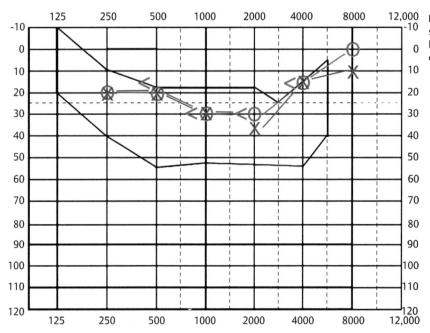

Fig. 64.4 Pure-tone audiogram of Hailey's older sister at age 8;11. O, right ear air conduction; X, left ear air conduction; <, right ear bone conduction.

A "minimal" hearing loss of any configuration can create difficulty hearing soft or distant speech. Moreover, the cookie-bite configuration of Hailey's hearing loss exacerbates listening in adverse situations such as in the presence of competing noise or reverberation—both of which are prevalent in a typical classroom setting. Hailey's close attention to visual cues accompanying vocal input (e.g., closely watching her mother's face) as a toddler reflects an attempt to gather multimodal sensory information to supplement an inadequate auditory signal, either in acuity or clarity. Amplification for minimal hearing losses affords adequate access to speech at both typical and lower intensities, an important undertaking because perception of "soft" speech has potential implications for acquisition of receptive and expressive language through both explicit and incidental learning.[2,3,4] Use of a remote microphone system may also prove to be beneficial.

A minimal bilateral sensorineural hearing loss also can have cascading effects on speech and language development. For example, inconsistent access to conversation can have negative influences on production of midfrequency speech sounds (e.g., /p/ and /h/), acquisition of morphology (e.g., word endings such as –s and –ed), and perception of unstressed syllables (e.g., articles such as *a* and *the*). This echoes the phonological errors Hailey exhibited, particularly final consonant deletion noted in her speech-language evaluation. Furthermore, children with bilateral minimal sensorineural hearing loss often exhibit delays in vocabulary comprehension, vocabulary expression, and storytelling abilities relative to hearing peers.[5,6] Quigley and Thomure estimate that an average hearing loss between 15 and 26 dB HL results in approximately a 1.2 year delay in language comprehension.[7] Although we do not have a measure of Hailey's receptive vocabulary, parent report and test results support a delay in both receptive and expressive language. She did not produce first words until 15 months of age and had the

expressive vocabulary of a 2-year-old at 4 years of age. Even participation in weekly speech-language therapy for nearly 2 years yielded little progress in communication milestones.

In addition to the direct effects of the hearing loss on Hailey's communication development, it also began to affect her psychosocial well-being. At age 4 years, Hailey expressed embarrassment about her speech production difficulties and inability to communicate effectively. Her self-awareness of her communication difficulties, paired with the disparity between her intellect and language abilities, could transition to poorer quality of life, particularly lower self-esteem, more behavioral problems, greater difficulty making and maintaining friendships, and higher stress, as seen historically in children with hearing loss.[6,8]

3. **Which type of special considerations might this child need relative to her social, communication, and academic needs?**
Professionals and parents working with children with minimal hearing loss need to consider the quality of life of a child with minimal hearing loss. First, we should consider Hailey's physical well-being. Having a hearing loss requires additional listening effort as well as additional cognitive energy needed to attend to and comprehend spoken language; the additional listening effort and expenditure of cognitive energy potentially lead to higher levels of fatigue. Listening effort increases with poor speech perception, difficult listening situations, and challenging or new content. This puts children with hearing loss at higher risk for fatigue. Greater fatigue also could negatively affect incidental learning, especially in a noisy classroom.[2,9] Although Hailey had not yet verbalized a sense of fatigue, parents and teachers should watch for signs of weariness and inattention, particularly in difficult listening situations or at the end of the day, to monitor Hailey's fatigue levels. As the intensity of school increases in later grades, educational personnel should pay attention to

Hailey's schedule to allow a mental rest between difficult core courses to reduce fatigue related to listening effort and facilitate her learning ability.

Second, we should consider Hailey's social well-being, particularly the quantity and quality of her peer relationships. Historically, children with hearing loss feel lonelier, are less socially accepted, and have more difficulty making and maintaining friends versus peers with typical hearing. A child with minimal sensorineural hearing loss may miss subtle conversation cues present in fast-paced peer interactions, which could create the perception of inappropriate or immature social skills among peers. In particular, Hailey's cookie-bite configuration may lead to accusations of "selective hearing" due to discrepancies in speech understanding in quiet versus noise. This may have significant effects in school because Hailey's hearing loss could create difficulties hearing in noisy cooperative learning situations (e.g., group activities), at lunchtime, or at recess, where complex noise environments make conversations more difficult. Signs of social problems may include avoidance of social events in difficult listening situations (e.g., school dance, cafeteria) or eschewing activities needing additional care of her hearing aids (e.g., connections to technology like Bluetooth; waterproof accessories). Hailey's development of peer relationships and interactions demands attention because social skills underlie academic and emotional development. Assessment of social skills can be addressed through both informal (i.e., case history) and formal (e.g., Behavior Assessment System for Children) metrics.

Third, professionals and parents need to consider academic implications of a minimal hearing loss. Children with minimal hearing loss historically lag behind hearing peers on academic achievement tests and overall educational performance, and have greater risk for academic failure.[4,5,6,10] By high school, the decline in academic performance may slow down, but this may relate to a student's selection of a less rigorous academic curriculum, which could have long-term effects on college admission, employability, and socioeconomic status in adulthood. Recommendations to combat academic deficits in children with minimal hearing loss, such as Hailey's, include a formal education plan that delineates (1) explicit instruction of sound–letter associations and subtle auditory discrimination skills necessary for reading; (2) preferential seating and use of a personal FM or DM system to decrease deleterious effects of noise and distance on access to a primary speech signal; and (3) consideration of special visual aids to enhance auditory and visual cues. Additionally, educational staff should participate in an in-service focused on behaviors and expectations of students with minimal hearing loss, including effects of hearing loss on listening effort and fatigue, effects of ambient classroom noise on speech understanding, and frustrations or behaviors that may be associated with difficulty in communication rather than a behavioral or attention deficit.

4. **What could have been done earlier?**

Hailey presented at an early age with signs of hearing loss—delayed word onset, slow vocabulary growth, poor progress in speech-language therapy, and increased visual attention when spoken to. The decision to dismiss hearing loss as a contributing factor stemmed from a "pass" on the otoacoustic emission screening at birth and minimal response levels in the sound field obtained at 2;6. A more comprehensive evaluation, including ear-specific information and diagnostic electrophysiologic measures, could have provided guidance in more systematic monitoring. Obtaining ear-specific information often involves multiple follow-up appointments with young children, particularly those with hearing loss, but affords confidence in ruling in or ruling out hearing loss. Additionally, diagnostic thresholds at 20 dB HL with insert earphones should not be considered within normal limits for a child. Although most audiograms mark 0 to 20 or 25 dB HL as typical hearing sensitivity, these reference levels reflect guidelines for adult hearing loss and its effect on worker's compensation.[11] **Children with thresholds exceeding 10 dB HL (i.e., 15 dB HL or more) can experience negative educational effects of hearing loss.** Therefore, the Joint Committee on Infant Hearing (JCIH) recommends follow-up every 3 months until a formal diagnosis of hearing loss is either confirmed or ruled out.

In addition, a good case history should have been completed earlier in the process. During our follow-up examination, a detailed history allowed us to observe a family history of language delay in Hailey's older sister and decreased hearing sensitivity in Hailey's mother. The combination of this information secured in a detailed, comprehensive case history leads to a successful diagnosis, intervention, and follow-up plan for Hailey.

64.5 Recommended Treatment

Hailey received bilateral hearing aids at 5 years of age.

64.6 Outcome

A hearing aid evaluation was completed in the office to assess the potential benefit of amplification. Aided versus unaided speech-in-noise testing was completed with a demonstration pair of hearing aids programmed using DSL prescription settings for Hailey's hearing loss. Hailey experienced immediate benefit from the hearing aids, evidenced by threshold responses (all 15 dB HL or better); quantitative performance on speech perception tasks, measured via accuracy and reaction time; and qualitative performance, observed as reduced frustration during the task itself. The immediate improvement in Hailey's performance led to the recommendation of a formal binaural hearing aid trial. Our recommendation of amplification was strengthened further by (1) the suggestion of hereditary, and possibly progressive, nature of her hearing loss; and (2) Hailey's limited progress in academic and language intervention strategies without amplification. At the recommendation of the clinical audiologist and agreement of her parents, Hailey received bilateral hearing aids at 5;6 years of age following medical clearance by her otorhinolaryngologist.

Receiver in the ear hearing aids with FM accessibility were fit binaurally. Traditionally, receiver in the ear hearing aids are not utilized for younger children due to concerns of durability and retention; however, these were recommended due to the size of Hailey's ear canal, the desire for a more "open" vent fitting strategy, and her comfort for wearing amplification. Durability was addressed by providing an additional receiver for the parents to troubleshoot at home if they suspected malfunction of the auditory technology.

Real-ear values were measured utilizing probe microphones and speech-mapping was completed to determine aided benefit for long-term average speech signals (▶ Fig. 64.5). Speech intelligibility index scores indicate significant improvement in access to speech, especially for soft input levels. Functional testing in sound field, completed using warbled tones, revealed excellent benefit with consistent aided responses at 10 to 15 dB HL between 500 and 4,000 Hz. Word recognition in quiet using Phonetically Balanced Kindergarten (PBK) lists also suggests good aided benefit at an average conversational level (45 dB HL) at a + 5 dB signal-to-noise ratio in the aided (100%) compared to unaided (72%) listening condition. Additionally, Hailey demonstrated noticeable improvement in her speech approximations

in her speech therapy appointments and progressed with articulation goals for the first time in over a year.

Follow-up audiometric assessment at age 6;1 revealed no more than a 5 dB shift in pure-tone thresholds between 500 and 4,000 Hz in either ear (▶ Fig. 64.6). Follow-up testing was recommended annually or more often if concerns in progress arise.

Pure-tone testing obtained at age 8;7 provided audiometric thresholds for a broader frequency range, from 250 to 8,000 Hz, including several interoctave bands (▶ Fig. 64.7). Results revealed a slight (5–10 dB) but insignificant shift in the midfrequencies relative to testing obtained at age 6;1. Speech recognition thresholds were in good agreement with pure-tone findings, suggesting good reliability. Word recognition testing, obtained at 50 dB HL using PBK word lists, revealed excellent (92–96% correct) abilities bilaterally. Additionally, Hailey competed sentence in noise testing using the Bamford–Kowal–Bench Speech in Noise test (BKB-SIN) at 60 dB HL. Results revealed a 3.7 dB signal-to-noise ratio unaided and a 1.7 dB signal-to-noise ratio aided.

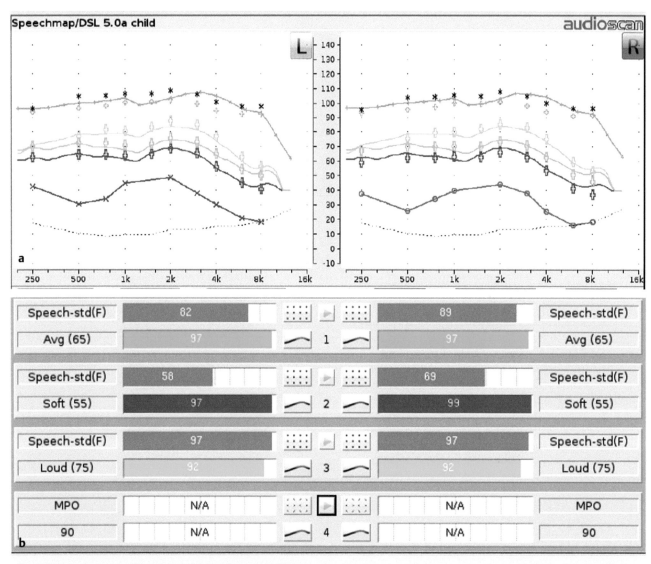

Fig. 64.5 Speech mapping from Hailey's bilateral hearing aid fitting.

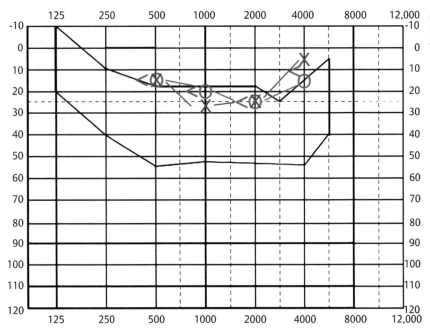

Fig. 64.6 Pure-tone threshold assessment for Hailey at 6;1. O, right ear air conduction; X, left ear air conduction; <, right ear bone conduction.

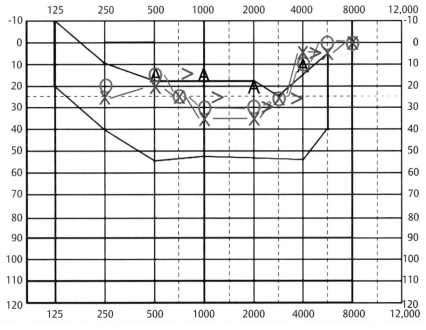

Fig. 64.7 Aided and unaided audiometric testing at 8;7. O, right ear air conduction; X, left ear air conduction; <, right ear bone conduction; A, binaural hearing aids behind the ear.

Parental interview at age 8;7 indicated Hailey enjoyed academic success in a mainstream classroom. She wore her bilateral hearing aids and used preferential seating during all instructional times. Per parent report, Hailey has a strong friend group and her speech intelligibility improved to levels approximating hearing age-mates. Hailey's older sister has also successfully been fitted with amplification based on her diagnosis and also has progressed to normal academic performance per parent report.

This case study supports a more assertive approach for children with minimal hearing loss compared to the historical perspective of waiting for them to fail before recommending intervention.[12] Focusing case history, auditory technology, and counseling has allowed Hailey—and her sister—to succeed personally and academically, in spite of their diagnosis of a minimal hearing loss with cookie-bite configuration.

References

[1] Duncan RD, Prucka S, Wiatrak BJ, Smith RJH, Robin NH. Pediatric otolaryngologists' use of genetic testing. Arch Otolaryngol Head Neck Surg. 2007; 133 (3):231–236

[2] Akhtar N, Jipson J, Callanan MA. Learning words through overhearing. Child Dev. 2001; 72(2):416–430

[3] Hart TR, Risley B. Meaningful Differences in the Everyday Experience of Young American Children. Baltimore, MD: Paul H. Brookes Publishing; 1995

[4] Suskind D, Leffel KR, Hernandez MW, et al. An exploratory study of "quantitative linguistic feedback:" Effect of LENA feedback on adult language production. Comm Disord Q. 2013; 34(4):199–209

[5] Bess FH, Dodd-Murphy J, Parker RA. Children with minimal sensorineural hearing loss: prevalence, educational performance, and functional status. Ear Hear. 1998; 19(5):339–354

[6] Davis JM, Elfenbein J, Schum R, Bentler RA. Effects of mild and moderate hearing impairments on language, educational, and psychosocial behavior of children. J Speech Hear Disord. 1986; 51(1):53–62

[7] Quigley SP, Thomure FE, eds. Some Effects of Hearing Impairment upon School Performance. Springfield, IL: Illinois Office of Education; 1968

[8] Guidelines for audiology services in the schools. Ad hoc committee on service delivery in the schools. American Speech-Language-Hearing Association. ASHA Suppl. 1993; 35(3, Suppl 10):24–32

[9] Bess FH, Hornsby BW. Commentary: listening can be exhausting–fatigue in children and adults with hearing loss. Ear Hear. 2014; 35(6):592–599

[10] Blair JC, Peterson ME, Viehweg SH. The effects of mild sensorineural hearing loss on academic performance of young school-age children. Volta Review. 1985; 87:87–93

[11] Shambaugh GE, Jr, American Academy of Ophthalmology and Otolaryngology. Guide for the classification and evaluation of hearing handicap. Trans Am Acad Ophthalmol Otolaryngol. 1965; 69:740–751

[12] Winiger AM, Alexander JM, Diefendorf AO. Minimal hearing loss: From a failure-based approach to evidence-based practice. Am J Audiol. 2016; 25 (3):232–245

Note: Page numbers set **bold** or *italic* indicate headings or figures, respectively.